Advancing Oral Health in America

Committee on an Oral Health Initiative

Board on Health Care Services

INSTITUTE OF MEDICINE
OF THE NATIONAL ACADEMIES

THE NATIONAL ACADEMIES PRESS
Washington, D.C.
www.nap.edu

THE NATIONAL ACADEMIES PRESS   500 Fifth Street, N.W.   Washington, DC 20001

NOTICE: The project that is the subject of this report was approved by the Governing Board of the National Research Council, whose members are drawn from the councils of the National Academy of Sciences, the National Academy of Engineering, and the Institute of Medicine. The members of the committee responsible for the report were chosen for their special competences and with regard for appropriate balance.

This study was supported by Contract No. HHSH25034003T between the National Academy of Sciences and the U.S. Department of Health and Human Services. Any opinions, findings, conclusions, or recommendations expressed in this publication are those of the author(s) and do not necessarily reflect the view of the organizations or agencies that provided support for this project.

International Standard Book Number-13: 978-0-309-18630-8
International Standard Book Number-10: 0-309-18630-7

Additional copies of this report are available from the National Academies Press, 500 Fifth Street, N.W., Lockbox 285, Washington, DC 20055; (800) 624-6242 or (202) 334-3313 (in the Washington metropolitan area); Internet, http://www.nap.edu.

For more information about the Institute of Medicine, visit the IOM home page at: www.iom.edu.

Cover art: Scientific micrograph of tooth enamel. Getty Images.

The serpent has been a symbol of long life, healing, and knowledge among almost all cultures and religions since the beginning of recorded history. The serpent adopted as a logotype by the Institute of Medicine is a relief carving from ancient Greece, now held by the Staatliche Museen in Berlin.

Suggested citation: IOM (Institute of Medicine). 2011. *Advancing Oral Health in America*. Washington, DC: The National Academies Press.

"Knowing is not enough; we must apply.
Willing is not enough; we must do."
—Goethe

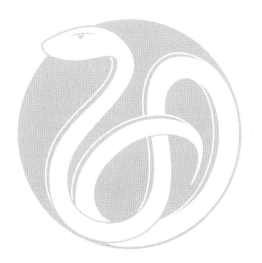

INSTITUTE OF MEDICINE
OF THE NATIONAL ACADEMIES

Advising the Nation. Improving Health.

THE NATIONAL ACADEMIES
Advisers to the Nation on Science, Engineering, and Medicine

The **National Academy of Sciences** is a private, nonprofit, self-perpetuating society of distinguished scholars engaged in scientific and engineering research, dedicated to the furtherance of science and technology and to their use for the general welfare. Upon the authority of the charter granted to it by the Congress in 1863, the Academy has a mandate that requires it to advise the federal government on scientific and technical matters. Dr. Ralph J. Cicerone is president of the National Academy of Sciences.

The **National Academy of Engineering** was established in 1964, under the charter of the National Academy of Sciences, as a parallel organization of outstanding engineers. It is autonomous in its administration and in the selection of its members, sharing with the National Academy of Sciences the responsibility for advising the federal government. The National Academy of Engineering also sponsors engineering programs aimed at meeting national needs, encourages education and research, and recognizes the superior achievements of engineers. Dr. Charles M. Vest is president of the National Academy of Engineering.

The **Institute of Medicine** was established in 1970 by the National Academy of Sciences to secure the services of eminent members of appropriate professions in the examination of policy matters pertaining to the health of the public. The Institute acts under the responsibility given to the National Academy of Sciences by its congressional charter to be an adviser to the federal government and, upon its own initiative, to identify issues of medical care, research, and education. Dr. Harvey V. Fineberg is president of the Institute of Medicine.

The **National Research Council** was organized by the National Academy of Sciences in 1916 to associate the broad community of science and technology with the Academy's purposes of furthering knowledge and advising the federal government. Functioning in accordance with general policies determined by the Academy, the Council has become the principal operating agency of both the National Academy of Sciences and the National Academy of Engineering in providing services to the government, the public, and the scientific and engineering communities. The Council is administered jointly by both Academies and the Institute of Medicine. Dr. Ralph J. Cicerone and Dr. Charles M. Vest are chair and vice chair, respectively, of the National Research Council.

www.national-academies.org

COMMITTEE ON AN ORAL HEALTH INITIATIVE

RICHARD D. KRUGMAN (*Chair*), Vice Chancellor for Health Affairs, School of Medicine, University of Colorado at Denver

JOSÉ F. CORDERO, Dean, Graduate School of Public Health, University of Puerto Rico

CLAUDE EARL FOX, Executive Director, Florida Public Health Institute; Research Professor, Miller School of Medicine, University of Miami

TERRY FULMER, Erline Perkins McGriff Professor and Dean, College of Nursing, New York University

VANESSA NORTHINGTON GAMBLE, University Professor of Medical Humanities, Professor of American Studies and Health Policy, The George Washington University

PAUL E. GATES, Chair, Department of Dentistry, Bronx-Lebanon Hospital Center; Chair, Department of Dentistry, Dr. Martin L. King, Jr. Community Health Center; Associate Professor, Albert Einstein College of Medicine

MARY C. GEORGE, Associate Professor Emeritus, Department of Dental Ecology, School of Dentistry, University of North Carolina at Chapel Hill

ALICE M. HOROWITZ, Research Associate Professor, School of Public Health, University of Maryland, College Park

ELIZABETH MERTZ, Assistant Professor in Residence, Preventive and Restorative Dental Sciences, School of Dentistry and Social and Behavioral Sciences, School of Nursing; Research Faculty, Center for the Health Professions, University of California, San Francisco

MATTHEW J. NEIDELL, Assistant Professor, Mailman School of Public Health, Columbia University; Faculty Research Fellow, National Bureau of Economic Research

MICHAEL PAINTER, Senior Program Officer, Robert Wood Johnson Foundation

SARA ROSENBAUM, Chair, Department of Health Policy; Harold and Jane Hirsh Professor of Health Law and Policy, The George Washington University School of Public Health and Health Sciences

HAROLD C. SLAVKIN, Professor, School of Dentistry, University of Southern California

CLEMENCIA M. VARGAS, Associate Professor, University of Maryland Dental School

ROBERT WEYANT, Associate Dean, Public Health and Outreach; Professor and Chair, Department of Dental Public Health and Information Management, School of Dental Medicine, University of Pittsburgh

Study Staff

TRACY A. HARRIS, Study Director
BEN WHEATLEY, Program Officer
MEG BARRY, Associate Program Officer
AMY ASHEROFF, Senior Program Assistant
REDA URMANAVICIUTE, Administrative Assistant (through December 2010)
JILLIAN LAFFREY, Administrative Assistant (from January 2011)
ROGER C. HERDMAN, Director, Board on Health Care Services

Reviewers

This report has been reviewed in draft form by individuals chosen for their diverse perspectives and technical expertise, in accordance with procedures approved by the National Research Council's Report Review Committee. The purpose of this independent review is to provide candid and critical comments that will assist the institution in making its published report as sound as possible and to ensure that the report meets institutional standards for objectivity, evidence, and responsiveness to the study charge. The review comments and draft manuscript remain confidential to protect the integrity of the deliberative process. We wish to thank the following individuals for their review of this report:

SUZANNE BOULTER, Concord Hospital Family Health Centers

JAMES J. CRALL, University of California, Los Angeles, and American Academy of Pediatric Dentistry

SUSAN J. CRIM, University of Tennessee Health Science Center

BURTON L. EDELSTEIN, Columbia University and Children's Dental Health Project

JOHN W. ERDMAN, JR., University of Illinois

ROBERT GENCO, University at Buffalo

HAROLD GOODMAN, Maryland Department of Health and Mental Hygiene

CATHERINE HAYES, Independent Consultant

AMID ISMAIL, Temple University

PAULA S. JONES, Private Practice

DUSHANKA KLEINMAN, University of Maryland

WILLIAM R. MAAS, Pew Center on the States
DONALD WAYNE MARIANOS, Consultant
R. GARY ROZIER, University of North Carolina at Chapel Hill
LISA A. TEDESCO, Emory University

Although the reviewers listed above have provided many constructive comments and suggestions, they were not asked to endorse the conclusions or recommendations, nor did they see the final draft of the report before its release. The review of this report was overseen by **HAROLD C. SOX,** Dartmouth Medical School (retired), and **GEORGES C. BENJAMIN,** American Public Health Association. Appointed by the National Research Council and the Institute of Medicine, they were responsible for making certain that an independent examination of this report was carried out in accordance with institutional procedures and that all review comments were carefully considered. Responsibility for the final content of this report rests entirely with the authoring committee and the institution.

Foreword

Oral health care is often excluded from our thinking about health. Taken together with vision care and mental health care, it seems that problems above the neck are commonly regarded as peripheral to health care and health care policy. This division is reinforced by the fact that dentists, dental hygienists, and dental assistants are separated from other health care professionals in virtually every way: where they are educated and trained, how their services are reimbursed, and where they provide oral health care. This separation is at odds with the fact that good oral health has been shown to directly affect a person's overall health.

The U.S. Department of Health and Human Services (HHS) is involved in oral health care in a variety of ways, from financing safety net care to developing the oral health workforce to providing public health surveillance. Previous efforts by HHS to improve oral health in America have produced some benefit, but not enough. Many populations, especially the most vulnerable and underserved populations, suffer significant oral health problems. Major barriers to care include low rates of dental insurance, high out-of-pocket payments (even for those with insurance), relative lack of training of the general health care workforce in oral health, and a lack of awareness about the importance of good oral health—both by health care professionals and the public.

The Health Resources and Services Administration asked the Institute of Medicine (IOM) to provide advice on where to focus its efforts in oral health. After the IOM convened the Committee on an Oral Health Initiative, HHS announced a broad Oral Health Initiative and expressed optimism that the committee's work would be able to inform this endeavor. The

IOM Committee on an Oral Health Initiative, led by Richard Krugman, was charged with assessing the current oral health care system, reviewing the elements of an HHS Oral Health Initiative and exploring ways to promote the use of preventive oral health interventions and improve oral health literacy. The committee worked in parallel with a second IOM committee that focused on issues of access to oral health care for underserved and vulnerable populations. Both of these IOM projects are included as official components of the HHS Oral Health Initiative.

The IOM's work in the area of oral health dates back more than 30 years. In 1980, the IOM released *Public Policy Options for Better Dental Health*, which argued that basic dental services should be broadly available and emphasized that any national health insurance plan should include dental services. The 1995 report *Dental Education at the Crossroads* called for numerous reforms in the system of education and training for dentists and other dental professionals. Most recently, in 2009, the IOM held a 3-day workshop on the *Sufficiency of the U.S. Oral Health Workforce in the Coming Decade*. The workshop focused on the connection between oral health and overall health, the challenges facing the current oral health system, and the roles various stakeholders can play in improving oral health care.

The Committee on an Oral Health Initiative reaffirms that oral health is an integral part of overall health and points to many opportunities to improve the nation's oral health. We issue this report in the hope that it will prove useful to responsible government agencies, informative to the health professions and public, and helpful in attaining higher levels of dental health.

Harvey V. Fineberg, M.D., Ph.D.
President, Institute of Medicine
April 2011

Preface

In 2009, the U.S. Department of Health and Human Services (HHS) asked the Institute of Medicine (IOM) to convene a panel to recommend strategic actions for HHS in oral health. Although HHS has been actively involved in oral health care for decades, many Americans continue to experience poor oral health and cannot access the oral health care system. In fact, like the overall health care system in many ways, the term *oral health care system* is a misnomer, as the delivery of oral health care occurs in multiple settings by various health care professionals without coordination or integration. To the extent that there is a system, it is fragmented into two tiers: one for those who can access traditional dental private practices and one for those who cannot, most often the vulnerable and underserved populations who are most in need of care.

HHS and others have documented the stark reality of the poor oral health status of many Americans. More than 10 years ago, the surgeon general called oral health disease a "silent epidemic." Unfortunately, the situation largely remains unchanged. Dental caries continues to be one of the most prevalent diseases of childhood.

While researchers have identified the multiple connections between oral health and overall health, oral health care remains artificially separated from the larger system of general health care. Many health professionals know little to nothing about oral health. Oral health is, for the most part, missing from the education and training of health care professionals such as nurses, pharmacists, physician assistants, physicians, and others. Instead of "oral health," many people continue to think about "dental health" as if it were separate from a person's general health.

HHS has sought to address many of these challenges and to fill some of the gaps in care nationwide. Its agencies currently perform the following:

- Finance oral health care services for millions of Americans through state Medicaid programs and the Children's Health Insurance Program (CHIP).
- Provide and oversee services through settings such as the Federally Qualified Health Centers (FQHCs).
- Support oral health workforce demonstration projects.
- Conduct oral health research and surveillance.
- Contribute in many other ways to the day-to-day functioning of the oral health care "system" in the United States.

However, HHS itself suffers from considerable fragmentation, given the multiple responsibilities and frequent lack of coordination among HHS agencies. In addition, while some notable progress has been made, previous HHS efforts to improve oral health have suffered from a lack of sufficient resources and high-level accountability.

In 2010, as this study was under way, HHS launched a cross-agency reform effort known as the Oral Health Initiative 2010, which seeks to improve coordination and integration among existing oral health-related programs within the department, and it included the launch of nine new initiatives, including this current study. The committee sought to frame and guide this effort by providing specific recommendations on the administration of the initiative and focused on issues that are particularly important for HHS to address. First is the need to focus on prevention. While effective preventive measures are well established, the oral health system continues to focus on the identification and treatment of existing disease. Second is the need to enhance the oral health workforce. The oral health system still largely depends on a traditional, isolated dental care model in the private practice setting—a model that does not always serve significant portions of the American population well. More needs to be done to support the education and training of all health care professionals in oral health care and to promote interdisciplinary, team-based approaches. HHS can also work to increase the racial and ethnic diversity of the oral health workforce and explore the use of new types of oral health professionals in nontraditional settings of care. In addition, HHS needs to explore new payment models that can help improve access and coverage. Finally, HHS needs to expand both primary and secondary research in oral health with a focus on developing a robust primary evidence base and coordinating federal data so it can be used for secondary research. In addition, because quality assessment and improvement efforts lag significantly behind those in the rest of health care, HHS can promote the development of oral health measures of quality.

And in all of these efforts, information and processes should be transparent and involve representation from multiple stakeholders.

This report calls upon HHS to capitalize on the work it has already done to improve oral health care in America. Currently, there is a confluence of high-level interest and passionate leadership. However, the committee recognizes that while HHS has a significant role to play as a leader in oral health care, it is just one part of a larger solution. HHS needs to work with stakeholders across the oral health care spectrum to focus on promoting oral health prevention, integrating oral health into overall health, and increasing access to oral health care for all Americans, including those who are not currently receiving the care they need. In essence, this report calls upon HHS to be a leader in helping to change our nation's way of thinking—to help leaders, health care professionals, and individuals to better understand that oral health and oral diseases are a *health care* problem, and not just a dental problem.

Richard D. Krugman, *Chair*
Committee on an Oral Health Initiative
April 2011

Acknowledgments

Many individuals and organizations contributed to this study. The Committee on an Oral Health Initiative takes this opportunity to recognize those who so generously gave their time and expertise to inform its deliberations.

The committee benefited from presentations made by a number of experts. The following individuals shared their experiences and perspectives during public meetings of the committee:

William Bailey, U.S. Public Health Service
Ann Battrell, American Dental Hygienists' Association
Cynthia Baur, Centers for Disease Control and Prevention
Marcia Brand, Health Resources and Services Administration
Jack Bresch, American Dental Education Association
Robin Brocato, Administration for Children and Families
James J. Crall, American Academy of Pediatric Dentistry
A. Conan Davis, Centers for Medicare and Medicaid Services
Bruce Dye, Centers for Disease Control and Prevention
Burton L. Edelstein, Columbia University
Isabel Garcia, National Institute of Dental and Craniofacial Research
Raymond Gist, American Dental Association
Karen Glanz, University of Pennsylvania
Christopher G. Halliday, Indian Health Service
David Halpern, Academy of General Dentistry
Rita Jablonski, The Pennsylvania State University
Laura Joseph, Farmingdale State College of New York

Dushanka Kleinman, University of Maryland
William Kohn, Centers for Disease Control and Prevention
Ann LaBelle
Susan Levy, University of Illinois at Chicago
William R. Maas, Pew Children's Dental Campaign
Richard J. Manski, Agency for Healthcare Research and Quality
Vincent C. Mayher, private practice
Marian Mehegan, Office on Women's Health
Lynn Douglas Mouden, Arkansas Department of Health
Wendy Mouradian, University of Washington
Linda Neuhauser, University of California, Berkeley
Rochelle Rollins, Office of Minority Health
John P. Rossetti
Rima Rudd, Harvard University
Mary Wakefield, Health Resources and Services Administration

The committee also thanks Kenneth Thorpe, Emory University, for his commissioned paper, *Financing Oral Health Care.*

We extend special thanks to the following individuals who generously gave their time and knowledge to further the committee's efforts:

Lewis N. Lampiris, American Dental Association
Scott L. Tomar, University of Florida
Richard W. Valachovic, American Dental Education Association

Many within the Institute of Medicine were helpful to the study staff. The staff would like to thank Pamella Atayi, Patrick Burke, Rosemary Chalk, Greta Gorman, Wendy Keenan, William McLeod, Janice Mehler, Abbey Meltzer, Patti Simon, and Lauren Tobias for their time and support to further the committee's efforts. We also thank Mark Goodin, copyeditor.

Finally, the committee gratefully acknowledges the assistance and support of two individuals instrumental in developing this project: Marcia Brand and Jeffrey Johnston, both of the Health Resources and Services Administration.

Contents

xvii

Summary

For decades, the U.S. Department of Health and Human Services (HHS) has shown a fluctuating commitment to making oral health a national priority. More than 10 years ago, the surgeon general's landmark report *Oral Health in America* described the poor oral health of our nation as a "silent epidemic." Today, oral diseases remain prevalent across the country, especially in vulnerable and underserved populations. Oral health has been shown to be inextricable from overall health, yet oral health care is still largely treated as separate and distinct from broader health care in terms of financing, education, sites of care, and workforce. While the surgeon general's report has been credited with raising awareness of the importance of good oral health, oral health still remains largely ignored in health policy.

STUDY CHARGE AND APPROACH

In 2009, the Health Resources and Services Administration (HRSA) approached the Institute of Medicine (IOM) to provide recommendations for a potential oral health initiative (Box S-1).

The committee recognized that many important factors influence the oral health of Americans, including settings of care, workforce, financing, quality assessment, access, and education, and focused attention to these areas on how they relate to possible or current HHS policies and programs. The committee was also cognizant of the sizable role that other non-HHS stakeholders play in the oral health care system, including those in the private sector and at the state and local levels. Consequently, the recommendations contained within this report will not on their own resolve many

---

BOX S-1
IOM Committee on an Oral Health Initiative
Statement of Task

- Assess the current oral health care system for the entire U.S. population.
- Examine preventive oral care interventions, their use and promotion.
- Explore ways of improving health literacy for oral health.
- Review elements of a potential HHS oral health initiative, including possible or current regulations, statutes, programs, research, data, financing, and policy.
- Recommend strategic actions for HHS agencies and, if relevant and important, other actors, as well as ways to evaluate this initiative.

---

of the problems that exist in the oral health care system. Instead, this report should be viewed as a complementary piece of a larger solution that will require efforts throughout the oral health community and beyond. This report therefore uses the term *oral health* in its most comprehensive sense—as the responsibility of the entire health care system.

Several major developments during the course of this study challenged the committee. In particular, after the project had already begun, HHS announced the launch of the Oral Health Initiative 2010 (OHI 2010), a cross-agency effort to improve coordination within HHS toward improving the oral health of the nation. HHS considers this current IOM study as part of the initiative. The committee decided to acknowledge the OHI 2010 but not to let its current structure limit their recommendations.

ORAL HEALTH TODAY

In recent decades, advances in oral health science broadened understanding not just of healthy teeth but of the health of the entire craniofacial-oral-dental complex and its relation to overall health. Scientifically, we have moved into a postgenomic era and expanded our understanding of oral conditions to also include their often complex, multigene, and hereditary bases. Despite these advances, *Oral Health in America* identified dental caries[1] as "the single most common chronic childhood disease." While

---

[1] The term *dental caries* is used in the singular and refers to the disease commonly known as tooth decay.

there have been notable successes, dental caries remains a common chronic disease across the life span in the United States and around the world. There is a measure of tragedy in this situation because dental caries is a highly, if not entirely, preventable disease.

There are a wide range of both acute and chronic conditions that manifest themselves in or near the oral cavity, including inherited, infectious, neoplastic, and neuromuscular diseases and disorders. This report focuses predominately on dental caries and periodontal diseases, which cause significant morbidity.

THE ORAL-SYSTEMIC CONNECTION

The surgeon general's report referred to the mouth as a mirror of health and disease occurring in the rest of the body in part because a thorough oral examination can detect signs of numerous general health problems, such as nutritional deficiencies, systemic diseases, microbial infections, immune disorders, injuries, and some cancers. In addition, there is mounting evidence that oral health complications not only reflect general health conditions but also exacerbate them. For example, periodontal disease may be associated with adverse pregnancy outcomes, respiratory disease, cardiovascular disease, coronary heart disease, and diabetes.

Popular attention to the connection between oral health and overall health increased dramatically in 2007 with the death of Deamonte Driver, a 12-year-old Maryland boy who died when bacteria from an untreated tooth infection spread to his brain. Driver's death transformed the oral health discussion as more people—including members of Congress—recognized the potential seriousness of untreated oral disease. His enduring story has contributed to the sustained interest in oral health seen in recent years.

THE CURRENT ROLE OF HHS

HHS' efforts to improve oral health and oral health care have been wide ranging, but the priority placed on these endeavors, including financial support, has been inconsistent. Enduring areas of attention include support for community water fluoridation, research on the etiology of oral diseases, dental education, oral health financing, workforce demonstrations, oral health surveillance, and recruitment of oral health care professionals[2] to work in underserved areas. For example, HHS oversees the provision of oral health care to select populations through the Indian Health Service

---

[2] In this report, the committee uses the term *oral health care professional* to refer to any health care professional who provides oral health care. This may include, but not be limited to, dental hygienists, dentists, nurses, physician assistants, and physicians.

and Federally Qualified Health Centers. The Centers for Medicare and Medicaid Services (CMS) finances oral health care through Medicaid and Children's Health Insurance Program (CHIP) programs. HHS supports the oral health workforce through school loan repayment programs and demonstration projects in innovative workforce models. HHS also monitors oral health and oral health care through surveys conducted by the Centers for Disease Control and Prevention (CDC) and the Agency for Healthcare Research and Quality (AHRQ), and it advances the scientific evidence base for oral and craniofacial health through the work of the National Institute of Dental and Craniofacial Research. HHS also plays a role in the assessment of evidence for preventive services, such as through AHRQ's convening of the U.S. Preventive Services Task Force and the CDC's convening of the Task Force on Community Preventive Services.

Despite the breadth of these efforts, it is often assumed that HHS has a fairly minor role in and very little leverage to influence the day-to-day functioning of the oral health care system in America. Data indicate that only 9 percent of dental expenditures come from public insurance (compared with 34 percent for physician and clinical services and 34 percent for prescription drugs). However, data on dental expenditures do not reflect the financial input of HHS in the broader definition of oral health since this calculation only reflects the services performed by dentists (as opposed to care provided by nondental health care professionals). In addition, those who are covered by public funds are often the most vulnerable populations; therefore, HHS' role is extremely important for those who cannot afford to pay for oral health care. Finally, as described previously, HHS has significant financial investments in other aspects of oral health beyond paying for services. So while the government does not currently have as large a role in financing oral health care services as for other health care services, it does, in fact, have a great role to play in the support of the overall oral health care system.

LEARNING FROM THE PAST

While the surgeon general's report was highly successful in many respects, it did not lead to a direct and immediate change in the government's approach to oral health. This may have been due to broader environmental factors, including immediate national crises; changes in the economy that affect state and federal budgets; competing health care priorities; a tendency to blame individual behaviors alone for poor oral health; a lack of political will; or simply the long-standing failure to recognize oral health as an integral part of overall health. Within HHS, changes in administrations, workforce turnover, lack of oral health champions, insufficient funding and staffing, and the overall lack of oral health parity may all have contributed to the disappointing results. Given that HHS' resources are currently limited, that the scope of the challenge is substantial, and that solutions will require the involvement of multiple stakeholders, one of the most important roles HHS can play is in providing leadership and direction for the country.

RECOMMENDATIONS

In considering a "potential HHS oral health initiative," the committee developed a set of organizing principles (see Box S-2) based on areas in greatest need of attention as well as approaches that have the most potential for creating improvements. It will be HHS' responsibility to adapt the current structure of the OHI 2010 to these principles and the recommendations that follow.

The committee outlines seven recommendations that as a whole comprise what will be referred to as the *new* Oral Health Initiative (NOHI) to distinguish it from and build upon the current initiative. The recommendations provide advice for setting intermediate, measurable goals, but the committee concluded that ultimately HHS should use the goals and objectives of *Healthy People 2020* as the continuing mission of the NOHI. *Healthy People 2020* is an existing and well-accepted set of benchmarks for the country and was developed by a strong collaboration of multiple partners. Creating a new set of goals would only contribute to the redundancy and fragmentation that is often criticized regarding government programming. The relevant goals and objectives are not just in the oral

---

BOX S-2
Organizing Principles for an HHS Oral Health Initiative

1. Establish high-level accountability.
2. Emphasize disease prevention and oral health promotion.
3. Improve oral health literacy and cultural competence.
4. Reduce oral health disparities.
5. Explore new models for payment and delivery of care.
6. Enhance the role of nondental health care professionals.[a]
7 Expand oral health research, and improve data collection.
8. Promote collaboration among private and public stakeholders.
9. Measure progress toward short-term and long-term goals and objectives.
10. Advance the goals and objectives of *Healthy People 2020*.

---

[a]*Nondental health care professionals* includes, but is not limited to, nurses, pharmacists, physician assistants, and physicians.

health section; the NOHI should embrace the goals and objectives of the health communication and health information technology section as well as oral health-related topics in other sections. Building upon *Healthy People 2020* gives the NOHI a foundation for sustainability and the ability to change goals and objectives depending upon achievements in improving oral health. More importantly, as better measures of quality in oral health are developed, more sophisticated goals can be set.

Establishing and Evaluating the Oral Health Initiative

The committee concluded that HHS has the ability and opportunity to play a vital role in the current oral health enterprise. This initiative can succeed if it has clearly articulated goals, is coordinated effectively, is adequately funded, and has high-level accountability.

> **RECOMMENDATION 1: The secretary of HHS should give the leader(s) of the new Oral Health Initiative (NOHI) the authority and resources needed to successfully integrate oral health into the planning, programming, policies, and research that occur across all HHS programs and agencies.**
> - **Each agency within HHS that has a role in oral health should provide an annual plan for how it will integrate oral health into existing programs within the first year.**
> - **Each agency should identify specific opportunities for public-private partnerships and collaborating with other agencies inside and outside HHS.**
> - **The leader(s) of the NOHI should coordinate, review, and implement these plans.**
> - **The leaders(s) of the NOHI should incorporate patient and consumer input into the design and implementation of the NOHI.**

The identification of specific leadership for the NOHI is necessary to establish accountability. Measurable objectives could focus on shorter-term or intermediate measures of departmental performance such as implementation of new programs and collaborations or demonstrated impact on oral health status and access. The leader(s) of the NOHI would be responsible for oversight of all of these plans, including looking for overarching areas for collaboration and learning both from within HHS and from external partners. Finally, the NOHI needs to ensure that patient and consumer perspectives are recognized and appreciated in future oral health planning.

Focusing on Prevention

Among the most important contributions HHS can make to improve oral health is to promote the use of regimens and services that have been shown to promote oral health, prevent oral diseases, and help manage those diseases. Too often, oral health care focuses more intently on treating disease once it has become manifest. A focus on prevention may help to reduce the overall need for treatment, reduce costs, and improve the capacity of the system to care for those in need.

The committee concluded that (1) preventive services have a strong evidence base for promoting oral health and preventing disease; and (2) HHS is a key provider of oral health care, especially for vulnerable and underserved populations through the safety net.

> **RECOMMENDATION 2:** All relevant HHS agencies should promote and monitor the use of evidence-based preventive services in oral health (both clinical and community based) and counseling across the life span by
> * Consulting with the U.S. Preventive Services Task Force and the Task Force on Community Preventive Services to give priority to evidentiary reviews of preventive services in oral health;
> * Ensuring that HHS-administered health care systems (e.g., Federally Qualified Health Centers, Indian Health Service) provide recommended preventive services and counseling to improve oral health;
> * Providing guidance and assistance to state and local health systems to implement these same approaches; and
> * Communicating with other federally administered health care systems to share best practices.

The committee emphasizes that preventive services should be provided by all types of health care professionals who are competent to do so, including nondental health care professionals. Assistance to state and local health systems could include both financial assistance and technical assistance. HHS will also need to evaluate the adequacy of and support needed for the public health infrastructure to carry out these activities—both at the federal and the state level.

Improving Oral Health Literacy

The public and health care professionals are largely unaware of the basic risk factors and preventive approaches for many oral diseases, and they do not fully appreciate the connection between good oral health and overall health and well-being. For example, the fact that dental caries is both infectious and preventable is not well known, and despite decades of robust evidence about the safety and efficacy of community water fluoridation, segments of the population remain wary of its use.

The committee concluded that the oral health literacy of individuals, communities, and all types of health care providers remains low. This includes lack of understanding about (1) how to prevent and manage oral diseases, (2) the impact of poor oral health, (3) how to navigate the oral health care system, and (4) the best techniques in patient–provider communication.

> **RECOMMENDATION 3:** All relevant HHS agencies should undertake oral health literacy and education efforts aimed at individuals, communities, and health care professionals. These efforts should include, but not be limited to:
> - Community-wide public education on the causes and implications of oral diseases and the effectiveness of preventive interventions;
>   - o Focus areas should include
>   - ▪ The infectious nature of dental caries,
>   - ▪ The effectiveness of fluorides and sealants,
>   - ▪ The role of diet and nutrition in oral health, and
>   - ▪ How oral diseases affect other health conditions.
> - Community-wide guidance on how to access oral health care; and
>   - o Focus areas should include using and promoting websites such as the National Oral Health Clearinghouse and www.health care.gov.
> - Professional education on best practices in patient–provider communication skills that result in improved oral health behaviors.
>   - o Focus areas should include how to communicate to an increasingly diverse population about prevention of oral cancers, dental caries, and periodontal disease.

The committee did not find enough evidence specifically in the oral health literacy and behavioral change literature to recommend exact strategies for delivering needed messages; the examples within the recommendation have the most evidence supporting the need for outreach and are therefore worthwhile areas for HHS to focus on. To be effective, literacy and education efforts should be carried out in accordance with standards for culturally and linguistically appropriate services.

Enhancing the Delivery of Oral Health Care

The adequacy of the oral health workforce, in terms of its size and capabilities, is difficult to assess. However, it is apparent that the current system is not meeting the needs of many citizens, particularly the most vulnerable populations. The nondental health care workforce has little education and training in the basics of oral health care and oral health literacy (e.g., being able to recognize oral diseases and disorders, teaching patients about self-care, understanding basic risk factors, applying topical fluorides). Dental professionals[3] and other health care professionals are trained separately and often do not learn how to work in collaborative teams, including the appropriate use of referrals in both directions. In addition, while professionals from underrepresented minority populations often care for, or are expected to care for, a larger proportion of underserved populations, efforts to increase the diversity of the dental professions have not had substantial impact. These and other challenges have resulted in persistent disparities in access to care along racial, socioeconomic, and urban and rural lines.

Oral health care is predominantly provided by dentists in the private practice setting. Efforts to use new sites of care or types of professionals have been controversial and polarizing. For example, the Indian Health Service recently gained some experience with using dental therapists to target populations that for a variety of reasons (e.g., geographic location) have difficulty accessing oral health care. While the most recent evaluation of these dental therapists was limited to five sites, early results have been promising in terms of the quality of care provided, improved access, and patient satisfaction. Concerns have been expressed about the quality of care provided in alternative settings or by new types of professionals, but data on the quality of care and long-term outcomes related to the provision of care by all types of oral health care professionals are almost wholly lacking. Without further research and evaluation on the delivery of oral health care by a variety of health care professionals, including a comparison of the quality of that care as compared to the care of dentists, better workforce models cannot be developed.

The committee concluded that (1) nondental health care professionals are well situated to play an increased role in oral health care, but they require additional education and training; (2) interprofessional, team-based care has the potential to improve care-coordination, patient outcomes, and produce cost savings, yet dental and nondental health care professionals are rarely trained to work in this manner; (3) new dental professionals and

---

[3] The term *dental professionals* is typically used to include dentists, dental hygienists, dental assistants, and dental laboratory technicians. It may also include new and emerging professionals as they become part of the health care workforce.

existing professionals with expanded duties may have a role to play in expanding access to care; and (4) efforts to broaden the diversity of the oral health care workforce have not produced marked changes.

RECOMMENDATION 4: HHS should invest in workforce innovations to improve oral health that focus on
- Core competency development, education, and training, to allow for the use of all health care professionals in oral health care;
- Interprofessional, team-based approaches to the prevention and treatment of oral diseases;
- Best use of new and existing oral health care professionals; and
- Increasing the diversity and improving the cultural competence of the workforce providing oral health care.

In addition to the training and composition of the oral health workforce, more needs to be done to improve the delivery and financing of oral health care. Significantly fewer Americans have dental coverage than health coverage, which is important because dental coverage is a major predictor of utilization. Challenges in federal financing include the almost complete exclusion of oral health care from the Medicare program and the limited numbers of professionals willing to care for Medicaid populations (often due to low reimbursement rates and high administrative burden). Many other Americans may be considered to be *underinsured*.

Because oral health care is integral to the overall health of individuals and the population, ideally it would be part of every health plan (e.g., Medicare); however, current political and economic barriers make this highly unlikely. Not enough research has been done to determine if alternative payment structures might offer incentives to deliver the most effective services efficiently, or to determine if coverage of preventive services results in long-term cost savings. In addition, as more members of the overall health care workforce become competent and licensed to deliver care, research will be needed for how they will work and be reimbursed.

The committee concluded that (1) distinct segments of the U.S. population have challenges with accessing care in typical settings of care; (2) lack of dental coverage contributes to access problems; (3) newer financing mechanisms might help contain costs and improve health outcomes; and (4) new delivery models need to be explored to improve efficiency.

RECOMMENDATION 5: CMS should explore new delivery and payment models for Medicare, Medicaid, and CHIP to improve access, quality, and coverage of oral health care across the life span.

One option for this endeavor is through the Center for Medicare and Medicaid Innovation that seeks to identify, support, and evaluate models of care that improve quality of care while also lowering costs.

Expanding Research

While much is known about the prevention and management of oral diseases, evidence is lacking for many important aspects of oral health. For example, not enough is known about the best ways to decrease the significant oral health disparities or the best ways to change oral health behaviors. In addition, very few quality measures exist for oral health care, leading to little evidence not only about the quality of the services themselves but also about their ultimate relationship to long-term improvements in oral health. Quality assessment efforts in oral health lag far behind analagous efforts in medicine, most notably in the lack of a universally accepted and used diagnostic coding system for dentistry.

Data sharing and surveillance activities are a central piece of what HHS can contribute to the U.S. oral health care system. Federal agencies, both inside and outside HHS, provide oral health services and collect data on oral health and oral health care; consolidating the data collected by all these sources would be useful in performing secondary research. However, much effort would be needed to make all of these data standardized and usable.

The committee concluded that a more robust evidence base in oral health is needed overall. Efforts are needed most toward (1) generating new evidence on best practices; (2) improving the usefulness of existing data; and (3) evaluating the quality of oral health care (including outcomes).

RECOMMENDATION 6: HHS should place a high priority on efforts to improve open, actionable, and timely information to advance science and improve oral health through research by
- Leveraging resources for research to promote a more robust evidence base specific to oral health care, including, but not limited to,
  - o oral health disparities, and
  - o best practices in oral health care and oral health behavior change;
- Working across HHS agencies—in collaboration with other federal departments (e.g., Department of Defense, Veterans Administration) involved in the collection of oral health data—to integrate, standardize, and promote public availability of relevant databases; and

- Promoting the creation and implementation of new, useful, and appropriate measures of quality oral health care practices, cost and efficiency, and oral health outcomes.

The committee supports the direction of new funding toward research, but in a time of limited resources, HHS needs to prioritize oral health research when deciding on distribution of existing resources.

Measuring Progress

Finally, the committee concluded that an effective NOHI needs an ongoing process for maintaining accountability and for measuring progress toward achieving specific goals of improved oral health.

RECOMMENDATION 7: To evaluate the NOHI the leader(s) of the NOHI should convene an annual public meeting of the agency heads to report on the progress of the NOHI, including
- Progress of each agency in reaching goals;
- New innovations and data;
- Dissemination of best practices and data into the community; and
- Improvement in health outcomes of populations served by HHS programs, especially as they relate to *Healthy People 2020* goals and specific objectives. HHS should provide a forum for public response and comment and make the final proceedings of each meeting available to the public.

This meeting can be an opportunity to report both on short-term and intermediate goals (as set by the individual agencies per Recommendation 1) and progress on *Healthy People 2020* goals and objectives (the overall mission of the NOHI). It is also a means to share best practices and new knowledge and to get public feedback. This meeting need not preclude additional meetings that HHS might hold internally without a public presence.

LOOKING TO THE FUTURE

As this committee looks to the future of HHS' involvement in oral health, questions arise regarding long-term viability both of maintaining oral health as a priority issue and the likelihood of the recommendations of this report coming to fruition. In this vein, the committee has identified three key areas that are needed for future success: strong leadership, sustained interest, and the involvement of multiple stakeholders.

The Importance of Strong Leadership

Compared to previous HHS efforts to improve oral health, the OHI 2010 involves many more HHS agencies and programs at multiple levels. The NOHI further calls for each agency to involve individuals at the staff level, a strategy that veterans of previous initiatives have said can be helpful. However, this also presents the challenge of organizing and directing multiple agencies that are highly autonomous and may not always act in concert. The NOHI presents an additional challenge in that it calls for the increased involvement of and collaboration with leaders from the private sector and other segments of the public sector. The committee believes that the current leadership at HHS is capable of meeting these challenges.

Sustaining Interest

Regardless of how an initiative is structured, much of its long-term viability depends on the interests and efforts of the individuals leading the agencies and HHS, which can change in unpredictable ways over time. For example, a key factor may be whether it can survive a change in presidential administrations, particularly one involving a change in parties. Long-term viability depends on HHS itself making and keeping oral health a priority issue. While the OHI 2010 reflects yet another attempt to enhance the prominence of oral health in HHS, several warning signs have arisen that could contribute to a loss of momentum. For example, in early 2011, the committee learned of the proposed downgrading of the CDC's Division of Oral Health into a branch of the Division of Adult and Community Health. In addition, despite the announcement of the OHI 2010, the CDC's Division of Adolescent and School Health does not list oral health among the "important topics that affect the health and well-being of children and adolescents" and the Administration on Aging does not have any specific initiatives related to the oral health of older adults. Similar to the need for consistent messages to patients and health care professionals about the importance of oral health, HHS needs consistent messaging within its own organization that oral health is a priority across the life span.

Involving Multiple Stakeholders

While HHS should look for ways to be a leader, a range of stakeholders have roles in the success of the NOHI. Collaboration with and learning from the private sector; other public sector entities at the local, state, and national levels; and patients themselves is essential toward achieving the goal of improving the oral health care and, ultimately, the oral health of the entire U.S. population.

CONCLUSION

In discussions with this committee, HRSA expressed a desire for recommendations that could be acted upon quickly, but also have enough flexibility to allow HHS to choose among several methods of implementation. The approach and details of the previously outlined recommendations do just this. Many of the recommendations are not necessarily "new"; as the title of this report suggests, the challenges and strategies illuminated by *Oral Health in America* remain the areas that have the strongest evidence for actions by HHS to advance oral health in America.

The recommendations provided in this report align with the current HHS Strategic Plan for Fiscal Years 2010–2015. Some of the specific objectives and strategies of this plan include ensuring access to quality, culturally competent care for vulnerable populations; strengthening oral health research; and promoting models of oral health care that use a variety of new and existing health care professionals. The recommendations of this report also align with the mission of HHS: "to enhance the health and well-being of Americans by providing for effective health and human services and by fostering sound, sustained advances in the sciences underlying medicine, public health, and social services."

Bringing disparate sectors together to effect significant change is a daunting task, but it is well suited to the mission and responsibilities of HHS. This report focuses on the role HHS can play in improving oral health and shaping oral health care in America—in particular, on the ways in which HHS can have the most impact. There are many reasons that HHS should seize this opportunity. However, most important is the burden that oral diseases are placing on the health and well-being of the American people.

1

Introduction

Can you imagine a time when we fully incorporate mental and dental health into our thinking about health? What is it about problems above the neck that seems to exclude them so often from policy about health care?

—Harvey V. Fineberg, President, Institute of Medicine
Institute of Medicine Annual Meeting, October 12, 2009
(Fineberg, 2009)

The history of efforts of the U.S. Department of Health and Human Services (HHS) to improve the oral health of the nation can probably be encapsulated by one central theme: the need for the mouth to rejoin the body. However, HHS' attempts to assume a leadership role in oral health over the last several decades have been challenged by ambiguous goal setting; a decreasing presence of dental leaders; and a lack of resources, accountability, and coordination among federal departments and agencies. The landmark surgeon general's report *Oral Health in America* was successful in raising the profile of oral health and expanding the conversation to include not just teeth but complete oral and craniofacial health as well (HHS, 2000). The report continues to be regarded as a benchmark for oral health care reform.

Despite numerous oral health initiatives, not enough has been done to address the "silent epidemic" the surgeon general described (HHS, 2000). *Oral Health in America* identified dental caries[1] as "the single most common chronic childhood disease (HHS, 2000)." Today, dental caries remains a common chronic disease across the life span in the United States as well as around the world (Dye et al., 2007; Petersen, 2008; WHO, 2007). Many Americans do not have access to oral health insurance or care. Oral health status among many population groups remains poor. Dentistry remains substantially separated from the rest of health care, and oral health is often overlooked in policy discussions about the nation's health care system. In its most recent attempt to provide leadership in improving the oral health of

---

[1] The term *dental caries* is used in the singular and refers to the disease commonly known as tooth decay (*Dorland's Illustrated Medical Dictionary*, 31st ed., s.v. "caries").

the United States, in 2010 HHS announced a department-wide Oral Health Initiative to create new initiatives in oral health and improve coordination (and align resources) among agencies with existing initiatives (HHS, 2010a,b). In launching this effort, HHS underscored the same key message: oral health is integral to overall health.

ORAL HEALTH AND OVERALL HEALTH

The surgeon general's report referred to the mouth as a mirror of health and disease occurring in the rest of the body in part because a thorough oral examination can detect signs of numerous general health problems, such as nutritional deficiencies and systemic diseases, including microbial infections, immune disorders, injuries, and some cancers (HHS, 2000). In addition, there is mounting evidence that oral health complications not only reflect general health conditions but also exacerbate and even initiate them. Periodontal disease has been associated with adverse pregnancy outcomes (Albert et al., 2011; Offenbacher et al., 2006; Scannapieco et al., 2003b; Tarannum and Faizuddin, 2007; Vergnes and Sixou, 2007), respiratory disease (Scannapieco and Ho, 2001), and cardiovascular disease (Blaizot et al., 2009; Janket et al., 2003; Scannapieco et al., 2003a; Slavkin and Baum, 2000). Periodontal disease has been also shown to affect glycemic control in patients with diabetes (Löe, 1993; Taylor, 2001; Teeuw et al., 2010).

Gies noted the seriousness of the oral-systemic connection nearly a century ago, stating "[c]ertain common and simple disorders of the teeth may involve prompt or insidious development of serious and possibly fatal ailments in other parts of the body" (Gies, 1926). Popular attention to oral health issues and the connection between oral health and overall health increased dramatically in 2007 with the death of Deamonte Driver, a 12-year-old Maryland boy who died when bacteria from an untreated tooth infection spread to his brain (Norris, 2007, 2010; Otto, 2007). Driver's death transformed the oral health discussion as more people—including members of Congress—have begun to recognize the potential seriousness of untreated oral disease. In fact, this tragedy is credited with spurring Congress to require that states provide dental services in their Children's Health Insurance Program (CHIP) benefit packages during the program's federal reauthorization (Iglehart, 2009). Unfortunately, Driver is not the only child to die directly as a result of oral infection (Casamassimo et al., 2009).

The impact of poor oral health is not limited to health alone. Costs of care can be high, and there are also costs related to lack of care, including lost work hours, lost school time, and increased cost of caring for advanced disease. In an often cited study based on the 1989 National Health Interview Survey (NHIS), the authors found that 164 million hours of work were missed annually as a result of dental visits or problems, with more hours being lost by lower-level workers (Gift et al., 1992). In addition, they found that 51 million hours of school were missed by school-age children for dental visits or problems, with the most hours being lost by female, Hispanic, lower-income, and uninsured children. Anecdotal evidence suggests that having visibly missing teeth may be associated with difficulties in finding a job, and a recent study suggests that fluoride exposure during childhood has a strong, statistically significant effect on women's earnings (Eckholm, 2006; Glied and Neidell, 2008; Hyde et al., 2006; Shipler, 2004). For over a century, poor oral health has been a factor in the readiness of military troops to be deployed (DOD, 2002; King and Hynson, 2007; Marburger et al., 2003; Teweles and King, 1987).

INFLUENCES ON ORAL HEALTH AND THE ORAL HEALTH CARE SYSTEM

A number of factors contribute to poor oral health, including the relative lack of attention to oral health among nondental health care professionals,[2] uneven and limited access to oral health care and dental coverage, social determinants of oral health, and the limited oral health literacy of the population. As poor oral health is a multifactorial problem, solutions will need to come from several different areas. In addition, appropriate quality measures in oral health care are necessary to reform the oral health care system to appropriately balance concerns for cost, quality, and access.

Absence from General Health Care

Oral health care has been largely absent from general health care. Nurses, physicians, and other health care professionals have generally not been trained in providing oral health services or screenings (Danielsen et al., 2006; Jablonski, 2010; Mouradian et al., 2005). In addition, dental professionals are generally educated and trained separately from other health care professionals, which reinforces the separation of care as well as lack of training in appropriate referrals between professionals (Mouradian et al., 2003; Pierce et al., 2002). Recently, several efforts have been made to introduce basic oral health care into primary health care.

---

[2] Dental professionals include dentists, dental hygienists, dental assistants, dental laboratory technicians, and new and emerging dental professionals (e.g., dental therapists). *Nondental health care professionals* refers to all other types of health care professionals, including, but not limited to, nurses, pharmacists, physician assistants, and physicians.

- The University of Washington Medical School developed and implemented an oral health curriculum for medical students that led to improvements in students' knowledge of and attitudes toward providing oral health care (Mouradian et al., 2006).
- Since 2006, all residencies in family medicine have been required to include formal training in oral health (Douglass et al., 2009).
- In 2005, New York University placed a college of nursing within the college of dentistry (Spielman et al., 2005). As part of the interdisciplinary educational model, pediatric nurse practitioner students work alongside dental students to provide care in school clinics and Head Start programs (Hallas and Shelley, 2009).

Lack of Coverage

Many people do not have dental coverage (Manski and Brown, 2007). Even with coverage, out-of-pocket costs can still be prohibitively expensive (Manski and Brown, 2007). Dental coverage is a major determinant of access to and utilization of oral health care (Brickhouse et al., 2008; Fisher and Mascarenhas, 2007, 2009; Manski and Brown, 2007).

Typical sources of health care insurance—Medicare, Medicaid, and employers—often do not cover oral health care. Medicaid and CHIP include comprehensive dental benefits for children, but coverage for adults is optional, covers only emergency care in most states, and is often cut when state budgets are tight (CMS, 2011; Veschusio, 2011). Many employers do not offer dental plans as a benefit; these plans are more likely to be offered in larger companies and to higher-wage employees (Ford, 2009). Most adults lose employer-sponsored dental benefits when they retire (Manski et al., 2009), and "routine dental care" is specifically excluded from the traditional Medicare benefits package.[3] The estimates of the number of Americans who are uninsured for dental care vary widely, but it is clear that the rate of dental uninsurance is much greater than that of medical uninsurance. For example, it has been estimated that as many as 130 million U.S. adults and children lack dental coverage (NADP, 2009).

Poor Oral Health Literacy and Communication

Nearly all aspects of oral health care require health literacy: scheduling a dental appointment, determining how much fluoride toothpaste to use on a toddler's toothbrush, understanding when to stop using a baby bottle, recognizing potential complications of a root canal, completing a Medicaid application, understanding media campaigns that promote community

---

[3] Social Security Act §1862(a)(12).

water fluoridation—some degree of literacy and knowledge is required for each task. Yet only 12 percent of the population has proficient health literacy (Kutner et al., 2006). Compounding the problem of low health literacy are the inadequate communication skills of health care professionals. Professionals use medical jargon, provide too much information at once, and fail to confirm that the patient understood the information provided (Williams et al., 2002). As the U.S. population grows more diverse, more will need to be understood about the importance of cultural competence in communication. For example, the cultural and linguistic misunderstandings in health care can be a contributing factor to adverse events such as unnecessary emergency room visits and longer hospital stays (OMH, 2001).

Social Determinants of Health

Aside from health literacy, other social determinants may also affect oral health and inequalities in oral health. The World Health Organization (WHO) describes social determinants of health as a combination of structural determinants ("the unequal distribution of power, income, goods, and services") and daily living conditions ("the conditions in which people are born, grow, live, work, and age") (CSDH, 2008). Commonly examined social determinants include factors such as income, education, occupation, community structure, cultural beliefs and attitudes, social networks, and availability of health services (Patrick et al., 2006). Social gradients in dental decay, periodontal disease, oral cancer, and tooth loss have all been reported (Dye and Thornton-Evans, 2010; Kwan and Petersen, 2010; Sondik et al., 2010). Recognizing the relationship between social determinants of health and oral health outcomes is important for developing interventions.

Limited and Uneven Access

Several factors described thus far, and other factors, contribute to limited and uneven access to oral health care. While access to oral health care has modestly improved over time, many people—typically those who are most vulnerable—still do not get the services they need. In 2007, only 5.5 percent of the population reported being unable to obtain, or had delays in receiving, needed dental care—but this was higher than the numbers that reported being unable to obtain, or had delays in receiving, needed medical care or prescription drugs (Chevarley, 2010). Accessing care is particularly difficult for certain populations, including people who live below the federal poverty line, African Americans, Hispanics, children insured by Medicaid and CHIP, residents of rural areas, people with disabilities, and migrant and seasonal farmworkers (Anthony et al., 2008; Glassman and Subar,

2008; Manski and Brown, 2007; Probst et al., 2007; Skillman et al., 2010; Stanton and Rutherford, 2003; Vargas et al., 2003).

Access to care is complex; it is not just a matter of having available services or being able to afford the care; it also requires having the health literacy, knowledge, and skills to perceive that care is needed as well as to understand how to navigate the oral health care system. Other factors include the availability of transportation and the availability of services provided during nonworking hours (Maserejian et al., 2008). For example, even when individuals have dental coverage, they often still do not receive needed services. Just over one-third of children insured by Medicaid received any dental care in 2004–2005, compared to more than half of children with private health insurance (GAO, 2008). A 2010 report from the U.S. Government Accountability Office (GAO) showed that in many states, most dentists treat few or no Medicaid or CHIP patients (GAO, 2010). The report also showed that "both health centers and the [National Health Service Corps] program report continued need for additional dentists and other dental providers to treat children and adults in underserved areas" (GAO, 2010).

Lack of Quality Assessment

Few quality measures are used in oral health, and no general standards exist for the quality assessment of oral health care (Bader, 2009). In part, quality assessment for oral health is limited by the absence of a universally accepted and used diagnostic coding system. By focusing on procedural codes instead, dental records and billing systems capture the number of oral health procedures conducted, but they do not provide any insight as to the diagnosis or oral health status of each patient. Quality assessment in oral health is also limited due to the absence of a strong evidence base for most treatments and therefore a lack of evidence-based practice guidelines. Oral health research is challenged in part because the typical dental practice design has only one or two dentists. As is the case in the overall health care system, it can be difficult to obtain outcomes data due to the need to gather data from multiple practices as well as the variety of forms that are used to collect the same data. Existing quality measurement tends to focus on patient perceptions and oral health-related quality of life but not treatment outcomes. Without quality measures linking provider interventions and patient outcomes, patients lack information to support decision making about their oral health care and research efforts into oral health best practices will continue to be limited.

STUDY CHARGE AND APPROACH

In February 2010, with support from the Health Resources and Services Administration (HRSA), the Institute of Medicine (IOM) formed the Committee on an Oral Health Initiative to assess the current oral health care system and to advise HHS on actions that should be taken for an HHS oral health initiative (see Box 1-1).

The committee met in person five times during the course of the study. It commissioned one technical paper and heard testimony from a wide range of experts during two public workshops. Staff and committee members also met with and received information from a wide variety of stakeholders and interested individuals.

Scope

While this report provides a brief description of oral health and oral health care in the United States overall, the report focuses mainly on the role HHS can play in shaping oral health in America and, in particular, on the ways in which HHS can have the most impact. There are a wide range of diseases and conditions that manifest themselves in or near the oral cavity—inherited, infectious, and neoplastic diseases and disorders (both acute and chronic). For the purposes of this report, the committee focused mainly on two classes of diseases and their sequelae that cause a great

---

BOX 1-1
The Committee on an Oral Health Initiative
Statement of Task

The IOM, Board on Health Care Services, in collaboration with the Board on Children, Youth, and Families, will undertake a study to

- Assess the current oral health care system for the entire U.S. population;
- Examine preventive oral care interventions, their use and promotion;
- Explore ways of improving health literacy for oral health;
- Review elements of a potential HHS oral health initiative, including possible or current regulations, statutes, programs, research, data, financing, and policy; and
- Recommend strategic actions for HHS agencies and, if relevant and important, other actors, as well as ways to evaluate this initiative.

amount of morbidity: dental caries and periodontal diseases. While HHS is not directly responsible for the functioning of the overall oral health system, it has the opportunity to serve as a leader in improving the oral health of the nation, and there is a need for it to rise to this opportunity.

The committee recognizes that many important factors influence the oral health of Americans, including social determinants, settings of care, workforce, financing, quality assessment, access, literacy, and education. A detailed examination of each of these areas is beyond the scope of this report. Therefore, the committee limited its examination of many of these issues and focused instead on how they relate to possible or current HHS policies and programs. Consequently, the findings, conclusions, and recommendations contained within this report are not exhaustive and will not on their own resolve many of the problems that exist in the nation's oral health care system. The committee is also cognizant of the sizable role that other stakeholders play in this system, including those at the state and local levels as well as private practitioners. This report should be viewed as a complementary piece of a larger solution that will require efforts from all members of the oral health community.

Use of the term *oral health* in this report is intended to promote this comprehensive view. For example, the term *oral health care professional* is used to refer to any health care professional who provides oral health care. This may include, but not be limited to, dental hygienists, dentists, nurses, physician assistants, and physicians. The term *dental* is used in (1) cases that apply only to the professions of dentists, dental hygienists, dental assistants, and, in some cases, dental laboratory technicians and newer dental professionals such as dental therapists; (2) cases in which it is historically accurate to use the term; and (3) cases of insurance coverage, in which *dental insurance or dental coverage* is used to refer to coverage for oral health care and *health insurance* is used to refer to all other health care (e.g., medical care).

In addition, the committee maintains that similar to criticisms of the overall "health care system," a true "oral health care system" does not exist—but is, in fact, a conglomeration of facilities and people that provide care in a variety of unrelated individual systems. This lack of a definable system has contributed, in part, to the existing burden of oral diseases. However, for the purposes of this report, the term *system* is used to describe this uncoordinated spectrum of individual systems of care.

It is also important to note that this report process occurred simultaneously with a report being produced by IOM's Committee on Oral Health Access to Services. While the two studies have related statements of task, the two projects had separate committees, meetings, and review processes. At the time of the writing of this report, the report from the Committee on Oral Health Access to Services was scheduled to be delivered approximately

2 months after this one. The two committees were not made aware of the other's conclusions or recommendations.

Previous IOM Work

More than 30 years have passed since the IOM's first significant look at oral health issues, *Public Policy Options for Better Dental Health* (IOM, 1980), which considered the inclusion of dental services under national health insurance plans. At that time, the IOM found that while methods to prevent and reduce disease were well known, there was a substantial unmet need for oral health care in the United States. The committee explicitly recognized the lack of a national plan for the prevention of disease, the significant financial barriers to access for many Americans, and the omission of oral health from larger public policy discussions. The IOM recommended the inclusion of oral health services in any national health insurance plan, the delivery of preventive services (at a minimum) to children in school-based settings, the use of dental hygienists and assistants (with appropriate training) to provide preventive care in school-based settings, the development of a system for quality and utilization review of dental services, and the institution of a population-based information system. Little has changed since that report both in regard to the need for oral health care as well as in the way that oral health care is delivered and paid for.

More than 15 years ago, the IOM focused on dental education issues in *Dental Education at the Crossroads* (IOM, 1995). In that report, the committee envisioned a future in which dentistry is more integrated in the overall health care system (e.g., education, research, and patient care); dental students have more diverse, hands-on clinical experiences; dental schools contribute to the larger health care community (e.g., research, technology transfer, service to community); dental leaders cooperate to reform accreditation and licensing; and stakeholders continue to test alternative models of education, practice, and performance assessment. The committee laid out four broad objectives: to improve knowledge of what works; to encourage prevention at both the individual and the community level; to reduce disparities; and to promote attention to oral health by those outside of the dental fields. The concerns articulated in that report largely remain, and the overall vision has yet to be realized.

In 2009, the IOM held a 3-day public workshop on the oral health workforce (IOM, 2009d). The first day focused on the connection between oral health and overall health and well-being, oral health needs and the status of access to care, demographics and trends of the oral health workforce, and delivery systems. The second day addressed challenges of the current system (e.g., financing, leadership, regulation, quality assessment), professional ethics, the international experience, and workforce strategies for improving access to oral health care. On the final day of the workshop, speakers and attendees discussed the role that each stakeholder has in improving access to oral health care.

Many other IOM studies that did not focus solely on oral health have highlighted particular oral health issues (e.g., the particular needs of adolescent populations, rural populations, and older adults) and made recommendations related to oral health (IOM, 1992, 2000, 2005b, 2008, 2009a). Previous IOM reports recommended that the National Institute of Dental and Craniofacial Research (NIDCR) of the National Institutes of Health (NIH) should implement programs to increase the number of dental school applicants interested in oral health research, should require that loan forgiveness recipients spend a significant amount of time on research, and should fund required years of the D.D.S./Ph.D. program (IOM, 2005a) and that the NIH should expand medical and dentist scientist training programs "specifically for training investigators in the skills of performing patient-oriented clinical research" (IOM, 1994). Among its most recent reports, the IOM found that the training of dentists and dental hygienists in the care of older adults is inadequate (IOM, 2008); that existing oral health services are generally insufficient to meet the needs of many adolescents (IOM, 2009a); that management of periodontal disease and the effectiveness of various delivery models in the prevention of dental caries in children ranked among the top 100 priority areas for comparative effectiveness research in health care (IOM, 2009c); and that the HHS and U.S. public health and health care workforces suffer from "shortages of primary care physicians and professionals in certain fields, such as oral health, mental health, and nursing (IOM, 2009b).

In 2009, the IOM produced the report *HHS in the 21st Century,* which provided a comprehensive examination of HHS' organization (IOM, 2009b). That committee assessed the overall structure of HHS in relation to its mission, activities, governance, and data collection efforts.

While not speaking explicitly to oral health care, many reports in IOM's history related to primary care, health literacy, access to care, diversity, nutrition, and improving public health have implications for all oral health care professionals (IOM, 1993, 1996, 1997, 2002, 2004a,b, 2005b). In 2002, the IOM examined the future health of the American public and stated:

> Adequate population health cannot be achieved without making comprehensive and affordable health care available to every person residing in the United States. It is the responsibility of the federal government to lead a national effort to examine the options available to achieve stable health care coverage of individuals and families and to assure the implementation of plans to achieve that result. (IOM, 2002)

In view of the strong links between oral health and overall health, the committee reaffirms the statement above in that the federal government (most notably HHS) has a real and pressing responsibility to help ensure that oral health care is comprehensive and available.

OVERVIEW OF THE REPORT

This chapter has provided a brief introduction of the poor oral health status of Americans and its causes, as well as an overview of the study charge and the committee's approach to the work. Chapter 2 broadens the discussion of the link between oral health and overall health and then provides a more detailed overview of the oral health status of Americans, including various subpopulations. The chapter then focuses on two important elements of the committee's charge—prevention and oral health literacy—both of which are central to improving oral health outcomes.

Chapter 3 describes the oral health care delivery and payment systems. It briefly discusses the predominant private practice model, as well as the provision of care through the oral health safety net. It discusses the financing of oral health care through private and public sources. The chapter also describes the oral health workforce, detailing the various professional types, including the nondental workforce and new and emerging members of the dental team. A brief discussion follows regarding how the health care workforce, particularly the dental workforce, is regulated. Finally, the chapter discusses the current and future roles of quality measurement to assess the quality of oral health care.

While Chapters 2 and 3 provide much of the background on the current status of oral health and oral health care overall in the United States, Chapter 4 expounds upon the role for HHS. It details historical and current efforts HHS has taken to reform oral health care, including the recent launch of the HHS Oral Health Initiative of 2010. It gives an overview of the department's wide-ranging activities directed to improving oral health care delivery and financing, including its role in the direct delivery of oral health care, health literacy, disease prevention, and education. The chapter also describes the general activities of other federal departments and agencies that are related to oral health care.

Chapter 5 contains the committee's blueprint for a new oral health initiative. The chapter begins with conclusions about lessons from past HHS oral health initiatives. It then discusses the committee's framework for devising a new oral health initiative. Next, the chapter describes the committee's major conclusions and final recommendations to HHS as to where HHS should place its efforts in improving the oral health of the nation. The report concludes with three key elements the committee believes are necessary for the success of the initiative.

In addition, the report contains four appendixes. Appendix A contains a list of key acronyms used throughout the report. Appendix B contains several organizational charts that describe where key oral health activities occur within HHS. Appendix C lists the agendas of the committee's workshops. Finally, Appendix D contains biographical sketches of the committee members and IOM project staff.

REFERENCES

Albert, D. A., M. D. Begg, H. F. Andrews, S. Z. Williams, A. Ward, M. Lee Conicella, V. Rauh, J. L. Thomson, and P. N. Papapanou. 2011. An examination of periodontal treatment, dental care, and pregnancy outcomes in an insured population in the United States. *American Journal of Public Health* 101(1):151-156.
Anthony, M., J. M. Williams, and A. M. Avery. 2008. Health needs of migrant and seasonal farmworkers. *Journal of Community Health Nursing* 25(3):153-160.
Bader, J. D. 2009. Challenges in quality assessment of dental care. *Journal of the American Dental Association* 140(12):1456-1464.
Blaizot, A., J. N. Vergnes, S. Nuwwareh, J. Amar, and M. Sixou. 2009. Periodontal diseases and cardiovascular events: Meta-analysis of observational studies. *International Dental Journal* 59(4):197-209.
Brickhouse, T. H., R. G. Rozier, and G. D. Slade. 2008. Effects of enrollment in Medicaid versus the State Children's Health Insurance Program on kindergarten children's untreated dental caries. *American Journal of Public Health* 98(5):876-881.
Casamassimo, P. S., S. Thikkurissy, B. L. Edelstein, and E. Maiorini. 2009. Beyond the DMFT: The human and economic cost of early childhood caries. *Journal of the American Dental Association* 140(6):650-657.
Chevarley, F. M. 2010. *Percentage of persons unable to get or delayed in getting needed medical care, dental care, or prescription medicines: United States, 2007.* Statistical Brief 282. Rockville, MD: Agency for Healthcare Research and Quality.
CMS (Centers for Medicare and Medicaid Services). 2011. *Medicaid dental coverage: Overview.* http://www.cms.gov/MedicaidDentalCoverage/ (accessed September 13, 2011).
CSDH (Commission on Social Determinants of Health). 2008. *Closing the gap in a generation: Health equity through action on the social determinants of health.* Geneva, Switzerland: World Health Organization.
Danielsen, R., J. Dillenberg, and C. Bay. 2006. Oral health competencies for physician assistants and nurse practitioners. *Journal of Physician Assistant Education* 17(4):12-16.
DOD (Department of Defense). 2002. *Policy on standardization of oral health and readiness classifications.* https://secure.ucci.com/non-ldap/forms/addp/forms/readiness-policy.pdf (accessed January 3, 2011).
Douglass, A. B., M. Deutchman, J. Douglass, W. Gonsalves, R. Maier, H. Silk, J. Tysinger, and A. S. Wrightson. 2009. Incorporation of a national oral health curriculum into family medicine residency programs. *Family Medicine* 41(3):159-160.
Dye, B., and G. Thornton-Evans. 2010. Trends in oral health by poverty status as measured by Healthy People 2010 objectives. *Public Health Reports* 125(6):817-830.
Dye, B. A., S. Tan, V. Smith, B. G. Lewis, L. K. Barker, G. Thornton-Evans, P. I. Eke, E. D. Beltran-Aguilar, A. M. Horowitz, and L. Chien-Hsun. 2007. *Trends in oral health status: United States, 1988-1994 and 1999-2004.* Hyattsville, MD: United States Department of Health and Human Services, National Center for Health Statistics.

Eckholm, E. 2006. America's "near poor" are increasingly at economic risk, experts say. *New York Times*, May 8. P A14.

Fineberg, H. V. 2009. *Health reform: Beyond health insurance*. Presentation at Institute of Medicine Annual Meeting, Washington, DC. October 12, 2009.

Fisher, M. A., and A. K. Mascarenhas. 2007. Does Medicaid improve utilization of medical and dental services and health outcomes for Medicaid-eligible children in the United States? *Community Dentistry and Oral Epidemiology* 35(4):263-271.

Fisher, M. A., and A. K. Mascarenhas. 2009. A comparison of medical and dental outcomes for Medicaid-insured and uninsured Medicaid-eligible children: A U.S. population-based study. *Journal of the American Dental Association* 140(11):1403-1412.

Ford, J. L. 2009. *The new health participation and access data from the national compensation survey*. http://www.bls.gov/opub/cwc/cm20091022ar01p1.htm (accessed December 27, 2010).

GAO (Government Accountability Office). 2008. *Extent of dental disease in children has not decreased, and millions are estimated to have untreated tooth decay*. Washington, DC: U.S. Government Accountability Office.

GAO. 2010. *Efforts under way to improve children's access to dental services, but sustained attention needed to address ongoing concerns*. Washington, DC: U.S. Government Accountability Office.

Gies, W. J. 1926. *Dental education in the United States and Canada*. New York: The Carnegie Foundation for the Advancement of Teaching.

Gift, H. C., S. T. Reisine, and D. C. Larach. 1992. The social impact of dental problems and visits. *American Journal of Public Health* 82(12):1663-1668.

Glassman, P., and P. Subar. 2008. Improving and maintaining oral health for people with special needs. *Dental Clinics of North America* 52(2):447-461.

Glied, S., and M. Neidell. 2008. The economic value of teeth. *NBER Working Paper Series* 13879.

Hallas, D., and D. Shelley. 2009. Role of pediatric nurse practitioners in oral health care. *Academic Pediatrics* 9(6):462-466.

HHS (Department of Health and Human Services). 2000. *Oral health in America: A report of the surgeon general*. Rockville, MD: Department of Health and Human Services.

HHS. 2010a. *HHS launches oral health initiative*. http://www.hhs.gov/ash/news/20100426.html (accessed November 17, 2010).

HHS. 2010b. *HHS oral health initiative 2010*. http://www.hrsa.gov/publichealth/clinical/oralhealth/hhsinitiative.pdf (accessed August 19, 2010).

Hyde, S., W. A. Satariano, and J. A. Weintraub. 2006. Welfare dental intervention improves employment and quality of life. *Journal of Dental Research* 85(1):79-84.

Iglehart, J. 2009. *Dental coverage in SCHIP: The legacy of Deamonte Driver*. http://healthaffairs.org/blog/2009/01/30/dental-coverage-in-schip-the-legacy-of-deamonte-driver/ (accessed August 19, 2010).

IOM (Institute of Medicine). 1980. *Public policy options for better dental health*. Washington, DC: National Academy Press.

IOM. 1992. *The second fifty years: Promoting health and preventing disability*. Washington, DC: National Academy Press.

IOM. 1993. *Access to health care in America*. Washington, DC: National Academy Press.

IOM. 1994. *Careers in clinical research: Obstacles and opportunities*. Washington, DC: National Academy Press.

IOM. 1995. *Dental education at the crossroads: Challenges and change*. Washington, DC: National Academy Press.

IOM. 1996. *Primary care: America's health in a new era*. Washington, DC. National Academy Press.

IOM. 1997. *Dietary reference intakes*. Washington, DC: National Academy Press.

IOM. 2000. *Extending Medicare coverage for preventive and other services*. Washington, DC: National Academy Press.

IOM. 2002. *The future of the public's health in the 21st century*. Washington, DC: The National Academies Press.

IOM. 2004a. *Health literacy: A prescription to end confusion*. Washington, DC: The National Academies Press.

IOM. 2004b. *In the nation's compelling interest: Ensuring diversity in the health-care workforce*. Washington, DC: The National Academies Press.

IOM. 2005a. *Advancing the nation's health needs: NIH research training programs*. Washington, DC: The National Acadmies Press.

IOM. 2005b. *Quality through collaboration: The future of rural health care*. Washington, DC: The National Academies Press.

IOM. 2008. *Retooling for an aging America*. Washington, DC: The National Academies Press.

IOM. 2009a. *Adolescent health services: Missing opportunities*. Washington, DC: The National Academies Press.

IOM. 2009b. *HHS in the 21st Century*. Washington, DC: The National Academies Press.

IOM. 2009c. *Initial national priorities for comparative effectiveness research*. Washington, DC: The National Academies Press.

IOM. 2009d. *The U.S. oral health workforce in the coming decade: Workshop summary*. Washington, DC: The National Academies Press.

Jablonski, R. 2010. *Nursing education and research (geriatrics)*. Presentation at meeting of the Committee on an Oral Health Initiative, Washington, DC. June 28, 2010.

Janket, S. J., A. E. Baird, S. K. Chuang, and J. A. Jones. 2003. Meta-analysis of periodontal disease and risk of coronary heart disease and stroke. *Oral Surgery, Oral Medicine, Oral Pathology, Oral Radiology, and Endodontics* 95(5):559-569.

King, J. E., and R. G. Hynson. 2007. *Highlights in the history of U.S. Army dentistry*. Falls Church, VA: U.S. Army.

Kutner, M., E. Greenberg, Y. Jin, and C. Paulsen. 2006. *The health literacy of America's adults: Results from the 2003 National Assessment of Adult Literacy*. Washington, DC: National Center for Health Statistics.

Kwan, S., and P. E. Petersen. 2010. Oral health: Equity and social determinants. In *Equity, social determinants and public health programmes*, edited by E. Blas and A. S. Kurup. Geneva, Switzerland: World Health Organization Press.

Löe, H. 1993. Periodontal disease. The sixth complication of diabetes mellitus. *Diabetes Care* 16(1):329-334.

Manski, R. J., and E. Brown. 2007. *Dental use, expenses, private dental coverage, and changes, 1996 and 2004*. Rockville, MD: Agency for Healthcare Research and Quality.

Manski, R. J., J. Moeller, J. Schimmel, P. A. St. Clair, H. Chen, L. Magder, and J. V. Pepper. 2009. Dental care coverage and retirement. *Journal of Public Health Dentistry* 70(1):1-12.

Marburger, T., J. Chaffin, and L. D. Fretwell. 2003. Dental class 3 intercept clinic: A model for treating dental class 3 soldiers. *Military Medicine* 168(7):548-552.

Maserejian, N. N., F. Trachtenberg, C. Link, and M. Tavares. 2008. Underutilization of dental care when it is freely available: A prospective study of the New England Children's Amalgam Trial. *Journal of Public Health Dentistry* 68(3):139-148.

Mouradian, W. E., J. H. Berg, and M. J. Somerman. 2003. Addressing disparities through dental-medical collaborations, part 1. The role of cultural competency in health disparities: Training of primary care medical practitioners in children's oral health. *Journal of Dental Education* 67(8):860-868.

Mouradian, W. E., A. Reeves, S. Kim, R. Evans, D. Schaad, S. G. Marshall, and R. Slayton. 2005. An oral health curriculum for medical students at the University of Washington. *Academic Medicine* 80(5):434-442.

Mouradian, W. E., A. Reeves, S. Kim, C. Lewis, A. Keerbs, R. L. Slayton, D. Gupta, R. Oskouian, D. Schaad, and T. Kalet. 2006. A new oral health elective for medical students at the University of Washington. *Teaching and Learning in Medicine* 18(4):336-342.

NADP (National Association of Dental Plans). 2009. *Dental benefits improve access to dental care.* http://www.nadp.org/Libraries/HCR_Documents/nadphcr-dentalbenefitsimprove accesstocare-3-28-09.sflb.ashx (accessed January 10, 2011).

Norris, L. 2007. *Testimony of the Public Justice Center on May 2, 2007 to the Subcommittee on Domestic Policy, Committee on Oversight and Government Reform, U.S. House of Representatives (110th Congress), on the story of Deamonte Driver and ensuring oral health for children enrolled in Medicaid.*

Norris, L. 2010. *Navigating the system: The patient's perspective.* Presentation at meeting of the Committee on Oral Health Access to Services, San Francisco, CA. July 27, 2010.

Offenbacher, S., D. Lin, R. Strauss, R. McKaig, J. Irving, S. P. Barros, K. Moss, D. A. Barrow, A. Hefti, and J. D. Beck. 2006. Effects of periodontal therapy during pregnancy on periodontal status, biological parameters, and pregnancy outcomes: A pilot study. *Journal of Periodontology* 77(12):2011-2024.

OMH (Office of Minority Health). 2001. *National standards for culturally and linguistically appropriate services in health care.* Washington, DC: U.S. Department of Health and Human Services.

Otto, M. 2007. For want of a dentist. *Washington Post*, February 28, P. B01.

Patrick, D. L., R. S. Y. Lee, M. Nucci, D. Grembowski, C. Z. Jolles, and P. Milgrom. 2006. Reducing oral health disparities: A focus on social and cultural determinants. *BMC Oral Health* 6(Supp. 1):S4.

Petersen, P. E. 2008. World Health Organization global policy for improvement of oral health—world health assembly 2007. *International Dental Journal* 58(3):115-121.

Pierce, K. M., R. G. Rozier, and W. F. Vann. 2002. Accuracy of pediatric primary care providers' screening and referral for early childhood caries. *Pediatrics* 109(5):e82.

Probst, J., S. Laditka, J.-Y. Wang, and A. Johnson. 2007. Effects of residence and race on burden of travel for care: Cross-sectional analysis of the 2001 U.S. National Household Travel Survey. *BMC Health Services Research* 7(1):40.

Scannapieco, F. A., and A. W. Ho. 2001. Potential associations between chronic respiratory disease and periodontal disease: Analysis of National Health and Nutrition Examination Survey III. *Journal of Periodontology* 72(1):50-56.

Scannapieco, F. A., R. B. Bush, and S. Paju. 2003a. Associations between periodontal disease and risk for atherosclerosis, cardiovascular disease, and stroke. A systematic review. *Annals of Periodontology* 8(1):38-53.

Scannapieco, F. A., R. B. Bush, and S. Paju. 2003b. Periodontal disease as a risk factor for adverse pregnancy outcomes. A systematic review. *Annals of Periodontology* 8(1):70-78.

Shipler, D. 2004. *Working poor: Invisible in America.* Westminster, MD: Alfred A. Knopf.

Skillman, S. M., M. P. Doescher, W. E. Mouradian, and D. K. Brunson. 2010. The challenge to delivering oral health services in rural America. *Journal of Public Health Dentistry* 70(Supp. 1):S49-S57.

Slavkin, H. C., and B. J. Baum. 2000. Relationship of dental and oral pathology to systemic illness. *Journal of the American Medical Association* 284(10):1215-1217.

Sondik, E. J., D. T. Huang, R. J. Klein, and D. Satcher. 2010. Progress toward the Healthy People 2010 goals and objectives. *Annual Review of Public Health* 31(1):271-281.

Spielman, A. I., T. Fulmer, E. S. Eisenberg, and M. C. Alfano. 2005. Dentistry, nursing, and medicine: A comparison of core competencies. *Journal of Dental Education* 69(11): 1257-1271.

Stanton, M. W., and M. K. Rutherford. 2003. *Dental care: Improving access and quality.* Rockville, MD: Agency for Healthcare Research and Quality.

Tarannum, F., and M. Faizuddin. 2007. Effect of periodontal therapy on pregnancy outcome in women affected by periodontitis. *Journal of Periodontology* 78(11):2095-2103.

Taylor, G. W. 2001. Bidirectional interrelationships between diabetes and periodontal diseases: An epidemiologic perspective. *Annals of Periodontology* 6(1):99-112.

Teeuw, W. J., V. E. A. Gerdes, and B. G. Loos. 2010. Effect of periodontal treatment on glycemic control of diabetic patients: A systematic review and meta-analysis. *Diabetes Care* 33(2):421-427.

Teweles, R. B., and J. E. King. 1987. Impact of troop dental health on combat readiness. *Military Medicine* 152(5):233-235.

Vargas, C. M., B. A. Dye, and K. L. Hayes. 2003. Oral health care utilization by U.S. rural residents, National Health Interview Survey 1999. *Journal of Public Health Dentistry* 63(3):150-157.

Vergnes, J. N., and M. Sixou. 2007. Preterm low birth weight and maternal periodontal status: A meta-analysis. *American Journal of Obstetrics and Gynecology* 196(2):135, e131-135, e137.

Veschusio, C. 2011. *Oral health update: Ten years after the surgeon general's report, a state perspective: South Carolina.* Paper presented at Presentation at National Health Policy Forum. January, 21, 2011.

WHO (World Health Organization). 2007. *Oral health—fact sheet No. 318.* http://www.who.int/mediacentre/factsheets/fs318/en/index.html (accessed February 17, 2011).

Williams, M. V., T. Davis, R. M. Parker, and B. D. Weiss. 2002. The role of health literacy in patient-physician communication. *Family Medicine* 34(5):383-389.

2

Oral Health and Overall Health and Well-Being

A number of factors influence oral health status and may act as obstacles to improving the oral health of the nation. Patients and health care professionals need to understand the importance of oral health, especially its connection to overall health, and apply that knowledge in practice. In addition, patients need to have the knowledge, understanding, ability, and means to access oral health care, and professionals must be available to provide care. Oral health may also be affected by several social determinants of health such as race, income, living conditions, and working conditions.

This chapter presents an overview of the inextricable link between oral health and overall health and well-being, as well as the many factors that can affect oral health improvement. First, the connection between oral health and overall health, including the implications of poor oral health, is briefly discussed. Next, the overall health status of the American population is reviewed, and the oral health status and utilization patterns of various vulnerable and underserved populations are considered. The chapter continues with the examination of preventive oral health interventions for many oral diseases. Finally, the chapter concludes with a discussion of basic health literacy issues (including oral health literacy), especially how they affect the ability of individuals, communities, and practitioners to improve oral health status. The specific roles of the U.S. Department of Health and Human Services (HHS) in health literacy and prevention are discussed in Chapter 4.

THE LINK BETWEEN ORAL HEALTH AND OVERALL HEALTH

For people suffering from dental, oral, or craniofacial pain, the link between oral health and general well-being is beyond dispute. However, for policy makers, payers, and health care professionals, a chasm dividing the two has developed over time and continues to exist today. In effect, the oral health care field has remained separated from general health care (e.g., medicine, pharmacy, nursing, allied health professions). Recently, however, researchers and others have placed a greater emphasis on establishing and clarifying the oral-systemic linkages.

The surgeon general's report *Oral Health in America* made it clear that oral health care is broader than dental care and that a healthy mouth is more than just healthy teeth (see Box 2-1). The report described the mouth as a mirror of health and disease occurring in the rest of the body, in part because a thorough oral examination can detect signs of numerous general health problems, such as nutritional deficiencies and systemic diseases, including microbial infections, immune disorders, injuries, and some cancers (HHS, 2000b). Oral lesions are often the first manifestation of HIV infection and may be used to predict progression from HIV to AIDS (Coogin et al., 2005). Sexually transmitted HP-16 virus has been established as the cause of a number of vaginal as well as oropharyngeal cancers (Marur et al., 2010; Shaw and Robinson, 2010). Dry mouth (xerostomia) is an early symptom of Sjogren's syndrome, one of the most common autoimmune disorders (Al-Hashimi, 2001), and is also a side effect for a large number

---

BOX 2-1
Dental, Oral, and Craniofacial

The word *oral* refers to the mouth. The mouth includes not only the teeth and the gums (gingiva) and their supporting tissues but also the hard and soft palate, the mucosal lining of the mouth and throat, the tongue, the lips, the salivary glands, the chewing muscles, and the upper and lower jaws. Equally important are the branches of the nervous, immune, and vascular systems that animate, protect, and nourish the oral tissues, as well as provide connections to the brain and the rest of the body. The genetic patterning of development in utero further reveals the intimate relationship of the oral tissues to the developing brain and to the tissues of the face and head that surround the mouth, structures whose location is captured in the word *craniofacial.*

SOURCE: HHS, 2000b

of prescribed medications (Nabi et al., 2006; Uher et al., 2009; Weinberger et al., 2010).

Further, there is mounting evidence that oral health complications not only reflect general health conditions but also exacerbate them. Infections that begin in the mouth can travel throughout the body. For example, periodontal bacteria have been found in samples removed from brain abscesses (Silva, 2004), pulmonary tissue (Suzuki and Delisle, 1984), and cardiovascular tissue (Haraszthy et al., 2000). Periodontal disease may be associated with adverse pregnancy outcomes (Offenbacher et al., 2006; Scannapieco et al., 2003b; Tarannum and Faizuddin, 2007; Vergnes and Sixou, 2007), respiratory disease (Scannapieco and Ho, 2001), cardiovascular disease (Blaizot et al., 2009; Janket et al., 2003; Paraskevas, 2008; Scannapieco et al., 2003a; Slavkin and Baum, 2000), coronary heart disease (Bahekar et al., 2007), and diabetes (Chávarry et al., 2009; Löe, 1993; Taylor, 2001; Teeuw et al., 2010). However, the relationship between periodontal disease and these systemic diseases is not well understood, and there is conflicting evidence about whether periodontal treatment affects outcomes for these systemic conditions (Beck et al., 2008; Fogacci et al., 2011; Jeffcoat et al., 2003; Lopez et al., 2002, 2005; Macones et al., 2010; Michalowicz et al., 2006; Newnham et al., 2009; Offenbacher et al., 2006, 2009; Paraskevas et al., 2008; Polyzos et al., 2009, 2010; Sadatmansouri et al., 2006; Simpson et al., 2010; Tarannum and Faizuddin, 2007; Teeuw et al., 2010; Uppal et al., 2010).

Although there is a wide range of diseases and conditions that manifest themselves in or near the oral cavity itself, discussions of oral health tend to focus on the diagnosis and treatment of two types of diseases and their sequelae: dental caries and periodontal diseases. The most common of those diseases, dental caries, is a common chronic disease in the United States (Dye et al., 2007) and among the most common diseases in the world (WHO, 2010e). As mentioned previously, periodontal disease has been associated with numerous systemic diseases throughout the body from heart disease to diabetes (Bahekar et al., 2007; Chávarry et al., 2009). There is some degree of tragedy in this situation because both dental caries and periodontal disease are highly preventable.

Dental caries was described in the surgeon general's report as "the single most common chronic childhood disease" (HHS, 2000b). Most people remain unaware that dental caries is caused by a bacterial infection (e.g., *Streptococcus mutans*) that is often passed from person to person (e.g., from mother to child). Aside from dental health implications, nontreatment of dental caries may be associated with several types of morbidity (both individual and societal), including loss of days from school (Gift et al., 1992, 1993), inappropriate use of emergency departments (Cohen et al., 2011; Davis et al., 2010), orofacial pain (Nomura et al., 2004; Traebert et al., 2005), and inability for military forces to deploy (Bray, 2006). In fact, while the death of Deamonte Driver made headlines and sparked a national debate about the importance of oral health care (Norris, 2007; Otto, 2007), there have been other similar cases in recent times (Casamassimo et al., 2009; Jackson, 2007). In spite of decades of knowledge of how to prevent dental caries, this disease remains a significant problem for all age groups.

OVERALL ORAL HEALTH STATUS

Evidence on how well the current oral health system is performing can be found in the mouths of the American people. And while evidence suggests that oral health has been improving in most of the U.S. population, many sub-groups are not faring as well (Dye et al., 2007).

The National Health and Nutrition Examination Survey

One of the most important functions HHS has performed over time has been monitoring the oral health status of the nation. The department has conducted a number of national data collection efforts through the National Center for Health Statistics of the Centers for Disease Control and Prevention (CDC), as well as other agencies within the department. The National Health and Nutrition Examination Survey (NHANES) is the main source for oral health information in the United States; data are collected from a representative sample of the civilian U.S. population through interviews and clinical examinations.

In April 2007, the National Center for Health Statistics released a comprehensive assessment of U.S. oral health status (Dye et al., 2007). Using data provided by two iterations of the NHANES (NHANES III, 1988–1994 and NHANES 1999–2004), the assessment concluded that most Americans experienced improvements in their oral health over the two time periods (Dye et al., 2007). Specifically, the report noted that among older adults, edentulism (complete tooth loss) and periodontitis (gum disease) had declined. Among adults, the CDC observed improvements in the prevalence of dental caries, tooth retention, and periodontal health. For adolescents and youths, dental caries decreased, while dental sealants (thin plastic coatings applied to the grooves on the chewing surfaces of the back teeth to protect them from dental caries) became more prevalent. Among poor Mexican-American children ages 6–11, untreated dental caries decreased from 51 to 42 percent (Dye et al., 2010). The proportion of adolescents age 12–19 with caries in their permanent dentition decreased (Edelstein and Chinn, 2009). More children have received at least one dental sealant on a permanent tooth; the prevalence increased from 22 to 30 percent among children ages 6–11 and from 18 to 38 percent in adolescents ages 12–19 (Dye et al.,

2007). Encouragingly, the increase was consistent among all racial and ethnic groups, although non-Hispanic black and Mexican-American children and adolescents continue to have a lower prevalence of sealants than do whites, and poor children receive fewer dental sealants than those who live above 200 percent of the federal poverty line (Dye et al., 2007).

While the data from the NHANES surveys showed improvements in oral health status across two intervals of time, the most current information on American oral health status was not especially favorable. For example, the latter survey found that more than a quarter of adults ages 20–64 and nearly one-fifth of respondents over age 65 were experiencing untreated dental caries at the time of their examination (Dye et al., 2007). Further, caries prevalence among preschool children increased between 1988–1994 and 1999–2004 (Dye et al., 2007). Based on the NHANES results, Table 2-1 provides an overview of the U.S. population's oral health status during the 1999–2004 time period. The percentage of persons with caries experience increases with age, in part because once cavitated, this is a nonreversible disease measured by active and treated disease. While a fifth of children 6–11 years of age have had caries, this proportion increases to more than half of children 12 to 19 years of age and to 90-plus percent of adults 20 years and over. Socioeconomic status, measured by poverty status in this case, is a strong determinant of oral health (Vargas et al., 1998). In every age group, persons in the lower-income group were more likely to have had caries experience and more than twice as likely to have untreated dental caries compared with their higher-income counterparts. Among persons age 65 and over, edentulism is more frequent among those living below the poverty level than among those living at twice the poverty level (Dye et al., 2007).

In addition, a significant proportion of the population continues to suffer from periodontal disease. According to the most recent NHANES survey, at least 8.5 percent of adults (ages 20–64) and 17.2 percent of older adults (age 65 and older) in the United States suffer from periodontal disease (NIDCR, 2011a,b), and in fact, the periodontal examination used in NHANES may have understated the true incidence of periodontal disease by 50 percent or more (Eke et al., 2010).

Healthy People

Since 1980, HHS has used the *Healthy People* process to set the country's health-promotion and disease-prevention agenda (Koh, 2010). *Healthy People* is a set of health objectives for the nation consisting of overarching goals for improving the overall health of all Americans and more specific objectives in a variety of focus areas, including oral health. Every 10 years, HHS evaluates the progress that has been made on *Healthy People* goals

TABLE 2-1
Prevalence of Caries Experience and Untreated Caries by Age
and Poverty Status (1999-2004)

Population Characteristics		Caries Prevalence	
		Caries Experience	Untreated Caries
Age and Dentition		**Percentage**	**Percentage**
2-11 primary teeth	*Total 2- to 11-year olds*	42.2	22.9
	2-5 years	27.9	20.5
	6-11 years	51.2	24.5
Poverty	< 100%	54.3	32.5
	100-200%	48.8	28.4
	> 200%	32.3	15.0
6-11 permanent teeth	*Total 6- to 11-year olds*	21.1	7.7
Poverty	< 100%	28.3	11.8
	100-200%	24.1	11.9
	> 200%	16.3	3.6
12-19 permanent teeth	*Total 12- to 19-year olds*	59.1	19.6
Poverty	< 100%	65.6	27.1
	100-200%	64.4	27.0
	> 200%	54.0	12.9
20-64 permanent teeth	*Total 20- to 64-year olds*	91.6	25.5
	20-34	85.6	27.9
	35-49	94.3	25.6
	50-64	95.6	22.1
Poverty	< 100%	88.7	43.9
	100-200%	88.9	39.3
	> 200%	93.1	18.0
65+ permanent teeth	*Total 65+*	93.0	18.2
Poverty	< 100%	83.5	33.2
	100-200%	90.9	23.8
	> 200%	95.5	14.2

SOURCE: Dye et al., 2007.

and objectives, develops new goals and objectives, and sets new bench-marks for progress. The objectives are drafted by relevant HHS agencies, with extensive input from external stakeholders and the public. The oral health objectives are developed by four co-lead agencies—the CDC, Health Resources and Services Administration (HRSA), the Indian Health Service, and the National Institutes of Health (NIH)—with input from the Office of Disease Prevention and Health Promotion, the Office of Minority Health, the Office on Women's Health, and the National Center for Health Statistics, as well as comments from dental professional organizations, including state and local dental directors (Dye, 2010). (See Chapter 4 for more on the history of *Healthy People* as well as a description of *Healthy People 2020* goals and objectives.)

Progress on the *Healthy People 2010* goals was mixed (Koh, 2010; Sondik et al., 2010; Tomar and Reeves, 2009). At the midcourse review in 2006, no oral health objectives had met or exceeded their targets (HHS, 2006). Encouragingly, however, progress was made in a number of categories, including decreasing caries among adolescents (although not among younger children), increasing the proportion of children with dental sealants, increasing the proportion of adults with no permanent tooth loss, and increasing the proportion of the population with access to community water fluoridation (HHS, 2006; Tomar and Reeves, 2009). In contrast, several objectives moved away from their targets. For example, the proportion of children age 2 to 4 years with dental caries increased from 18 to 22 percent, and the proportion of untreated dental caries in this population increased from 16 to 17 percent (HHS, 2006). In addition, the number of oral and pharyngeal cancers detected at an early stage decreased.

Oral Health Status: Beyond the Teeth

Oral health is more than healthy teeth, and oral diseases and disorders are more than caries and periodontal disease. Oral diseases and disorders can be either acute (e.g., broken tooth) or chronic (e.g., caries) and have a number of different causes, including inheritance (e.g., cleft lip and palate), infection (e.g., caries), neoplasia (e.g., oral, nasal, and pharyngeal cancers), and neuromuscular (e.g., temporomandibular joint disorder). Although caries and periodontal disease are the most commonly discussed oral diseases, other oral diseases also have a significant burden. Between 1999 and 2001, the annual prevalence of cleft lip in the United States was approximately 1 in 1,000 live births (NIDCR, 2010). The overall incidence of head and neck cancers is falling due to declining use of cigarettes and other tobacco products; however, an increasing number of younger women without the typical risk factors (tobacco and alcohol use) have been diagnosed with oral cancers, causing speculation about the relationship between human papilloma virus and oral cancer (D'Souza et al., 2007; Mork et al., 2001; Sturgis and Cinciripini, 2007). In 2010, there were more than 36,000 new cases of oral and pharyngeal cancer (Altekruse et al., 2010). Although early-stage oral cancers are treatable, the mortality rate is relatively high because most oral cancers are diagnosed at a later stage (HHS, 2000b). This problem is particularly acute for African Americans, who are more likely to be diagnosed at a late stage and who have a much lower 5-year survival rate than whites do (about 42 percent for African Americans compared to about 63 percent for whites) (Altekruse et al., 2010).

ORAL HEALTH STATUS AND ORAL HEALTH CARE UTILIZATION BY SPECIFIC POPULATIONS

While some data show improvements in the U.S. oral health status overall, underserved and vulnerable populations continue to suffer disparities in both their disease burden and access to needed services. Dental caries remains a significant problem in certain populations such as poor children and racial and ethnic minorities of all ages (Dye, 2010; Dye et al., 2007). In addition, limited and uneven use of oral health care services contributes to both poor oral health and disparities in oral health. More than half of the population (56 percent) did not visit a dentist in 2004 (Manski and Brown, 2007), and in 2007, 5.5 percent of the population reported being unable to get or delaying needed dental care, higher than the percentage that reported being unable to get or delaying needed medical care or prescription drugs (Chevarley, 2010). In this section, the particular issues of some underserved populations are highlighted. The specific challenges of these populations and others are being examined more in depth by the IOM Committee on Oral Health Access to Services.

Age Groups

Dental disease is also a problem across the age spectrum. In this section, special challenges for children, adolescents, and older adults are highlighted.

Children

Over the decades, many different sources have noted the burden of dental disease on children. The surgeon general's report identified dental caries as "the single most common chronic childhood disease—five times more common than asthma and seven times more common than hay fever" (HHS, 2000b). Over 27 percent of children ages 2 to 5 have early childhood caries (defined as caries in children ages 1 to 5 years old), and more than 50 percent of children ages 6 to 11 have caries in their primary teeth (Dye et al., 2007; Ismail and Sohn, 1999). More than 20 percent of those caries are untreated (Dye et al., 2007). The lack of adequate dental treatment may affect children's speech, nutrition, growth and function, social development, and quality of life (HHS, 2000b). For school-age children in particular, oral disease can impose restrictions in their daily activities; in excess of 51 million school hours are lost each year due to dental-related illness (HHS, 2000b). In addition, 14 percent of children 6–12 years old have had toothache severe enough during the past six months to have complained to their parents, and many others may have suffered silently with the same symptoms (Lewis and Stout, 2010).

Adolescents

Adolescents, generally those age 10–19 (IOM, 2009), have risk factors for dental caries similar to those for other age groups, but adolescents' risk for oral and perioral injury is especially exacerbated by behaviors such as the use of alcohol and illicit drugs, driving without a seat belt, cycling without a helmet, engaging in contact sports without a mouth guard, and using firearms (IOM, 2009). Other concerns among adolescent populations (that may be similar to those of other age groups) include damage caused by the use of all forms of tobacco, erosion of teeth and damage to soft tissues caused by eating disorders, oral manifestations of sexually transmitted infections (e.g., soft tissue lesions) as a result of oral sex, and increased risk of periodontal disease during pregnancy.

Adults

Adults ages 20 to 64 have similar risk factors for oral disease as other age groups, although because oral disease accumulates with age, adults generally have more oral disease than do their younger cohorts. In addition, adults may have difficulty obtaining dental insurance, because many states offer limited or no dental benefits to adults through Medicaid (Kaiser Family Foundation, 2011). In 2007, 5 percent of adults were covered by public dental insurance, an additional 65.5 percent had private coverage, and 35.5 percent lacked dental insurance altogether (Manski and Brown, 2010).

Older Adults

Both the prevalence of periodontal disease and the percentage of teeth with caries increase as the population ages (Dye et al., 2007; Vargas et al., 2001). Older adults often have chronic diseases that may exacerbate their oral health, and vice versa. Older adults are more likely to have serious medical issues and functional limitations, which can deter them from seeking dental care (Dolan et al., 1998; Kiyak and Reichmuth, 2005). Older adults who spend more on medication and medical visits are less likely to use dental services (Kuthy et al., 1996). Moreover, dental insurance is generally linked to employment, and upon retirement, most older adults lose their dental insurance (Manski et al., 2010). Despite these challenges, the oral health of older adults is improving: between NHANES III and NHANES 1999–2004, the prevalence of caries, periodontal disease, and edentulism among older adults all decreased (Dye et al., 2007).

While federal law requires long-term care facilities that receive Medicare or Medicaid funding to provide access to dental care, only 80 percent of facilities report doing so (Dolan et al., 2005). Even when dental care is available, many residents do not regularly receive dental care, and many oral health problems go undetected (Dolan et al., 2005). Only 19 percent of dentists report providing treatment in long-term care facilities in the past, and only 37 percent showed interest in doing so in the future (Dolan et al., 2005). In the absence of dentists, nursing home staff must identify residents' oral health needs, but nurses (as well as many other health professionals) are not adequately trained to identify or treat many oral health issues (Dolan et al., 2005; IOM, 2008).

People with Special Health Care Needs

It appears that people with special health care needs[1] have poorer oral health than the general population has (Anders and Davis, 2010; Owens et al., 2006). Most, though not all, studies indicate that the overall prevalence of caries in people with special needs is either the same as the general population or slightly lower (Anders and Davis, 2010; López Pérez et al., 2002; Seirawan et al., 2008; Tiller et al., 2001). But, available data indicate that people with special needs suffer disproportionately from periodontal disease and edentulism, have more untreated caries, have poorer oral hygiene, and receive less care than the general population does (Anders and Davis, 2010; Armour et al., 2008; Havercamp et al., 2004; Owens et al., 2006). However, high-quality data on the oral health of people with special needs in the United States is scarce (Anders and Davis, 2010). People with special health care needs are a difficult population to reach, in part because of their diversity, and also because they are geographically dispersed. Moreover, it is also difficult to analyze national data on this population because their numbers are not large enough to produce reliable statistics. Many of the

---

[1] For the purpose of this report, people with special health care needs are people who have difficulty accessing oral health care due to complicated medical, physical, or psychological conditions (Glassman and Subar, 2008).

available studies of people with special health care needs were conducted with populations that are not representative of the special needs community as a whole (Feldman et al., 1997; Owens et al., 2006; Reid et al., 2003).

Disparities in oral health for people with special needs are due to a variety of reasons. People with special needs often take medications that cause a reduced saliva flow, which promotes caries and periodontal disease (HHS, 2000b). Additionally, people with special needs often have impaired dexterity and thus rely on others for oral hygiene (Shaw et al., 1989). They also face systematic barriers to oral health care such as transportation barriers (especially for those with physical disabilities), cost, and health professionals that are not trained to work with special needs patients or dental offices that are not physically suited for them (Glassman and Subar, 2008; Glassman et al., 2005; Stiefel, 2002; Yuen et al., 2010).

Poor Populations

Poor children are more likely to have untreated dental caries and less likely to receive sealants than nonpoor children, despite having almost universal access to dental insurance through Medicaid (Dye et al., 2007; HHS, 2000b). Poor children and adults receive fewer dental services than does the population as a whole (Dye et al., 2007; Lewis et al., 2007; Stanton and Rutherford, 2003). Encouragingly, however, a recent analysis of NHANES data indicated that the largest increase in dental sealant use occurred among poor children, although they continue to lag behind higher-income children (Dye and Thornton-Evans, 2010). The increase among poor children may be due to school-based sealant programs, which in 17 states reach children in 25 percent or more of schools serving low-income families (Pew Center on the States, 2010). The likelihood of visiting a dentist decreases with decreasing income, and people from poor families are less likely to have visited a dentist within the previous year and less likely to have a preventive dental visit (Manski and Brown, 2007; Stanton and Rutherford, 2003).

Pregnant Women and Mothers

The oral health care of women is important for the health of the women as well as for the effects it has on their children. The oral health status of children has been linked both with the oral health status of their mother as well as their mother's educational level (Fisher-Owens et al., 2007; Ramos-Gomez et al., 2002; Weintraub, 2007; Weintraub et al., 2010). For some populations of children, evidence suggests that children's use of oral health care services is higher when their mothers have regular access to care (Grembowski et al., 2008; Isong et al., 2010). Arguably, the oral health care of children begins during pregnancy. For example, use of folic acid supplements during pregnancy may reduce the risk for isolated cleft lip (with or without cleft palate) by about one-third (Wilcox et al., 2007). In addition, periodontal disease in pregnant women has been associated with adverse pregnancy outcomes such as preterm low birth weight (Offenbacher et al., 2006; Scannapieco et al., 2003b; Tarannum and Faizuddin, 2007; Vergnes and Sixou, 2007), and use of preventive dental care during pregnancy is associated with lower incidence of adverse birth outcomes (Albert et al., 2011). After birth, the bacteria responsible for causing dental caries in children, *mutans streptococci*, appears to be transmissible from caregivers, especially mothers, to children (Berkowitz, 2006; Douglass et al., 2008; Li and Caufield, 1995; Slavkin, 1997).

Obstetricians and gynecologists need to be aware of how oral health has a particular interaction with the overall health of pregnant women. For example, hormonal changes during pregnancy put pregnant women at higher risk of developing oral diseases, most commonly gingivitis, which affects 30–75 percent of pregnant women (Silk et al., 2008; Steinberg et al., 2008). Oral health services for pregnant women and mothers may include education and counseling about how their own oral health relates to their children's oral health, as well as how to prevent dental caries in their young children. Although oral health care for pregnant women is safe and effective, less than half of women receive oral care or counseling during pregnancy (ACOG, 2004; CDA, 2010; Gaffield et al., 2001; Hwang et al., 2010; Michalowicz et al., 2008; New York State Department of Health, 2006; Newnham et al., 2009). In addition, there are significant racial and ethnic disparities in the oral health care of pregnant women (Hwang et al., 2010). The reasons for low use of oral care during pregnancy are similar to those for other populations, such as cost and low reimbursement for dentists, but reasons also include incorrect knowledge by both professionals and patients about the safety of dental care for pregnant women (Al Habashneh et al., 2005; Detman et al., 2010; Huebner et al., 2009; Hughes, 2010; Lee et al., 2010; Russell and Mayberry, 2008). In addition, while health care professionals may be aware of the importance of oral health care during pregnancy, they often still do not address it with their patients (Morgan et al., 2009).

Racial and Ethnic Minorities

Hispanics and African Americans have poorer oral health than whites have (Dietrich et al., 2008; Dye et al., 2007; Vargas and Ronzio, 2006). These disparities exist independently of income level, education, dental insurance status, and attitude toward preventive dental care, and they persist throughout the life cycle, from childhood through old age (Dietrich et al., 2008; Dye et al., 2007; Kiyak and Reichmuth, 2005). Minority children are more likely to have dental caries than are white children, and their decay is more severe (Vargas and Ronzio, 2006). American Indians and Alaska Natives (AI/AN) have poorer oral health than does the overall U.S. population throughout the life cycle (IHS, 2002; Jones et al., 2000). The prevalence of tooth decay in AI/AN children ages 2 to 5, for example, is nearly three times the U.S. average, and more than two-thirds of AI/AN children ages 2 to 5 have untreated dental caries (Dye et al., 2007; IHS, 2002).

Hispanics and African Americans receive fewer dental services compared to white populations. They are less likely to report any dental visit in the past year, either for preventive, restorative, or emergency care (Dietrich et al., 2008; Manski and Brown, 2007; Manski and Magder, 1998). When migrant and seasonal farmworkers were asked which health care service would benefit them the most, the most common response was dental services, ahead of pediatric care, transportation, and interpretation, among other services (Anthony et al., 2008).

Assurance of equal access to dental care can markedly reduce some oral health disparities. A study of the oral health of military personnel found "the disparities between black and white adults in untreated caries and recent dental visits that are seen in the U.S. civilian population were absent among military personnel. Racial disparities in missing teeth persisted among military personnel, though they were much smaller than those seen in their civilian counterparts" (Hyman et al., 2006).

Rural Populations

About 17 percent of the U.S. population lives in rural areas, and this is expected to increase dramatically with the aging of the baby boom population (Cromartie and Nelson, 2009; USDA, 2009). In general, rural residents have significantly poorer oral health than urban residents have throughout the life cycle (Vargas et al., 2002, 2003a,b,c). Residents of rural areas are less likely than urban residents to have visited a dentist in the past year and more likely to have unmet dental needs (Vargas et al., 2003a,b,c). A number of factors contribute to these problems. The supply of dentists in rural counties is less than half that of urban counties, with 29 dentists per 100,000 residents in the most rural counties compared to 61–62 dentists per 100,000 residents in large metropolitan areas (Eberhardt et al., 2001). Residents of rural areas must travel further than urban residents do to reach dental care (Probst et al., 2007). In addition, a smaller proportion of rural residents have dental insurance, which is predictive of oral health care use (DeVoe et al., 2003; Lewis et al., 2007). Rural populations are also less likely to have access to fluoridated community water supplies and have higher rates of tobacco use (Skillman et al., 2010), both of which are directly related to the development of oral diseases.

PREVENTION OF ORAL DISEASES

The World Health Organization defines oral health as "a state of being free from chronic mouth and facial pain, oral and throat cancer, oral sores, birth defects such as cleft lip and palate, periodontal (gum) disease, tooth decay and tooth loss, and other diseases and disorders that affect the oral cavity. Risk factors for oral diseases include unhealthy diet, tobacco use, harmful alcohol use, and poor oral hygiene" (WHO, 2010a).

The term *prevention* has been applied in a number of ways. In oral health care, the term can refer to brushing with fluoride toothpaste, flossing, oral health screenings by a health care professional, and the professional application of fluorides, but it might also be applied to drilling and filling a tooth to prevent loss of function. So the term *prevention* can be applied at various stages of the disease process. For example, a 2005 IOM report on childhood obesity adopted the public health definition of prevention, saying that

> With regard to obesity, primary prevention represents avoiding the occurrence of obesity in a population; secondary prevention represents early detection of disease through screening with the purpose of limiting its occurrence; and tertiary prevention involves preventing the sequelae of obesity in childhood and adulthood. (IOM, 2005)

This definition has been used regularly in the context of oral health (Dunning, 1986; HHS, 2000b).

In this chapter, the committee will focus on primary prevention. This is fitting, given the highly preventable nature of oral diseases, including dental caries and periodontal disease. The objective of oral health promotion and disease prevention is to promote the optimal state of the mouth and the normal functioning of the organs of the mouth without evidence of disease. While secondary and tertiary prevention will not be discussed extensively in this report, the committee recognizes that they are important in overall oral health. For example, secondary prevention may be considered through improving the education and training of primary health care providers to look for early signs of oral disease during routine health examinations (discussed more in Chapter 3), and tertiary prevention may include interventions by oral health care providers to manage oral diseases once present, including the prevention of further decay and infection.

Dental Caries and Periodontal Disease: The Disease Process

The basic etiology of dental caries and periodontal disease has been understood for many years. Teeth are normally covered in biofilms (also known as dental plaque) that consist of complex microbial communities (Marsh, 2006). The composition of this dental plaque is exquisitely sensitive to its environment, and both diseases result from alterations in the ecology in ways that allow virulent species to become predominant (Marsh, 2006). Unlike other bacterial pathologies such as *E. coli* and *salmonella,* in which the bacterial pathogens are exogenous, in the case of oral disease, the bacteria involved are indigenous to the mouth. This habitat is significantly influenced by saliva, food, fluoride, toothbrushing and dental flossing, and when present, to smoke, tobacco, alcohol, and other noxious agents.

For example, excessive exposure to sugar can lead to dental caries as the bacterial composition of the plaque changes from a healthy state to one that is overly acidic and consequently pathologic (cariogenic). At that point, the predominant bacteria in the biofilm on the teeth begin to transition to species that are acidogenic and aciduric (primarily *S. mutans*), and the biofilm becomes cariogenic (Marsh, 2006). A similar transition occurs in the biofilm associated with periodontal disease (Pihlstrom et al., 2005). In susceptible individuals, when the biofilm remains undisturbed by failing to maintain adequate oral hygiene, the plaque transitions from one characterized by gram-positive aerobic species to one that is composed of gram-negative anaerobic species (Marsh, 2003). This ecological shift in the biofilm leads to periodontal disease, a condition that eventually destroys the tooth's attachment to the gums and leads to tooth loss.

Effective Interventions

Many oral diseases can be prevented through a combination of steps taken at home, in the dental office or other care locations, or on a community-wide basis. For example, caries incidence can be reduced through water fluoridation at the community level, topical fluoride treatments can be applied by health care professionals in a wide variety of settings, and fluoridated toothpaste can be used in the home. This section does not include an exhaustive list of oral health preventive measures, but it does describe a range of interventions for which evidence is strong.

The value of preventive services has been recognized for decades. For example, in 1969, Harold L. Applewhite (D.D.S., M.P.H.) stated:

> At present, public and professional response to preventive measures lags behind scientific knowledge[. . . .] So far, our present preoccupation with repairing, removing, and replacing teeth have not proven to be successful in the clinical treatment of oral diseases. The rapid changes in the political and socioeconomic situation, and the rapid increase in knowledge of causative factors and preventive measures in oral diseases, do call for a new approach. (Applewhite, 1969)

It has been known for some time that dental caries, like most diseases, has a multifactorial causal pathway, which also provides multiple points at which the disease process could be curtailed (Featherstone, 2004). While there is always room for improvement and advancement, dentistry now has a very effective armamentarium to prevent dental caries. Those preventive interventions include a wide range of fluorides, which generally inhibit the caries process by reducing the rate of enamel demineralization and promoting remineralization. Some modes of fluoride delivery to whole communities involve the addition of very low levels of fluoride to public water systems, salt, or milk (Griffin et al., 2001a). Other forms of fluoride are applied personally or by a caretaker, including fluoride toothpaste and fluoride mouthwashes. Finally, some types of high concentration topical fluoride products are applied by a health care professional. Fluoride supplements, such as drops and chewable tablets, also may be prescribed or dispensed by health care professionals to high-risk children in communities whose water supply is not fluoridated.

Professionally delivered preventive measures also include the application of dental pit and fissure sealants to susceptible tooth surfaces to provide a physical barrier to cariogenic bacteria and their nutrients. Health care professionals may prescribe or dispense antibacterial rinses such as chlorhexidine for bacterial plaque control. Health care professionals also can remove plaque and other deposits from tooth surfaces, provide dietary counseling, and provide or recommend other measures that may prevent or control dental caries.

Aside from clinical effectiveness, many studies support the cost-effectiveness of preventive dental care, often due to the avoided expensive treatments associated with severe dental disease (CDC, 1999c; Lee et al., 2006; Quiñonez et al., 2005; Ruddy, 2007; Weintraub et al., 2001).

Fluoride

The oral health benefits of fluoride have been well known for more than 75 years (CDC, 2010a). Fluoride reduces the risk of caries in both children and adults (Griffin et al., 2007; IOM, 1997; Marinho, 2009; Marinho et al., 2002, 2003a; NRC, 1989; Twetman, 2009; WHO, 2010d). Fluoride works through a variety of systemic and topical mechanisms, including incorporating into enamel before teeth erupt, inhibiting demineralization and enhancing remineralization of teeth, and inhibiting bacterial activity in dental plaque (CDC, 2001; HHS, 2000b). Sources of fluorides include, but are not limited to fluoridated drinking water, mouthwash, toothpaste, and professionally applied fluorides (e.g., fluoride varnish). The broad availability of fluoride products produces a risk for overconsumption of fluoride, which can result in fluorosis, a broad term used to describe the tooth discoloration associated with excess fluoride intake during the tooth-forming years (0–8 years) (CDC, 2001; HHS, 2000a). The mild fluorosis occasionally caused by fluoride consumption, however, is rarely cause for aesthetic concern let alone health concern, and the risk of fluorosis can be minimized with appropriate use of fluoride products (Alvarez et al., 2009; HHS, 2000b; National Health and Medical Research Council, 2007; Newbrun, 2010).

Fluoridated Water

Community water fluoridation is credited with significantly reducing caries incidence in the United States, and it was recognized as one of the 10 great public health achievements of the 20th century (CDC, 1999b). Evidence continues to show that community water fluoridation is effective, safe, and inexpensive, and it is associated with significant cost savings (CDC, 1999c, 2001; Griffin et al., 2001a,b; HHS, 2000b; Horowitz, 1996; Kumar et al., 2010; O'Connell et al., 2005; Parnell et al., 2009; Yeung, 2008). The Task Force on Community Preventive Services recommends community water fluoridation, and it is supported by most health professional associations (ADA, 2010; APHA, 2008; Task Force on Community Preventive Services, 2002).

The National Institute of Dental and Craniofacial Research (NIDCR) at the NIH was founded in 1931 as the Dental Hygiene Unit, with the mission of investigating the connection between naturally occurring fluoride in water supplies and mottled teeth (i.e., fluorosis) in children (CDC, 1999a). The results of that research indicated children living in areas with high concentrations of fluoride in the water had more "mottled teeth," but also lower incidence of dental caries (CDC, 1999a). Later field studies established optimal fluoride levels that maximize the oral health benefits while minimizing the fluorosis effects (CDC, 1999b). HHS continues to make recommendations to balance the benefits of preventing tooth decay while limiting any unwanted health effects; the agency recently proposed focusing the optimal fluoride concentration to 0.7 mg of fluoride per liter of water from the original range, set in 1962, of 0.7–1.2 mg/L (HHS, 2011). HHS cited "scientific evidence related to effectiveness of water fluoridation on caries prevention and control across all age groups; fluoride in drinking water as one of several available fluoride sources; trends in the prevalence and severity of dental fluorosis; and current evidence on fluid intake across various ambient air temperatures" as the justification for this change (HHS, 2011).

An increasing number of Americans have access to fluoridated water. The most recent data show that in 2008, more than 72 percent of people who are served by public water systems (64 percent of the entire population) had access to optimally fluoridated water (CDC, 2010b), just shy of the *Healthy People 2010* goal of 75 percent (HHS, 2000a). Individually, 27 states and the District of Columbia have already reached this goal (NCHS, 2011). However, there is a perception in some communities (e.g., among Hispanics) that public water sources are not safe, and thus they frequently substitute bottled water; these individuals are often unaware of whether the bottle water is fluoridated (Hobson et al., 2007; Napier and Kodner, 2008; Scherzer et al., 2010; Sriraman et al., 2009; Weissman, 1997). The clinical effects related to increases in consumption of bottled water are unknown (Newbrun, 2010).

Fluoridated Toothpaste

As with the use of fluoridated water, the efficacy of fluoride toothpastes in preventing dental caries has been well established for decades. In 1960, Crest became the first brand of toothpaste to receive endorsement from the American Dental Association (ADA) for its effectiveness in preventing dental caries (Miskell, 2005). There is strong evidence that daily use of fluoride toothpaste reduces the incidence of caries in children (CDC, 2001; Marinho et al., 2003b; Twetman, 2009). The caries preventive effects are greater with more frequent brushing and when parents supervise (Marinho et al., 2003b). The preventive effects of fluoride toothpaste are likely similar in adults, although few studies have used adults as subjects (CDC, 2001). The evidence for the use of fluoridated toothpaste is high quality, and its use is recommended for all populations (CDC, 2001).

Professionally Applied Fluorides

Fluorides can be professionally applied in the form of varnish or gel. Varnishes are brushed onto clean, dry teeth (Bawden, 1998). The application takes about 1 minute, and the varnish sets quickly. To keep the varnish on the teeth for a number of hours, patients are told to eat soft foods and avoid brushing and flossing for the remainder of the day (Bawden, 1998). Gels are applied to the teeth using gel trays, which must stay on the patient's teeth for approximately 4 minutes (Bawden, 1998). Increasingly, varnishes are used instead of gels due to the ease of application and low risk of ingestion, especially for younger children (Bawden, 1998). Varnishes and gels are equally effective at preventing caries (Seppä et al., 1995).

Fluoride varnish has been shown to be effective in the prevention of caries in both deciduous and permanent teeth (Marinho et al., 2002). The interval for frequency of application of fluoride varnish varies depending on the risk of the patient—more frequently for children with higher risk (ADA, 2006; Azarpazhooh and Main, 2008). Although use of fluoride varnish for caries prevention is technically considered an "off-label" use, there is a robust evidence base for the efficacy of varnish at preventing caries (Beltran-Aguilar et al., 2000; Marinho et al., 2002; Weintraub et al., 2006).

Dental Sealants

Dental sealants prevent caries from developing in the pits and fissures of teeth, where caries are most prevalent (Ahovuo-Saloranta et al., 2008). A dental sealant is a thin, protective coating of plastic resin or glass ionomer that is applied to the chewing surfaces of teeth to prevent food particles and bacteria from collecting in the normal pits and fissures and developing into caries. A Cochrane review of sealant studies found that resin-based sealants were effective at preventing caries, ranging from an 87 percent reduction in caries after 12 months to 60 percent at 48–54 months (Ahovuo-Saloranta et al., 2008). Sealants are most effective when placed on fully erupted molars (Dennison et al., 1990). Sealants can also be placed over noncavitated carious lesions to reduce the progression of the lesions (Griffin et al., 2008).

Despite their effectiveness, few children receive sealants. The most recent NHANES (1999–2004) data indicate that 32 percent of 8-year-olds and 21 percent of 14-year-olds have sealants on their permanent molars (Dye et al., 2007). While this is a significant increase over the 23 percent of 8-year-olds and 15 percent of 14-year-olds with sealants in 1988–1994, it falls short of the *Healthy People 2010* goal of 50 percent of both groups (Dye et al., 2007; HHS, 2000a). Unfortunately, low-income children, who are most likely to have caries, are the least likely to receive sealants (Dye et al., 2007).

Sealants can be applied in a dental office or in a community-based program, such as school-based sealant programs. Many sealant programs strive to target high-risk populations because this has proven to be effective for the prevention of caries as well as to demonstrate cost savings (Kitchens, 2005; Pew Center on the States, 2010; Weintraub, 1989, 2001; Weintraub et al., 1993, 2001). The evidence that school-based sealant programs decrease decay is strong, and they are recommended by the Task Force on Community Preventive Services (see Chapter 4). However, evidence is insufficient to comment on the effectiveness of less targeted state- or community-wide programs (Truman et al., 2002).

Personal Health Behaviors

While community- and dental-office-based interventions are important for preventing oral diseases, personal behaviors also play an important role in oral health. A healthy diet is important for maintaining oral health, because it reduces the risk for dental caries and oral cancers (Mobley et al., 2009; Moynihan and Petersen, 2004) and potentially periodontal disease (Merchant et al., 2006; Nishida, 2000a,b; Pihlstrom, 2005). Tobacco and alcohol use are risk factors for oral cancers and periodontal disease (Rethman et al., 2010). Good personal hygiene, including toothbrushing with fluoridated toothpaste, reduces the risk for dental caries (Twetman, 2009). However, changing personal behaviors is a complex task (see discussion later in this chapter about health care behavior change).

Nutrition and Diet

Nutrition and oral health have a two-way relationship: poor nutrition promotes oral diseases, and poor oral health can adversely affect nutrition. For example, studies suggest that loss of teeth is associated with poorer nutritional intake, which may put individuals at risk for other systemic diseases (Hung et al., 2003; Joshipura and Ritchie, 2005). In addition, an insufficient level of folic acid is a risk factor in the development of birth defects such as cleft lip and palate (HHS, 2000b). Dietary carbohydrates are a necessary ingredient in the formation of dental caries (HHS, 2000b; Moynihan and Petersen, 2004), and consuming sugar-rich foods and drinks significantly increases the risk for dental caries (Burt et al., 1988; Grindefjord et al., 1996; Heller et al., 2001; Marshall et al., 2005; Sundin et al., 1992; WHO, 2010b). Carbonated beverages also promote dental erosion due to high acid levels (Ehlen et al., 2008; Kitchens and Owens, 2007). Fruits and vegetable consumption, however, can protect against oral cancers (HHS, 2000b; Pavia et al., 2006; WHO, 2010b).

Tobacco and Alcohol Use

Tobacco is a primary risk factor for oral cancers, the development and progression of periodontal disease, oral cancer recurrence, and congenital birth defects such as cleft lip and palate (Bergström, 2003; Gelskey, 1999; HHS, 2000b; Lebby et al., 2010; WHO, 2010c; Wyszynski et al., 1997). Excessive consumption of alcohol is a risk factor for precancerous and neoplastic lesions as well as oral cancers (HHS, 2000b; WHO, 2010b). When used together, alcohol and tobacco are synergistic in their risk for oral cancers (Rothman and Keller, 1972). Tobacco use and excessive alcohol consumption account for 90 percent of all oral cancers (Truman et al., 2002). Studies have shown that oral health professionals have a role to play in tobacco cessation programs (Albert et al., 2006; Gordon et al., 2010). However, one survey showed that most dentists do not ask their patients about their tobacco use (Albert et al., 2005).

Personal Hygiene

Individuals can also reduce the risk of developing oral disease through personal hygiene, including toothbrushing and flossing. For example, regular toothbrushing with fluoridated toothpaste reduces both caries risk and gingival inflammation (Deery et al., 2004; Marinho, 2009; Marinho et al., 2003a,b; Robinson et al., 2005; Walsh et al., 2010). Some steps that patients can take to improve their own (or their children's) care include

- Use of topical fluorides including toothpastes and rinses,
- Consumption of fluoridated water,
- Reducing sugar consumption,
- Reducing the numbers of sugar exposures each day (i.e., eliminating or minimizing snacks and/or changing the type of snack food to noncariogenic), and
- Not putting an infant or child to bed with a bottle that contains anything but water.

ORAL HEALTH LITERACY

Nearly all aspects of oral health care use require literacy. Beyond just the ability to read, write, and communicate effectively, literacy addresses the patient's ability to successfully navigate the health care system to obtain needed care services or perform self-care. Examples include completing a Medicaid application, scheduling a dental appointment, determining how much fluoride toothpaste to use on a toddler's toothbrush, understanding media campaigns, and weighing the potential complications of a root canal. While there is ample evidence supporting the association between general health and health literacy, very little research has been done specifically in oral health literacy. The role and current activities of HHS related to health literacy are discussed in Chapter 4.

What Is Oral Health Literacy?

Consensus has developed around the National Library of Medicine's definition of health literacy (IOM, 2004; Selden et al., 2000), which has been adapted for oral health: "Oral health literacy is the degree to which individuals have the capacity to obtain, process, and understand basic oral and craniofacial health information and services needed to make appropriate health decisions" (NIDCR, 2005). This definition excludes both provider and system-level contributions to oral health literacy, but despite these limitations, the IOM Committee on Health Literacy, *Healthy People*

2010, and the NIDCR all use this definition of oral health/health literacy (HHS, 2000a; IOM, 2004; NIDCR, 2005).

An individual's success at making these oral health-related decisions is based partially on his or her own literacy, but most experts agree that an individual's health literacy depends heavily on system-level contributions. Three sectors are responsible for and have the potential to build health literacy: culture and society, the health system, and the educational system (IOM, 2004). The interaction between these sectors and health literacy is illustrated in Figure 2-1.

Culture and Society

Health literacy is inextricably linked with culture and society, which includes factors such as race, ethnicity, native language, socioeconomic status, gender, and age, as well as influences such as media, advertising, marketing, and the Internet. Culture provides the context for understanding illness, di-

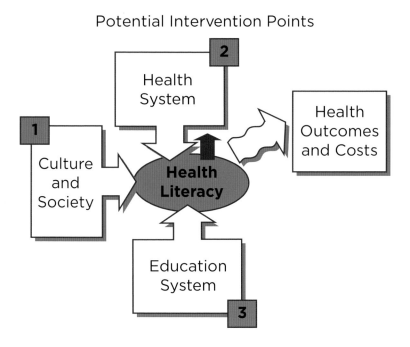

FIGURE 2-1
Intervention points for health literacy.
SOURCE: IOM, 2004.

agnoses, and health care messages. Different cultures use different communication styles, ascribe different meaning to words and gestures, and have different comfort levels in discussing the body, health, and illness (IOM, 2004). Health literacy requires communication and mutual understanding between patients and their families and health care professionals and staff about these differences (IOM, 2004). Cultural competence training may be an important step in improving health outcomes, although evidence has not yet established that link (Betancourt and Green, 2010; Hewlett et al., 2007; Novak et al., 2004; Pilcher et al., 2008; Wagner and Redford-Badwal, 2008; Wagner et al., 2007, 2008). Cultural competence includes linguistic competence—health professionals must also address language barriers for patients who have limited English proficiency (IOM, 2004). Recognizing the importance of culture on health literacy and health care outcomes,in 2001 HHS published National Standards on Culturally and Linguistically Appropriate Services (CLAS standards) in health care (OMH, 2001). These standards are discussed in further detail in Chapter 4.

The Health System

The organization of the health system can also enhance or inhibit health literacy. Currently, the literacy demands in the U.S. health care system exceed the health literacy skills of most adults (IOM, 2004). Navigating the system requires understanding complicated bureaucracy, a fragmented delivery system, and complex medical jargon. Even highly literate individuals struggle to make sense of the large amounts of information required to function effectively in the health care system. The problem of low health literacy is exacerbated and is becoming more apparent by the increasing prevalence of chronic diseases, including dental caries, that require long-term self-management by patients and the limited amount of time professionals have to spend with patients (OMH, 2001).

Individual practitioners, health organizations, and HHS can all take action to mitigate the effects of low health literacy. Health care professionals can make an effort to use plain language, slow down, show drawings or pictures, limit the amount of information provided and repeat it, use the teach-back method, and create an environment where patients feel comfortable asking questions (Schwartzberg et al., 2007; Weiss, 2007). Organizations can improve the readability of written materials, standardize medication labels and information, follow up with patients by phone, train health care professionals in communication skills and cultural competence, help patients navigate through the system, and coordinate care across multiple providers (DeWalt et al., 2006, 2010; Rothman et al., 2004; Sudore and Schillinger, 2009). Health professional schools and licensing bodies can teach evidence-based and culturally competent communication skills in schools and continuing medical education courses (Cannick et al., 2007; Carey et al., 2010; Eiser and Ellis, 2007; IOM, 2003). Health care professionals and provider organizations must recognize and address literacy, culture, and native language in their health literacy efforts. HHS can sponsor, conduct, and disseminate research on interventions to improve communication for patients with low health literacy, since few techniques have been rigorously evaluated.

The Education System

The education system is where most individuals develop both basic literacy skills and health knowledge, and therefore it plays a critical role in developing health literacy. Students learn health knowledge through health education programs provided in elementary, middle, and high schools. See Chapter 4 for more on the role of public education in improving health literacy.

Knowledge

Knowledge about health care topics is sometimes included in the definition of health literacy (IOM, 2004), and sometimes it is regarded as a resource that facilitates literacy (Baker, 2006). In either case, correct, evidence-based knowledge about health topics allows individuals and health care professionals to make informed health care decisions and recommendations, and to interact more effectively in health care contexts.

The Importance of Health Literacy

Health literacy is important because it can affect health care use, patient outcomes, and overall health care costs. Adults with limited health literacy have less knowledge of disease management and of health-promoting behaviors, report poorer health status, and are less likely to use preventive services (Arnold et al., 2001; DeWalt et al., 2004; IOM, 2004; Scott et al., 2002; Williams et al., 1998). People with low health literacy have adverse health outcomes (DeWalt et al., 2004; Mancuso and Rincon, 2006; Wolf et al., 2005). In addition, parents with low literacy make health care decisions that are less advantageous to their children, and their children have poorer health outcomes (DeWalt and Hink, 2009; Miller et al., 2010; Sanders et al., 2009). Currently, there is little consensus about the best ways to improve health outcomes for people with low health literacy (Pignone et al., 2005). Medical errors can occur when patients do not understand instructions provided by a doctor. In fact, one study found that nearly half of all pediatricians surveyed reported being aware of a communication-related medical error in the past 12 months (Turner et al., 2009). The HHS Office of Minority Health noted in the final report on CLAS standards that "[e]rrors made due to cultural or linguistic misunderstandings in health care encounters can lead to repeat appointments, extra time spent rectifying misdiagnoses, unnecessary emergency room visits, longer hospital stays, and canceled diagnostic or surgical procedures" (OMH, 2001). Poor health literacy is also expensive; it contributes significantly to both overall health care costs and individual expenditures (Eichler et al., 2009; Howard et al., 2005; Vernon et al., 2007; Weiss and Palmer, 2004).

Not enough is known specifically about oral health literacy. The NIDCR Workgroup on Oral Health Literacy proposed a research agenda for oral health literacy in 2005 (NIDCR, 2005). Progress has been slow; researchers have developed instruments to measure oral health literacy, although more work must be done to assess their validity (Atchison et al., 2010; Gong et al., 2007; Lee et al., 2007; Richman et al., 2007; Sabbahi et al., 2009).

Oral Health Literacy of the Public

All available measures indicate that the public's health literacy in general and oral health literacy in particular is poor. In 2003, the National Assessment of Adult Literacy assessed the health literacy of adult Americans on a large scale for the first time. It determined that only 12 percent of adults had proficient health literacy (Kutner et al., 2006). One study that specifically investigated the oral health literacy of patients in a clinical setting found poor oral health literacy was strongly associated with self-reported poor oral health status and lower dental knowledge (Jones et al., 2007).

The public has little knowledge about the best ways to prevent oral diseases. Fluoride and dental sealants (for children) have long been acknowledged as the most effective ways to prevent dental caries, yet the public consistently answers that toothbrushing and flossing are more effective (Ahovuo-Saloranta et al., 2008; Gift et al., 1994; Marinho et al., 2003a). When asked to choose the best way to prevent tooth decay from five options, only 7 percent of respondents to the National Health Interview Survey correctly answered using fluoride, while 70 percent answered that brushing and flossing were most effective (Gift et al., 1994). Further, only 23 percent of respondents knew the purpose of dental sealants. Other studies show that the public remains generally unaware of the transmissible, infectious nature of dental caries, including that the bacteria involved in the etiology of the disease can be passed from caretaker to child through the sharing of food and utensils and by kissing (Gussy et al., 2008; Sakai et al., 2008).

Much of the oral health literacy literature focuses on knowledge (or lack of knowledge) about oral and pharyngeal cancer. Although each year more than 30,000 Americans are diagnosed with these cancers and nearly 8,000 people die from them, the public's knowledge about the risk factors and symptoms of oral cancers is low (ACS, 2009; Cruz et al., 2002; Horowitz et al., 1998, 2002; Patton et al., 2004). While 85 percent of respondents to a telephone survey had heard of oral cancer, only 23 percent of those could name one early symptom (Horowitz et al., 1998). Many people also could not identify common risk factors for oral cancer. Although 67 percent of adults responding to the 1990 National Health Interview Survey knew that tobacco use is a risk factor for oral cancer, very few respondents knew about any other risk factors (Horowitz et al., 1995).

Oral Health Literacy of Health Care Professionals

All health care professionals can facilitate literacy by communicating clearly and accurately. This requires them to have good communication skills and knowledge related to oral health. Recognizing literacy as an important issue in oral health, the ADA recently developed a strategic action plan that provides guidance (but not requirements) on principles, goals, and strategies to improve health literacy in dentistry (ADA, 2009). Strategies include facilitating the development, testing, distribution, and evaluation of a health literacy training program for dentists and other members of the oral health team, investigating the feasibility of a systematic review of the health literacy literature, and encouraging oral health education in schools (ADA, 2009).

Communication Skills

In general, health care professionals can help by assessing patients' health literacy and communicating at an appropriate level of complexity. However, health care professionals are generally not trained in how to perform such an assessment and do not account for the low health literacy of patients when communicating health information. Practitioners often use medical jargon, provide too much information at once, and fail to confirm that the patient understood the information provided (Williams et al., 2002). While nearly all professionals surveyed report using at least one technique to improve communication with patients, fewer than half use the techniques shown to be most effective—indicating key points on written materials and the "teach-back" method, where professionals ask patients to repeat back the information (Schwartzberg et al., 2007; Turner et al., 2009).

At this IOM committee's second meeting, the ADA presented preliminary findings of a survey on the communication skills of members of the dental team (Neuhauser, 2010). This study aimed to determine the techniques that are used by dentists and dental team members to communicate effectively with their patients; examine variation in the use of these techniques; and explore the different variables that might be targeted in the future to improve communication and dental practices. Findings included a high amount of variation in the type and number of communication techniques used, and the use of more techniques by older dentists, by dentists from racial and ethnic populations, and by dentists who are specialists (e.g., oral surgeons). Routine use of communication techniques is low among dentists, especially some techniques such as the teach-back method, thought to be most effective with patients with low literacy. Nearly two-thirds of the dentists said they did not have training in health literacy and clear communication.

Improving the communication skills of oral health care professionals may require curricular changes in both health professional schools and continuing dental education programs. The Commission on Dental Accreditation (the accrediting body for dental schools) requires schools to ensure that dental students "have the interpersonal and communications skills to function successfully in a multicultural work environment" (CODA, 2010). In addition, the American Dental Education Association (the professional organization for dental education schools) has established competencies for the new general dentist that include "apply[ing] appropriate interpersonal and communication skills, apply[ing] psychosocial and behavioral principles in patient-centered health care, and communicat[ing] effectively with individuals from diverse populations" (ADEA, 2009). Despite these standards, few schools have adopted a competency exam for communication (Cannick et al., 2008). Further, unlike in medicine, the national dental licensing exam does not include a clinical component that assesses communication skills (JCNDE, 2011; USMLE, 2010). Continuing education courses can also improve the communication skills of providers (Barth and Lannen, 2010; Levinson and Roter, 1993), yet at least one state does not allow continuing education credit for courses taken in communication.[2]

Oral Health Knowledge

As patients of all ages often visit primary care professionals more frequently than they visit dentists, these practitioners are in a good position to provide basic oral health education. For example, 90-plus percent of practicing pediatricians think they play an important role in identifying oral health problems and counseling parents about the importance of oral health (Lewis et al., 2000). Even more dramatically, nearly all (99 per-

---

[2] 49 Pa. Cons. Stat. §33.402 (2011).

cent) of the residents graduating from pediatric residency programs believe pediatricians should educate parents about the effects of their children sleeping with a baby bottle and drinking juice and carbonated beverages, and a significant percentage think pediatricians should identify cavities (89 percent), and teach patients how to brush correctly (86 percent) (Caspary et al., 2008). Despite this, pediatricians lack the necessary knowledge about basic oral health to educate patients about oral health issues or screen for oral disease. Thirty-five percent of pediatric residents receive no oral health training during their residency, and 73 percent of those who do receive training spend less than 3 hours on oral health (Caspary et al., 2008). This is significant because physicians' oral health care practices improve with training. Graduating residents with more than 3 hours of oral health training were significantly more likely to feel confident performing oral health education and assessments (Caspary et al., 2008). Additionally, osteopathic medical students who received 2 days of oral health education showed dramatically improved oral health knowledge (Skelton et al., 2002). (The education and training of health care professionals in oral health is discussed further in Chapter 3.)

Similar patterns are seen in other types of health care professionals as well as for other oral diseases. For example, one study of internal medicine trainees showed that only 34 percent correctly answered all five general knowledge questions on periodontal disease; 90 percent of the trainees stated they did not receive any training regarding periodontal disease during medical school (Quijano et al., 2010). In a 2009 study by Applebaum et al., only 9 percent of primary care physicians could identify the two most common sites for oral cancers, and only 24 percent knew the most common symptom of early oral cancer (Applebaum et al., 2009). In a survey of nurse practitioners, only 35 percent identified sun exposure as a risk for lip cancer, and only 19 percent thought their knowledge of oral cancers was current (Siriphant et al., 2001). A survey of nursing assistants in nursing homes found that the nursing assistants generally regarded tooth loss as "a natural consequence of aging" (Jablonski et al., 2009).

The few surveys that have investigated the oral health knowledge of dentists and hygienists have found it lacking. In a national survey, fewer than 50 percent of dental hygienists knew that dental caries was a chronic infectious disease, and many did not recognize the value of fluoride in preventing dental caries (Forrest et al., 2000). In a survey about knowledge of oral cancer risk factors, dentists averaged 8.4 correct answers out of 14, and hygienists averaged 7.9 correct answers (Yellowitz et al., 2000). When asked about oral cancer diagnostic procedures; dentists averaged six correct answers out of nine, but more than one-third answered four or fewer answers correctly (Yellowitz et al., 2000). In the above-cited study by Applebaum et al. (2009), 39 percent of dentists could identify the two most common oral cancer sites and 57 percent could identify the most common symptom of early oral cancer (Applebaum et al., 2009). Although 98 percent of dental hygienists responded that adults over age 40 should receive an oral cancer examination annually, only 66 percent report providing the exam all of the time, and an additional 10 percent report doing so some of the time (Forrest et al., 2001).

Behavior Change

While a full examination of the evidence base and approaches for behavior change is beyond the scope of this report, it is important to note that improving health literacy is just the beginning of the behavioral change process. A number of factors make behavior change very difficult, including cultural norms, individual preferences, economic factors, and the role of the larger society (Glanz and Bishop, 2010; IOM, 2000; McLeroy et al., 1988). Simply providing information is generally not sufficient to modify patients' behaviors or change their attitudes (Freeman and Ismail, 2009; Satur et al., 2010). A 2000 IOM report on social and behavioral research stated:

> To prevent disease, we increasingly ask people to do things that they have not done previously, to stop doing things they have been doing for years, and to do more of some things and less of other things. Although there certainly are examples of successful programs to change behavior, it is clear that behavior change is a difficult and complex challenge. It is unreasonable to expect that people will change their behavior easily when so many forces in the social, cultural, and physical environment conspire against such change. (IOM, 2000)

In oral health care, behavior change requires attention to individuals (e.g., personal health behaviors), families (e.g., family stress, social support), health care professionals (e.g., appropriate counseling techniques), the environment (e.g., accessibility to oral health care, status of community water fluoridation), and cross-cutting issues (e.g., racial and ethnic health disparities, cultural preferences) (Finlayson et al., 2007; Glanz, 2010; Kelly et al., 2005; Quinoñez et al., 2000). This is illustrated graphically in Figure 2-2. Despite the difficulties in influencing health behaviors, there are promising behavioral change models. One example is motivational interviewing, a "directive, client-centered counseling style for eliciting behavior change by helping clients to explore and resolve ambivalence" (Rollnick and Miller, 1995). Motivational interviewing has been shown to improve a variety of health behaviors and conditions, including smoking cessation and dental caries (Freudenthal and Bowen, 2010; Lai et al., 2010; Miller, 1983; Naar-King et al., 2009; Rubak et al., 2005; Weinstein et al., 2006).

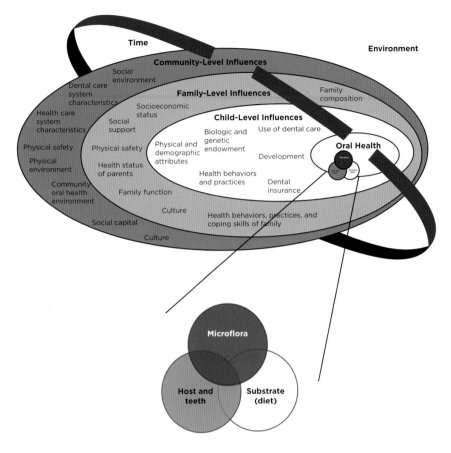

FIGURE 2-2
Conceptual of model of oral health and the influences on oral health.
SOURCE: Fisher-Owens et al., 2007. Reproduced with permission from *Pediatrics*, Vol. 120, Pages 510–520, Copyright © 2007 by the American Academy of Pediatrics.

KEY FINDINGS AND CONCLUSIONS

The committee noted the following key findings and conclusions:

Oral Health and Overall Health

- Oral health is inextricably linked to overall health.

Oral Health Status

- The overall oral health status of the U.S. population is improving, but significant disparities remain for many vulnerable populations. Therefore, HHS' efforts need to focus on populations with the greatest need.
- Discrete segments of the U.S. population have difficulty accessing oral health care services.
- Fourteen percent of children 6–12 years old have had toothache severe enough during the past 6 months to have complained to their parents.

Prevention

- Seventy-two percent of people who are served by public water systems (64 percent of the entire population) have access to optimally fluoridated water.
- There is a strong evidence base to support the effectiveness many oral disease prevention interventions (e.g., community water fluoridation, fluoride varnish, and sealants).
- The public and many health care professionals are generally unaware of the causes and consequences of oral diseases and the ways in which these diseases can be prevented.

Health Literacy

- Oral health care professionals often do not use the best techniques to communicate with their patients. Oral health care professionals need to be be trained in effective communication and cultural competence.
- Further improvements to the oral health of the U.S. population will require behavior change at many levels (e.g., individual, families, communities, and nationally), but little is known about the best ways to encourage those changes.
- Poor oral health literacy contributes to poor access because individuals may not understand the importance of oral health care or their options for accessing such care.

REFERENCES

ACOG (American Congress of Obstetricians and Gynecologists). 2004. Guidelines for diagnostic imaging during pregnancy. *Obstetrics and Gynecology* 104(3):647-651.

ACS (American Cancer Society). 2009. *Cancer facts and figures 2009*. Atlanta, GA: American Cancer Society.

ADA (American Dental Association). 2006. Professionally applied topical fluoride: Evidence-based clinical recommendations. *Journal of the American Dental Association* 137(8):1151-1159.

ADA. 2009. *Health literacy in dentistry action plan 2010-2015.* Chicago, IL: American Dental Association.

ADA. 2010. *Fluoride & fluoridation.* http://www.ada.org/2467.aspx (accessed September 16, 2010).

ADEA (American Dental Education Association). 2009. Competencies for the new general dentist. *Journal of Dental Education* 73(7):866-869.

Ahovuo-Saloranta, A., A. Hiiri, A. Nordblad, H. Worthington, and M. Mäkelä. 2008. Pit and fissure sealants for preventing dental decay in the permanent teeth of children and adolescents. *Cochrane Database of Systematic Reviews* (4):CD001830.

Al Habashneh, R., J. M. Guthmiller, S. Levy, G. K. Johnson, C. Squier, D. V. Dawson, and Q. Fang. 2005. Factors related to utilization of dental services during pregnancy. *Journal of Clinical Periodontology* 32(7):815-821.

Al-Hashimi, I. 2001. The management of Sjögren's syndrome in dental practice. *Journal of the American Dental Association* 132(10):1409-1417.

Albert, D. A., H. Severson, J. Gordon, A. Ward, J. Andrews, and D. Sadowsky. 2005. Tobacco attitudes, practices, and behaviors: A survey of dentists participating in managed care. *Nicotine and Tobacco Research* 7(Supp. 1):S9-S18.

Albert, D. A., H. H. Severson, and J. A. Andrews. 2006. Tobacco use by adolescents: The role of the oral health professional in evidence-based cessation programs. *Pediatric Dentistry* 28(2):177-187.

Albert, D. A., M. D. Begg, H. F. Andrews, S. Z. Williams, A. Ward, M. Lee Conicella, V. Rauh, J. L. Thomson, and P. N. Papapanou. 2011. An examination of periodontal treatment, dental care, and pregnancy outcomes in an insured population in the United States. *American Journal of Public Health* 101(1):151-156.

Altekruse, S. F., C. L. Kosary, M. Krapcho, N. Neyman, R. Aminou, W. Waldron, J. Ruhl, N. Howlader, Z. Tatalovich, H. Cho, A. Mariotto, M. P. Eisner, D. R. Lewis, K. Cronin, H. S. Chen, E. J. Feuer, D. G. Stinchcomb, and B. K. Edwards. 2010. *SEER cancer statistics review, 1975-2007.* Bethesda, MD: National Cancer Institute.

Alvarez, J. A., K. M. P. C. Rezende, S. M. S. Marocho, F. B. T. Alves, P. Celiberti, and A. L. Ciamponi. 2009. Dental fluorosis: Exposure, prevention and management. *Journal of Clinical and Experimental Dentistry* 1(1):e14-e18.

Anders, P. L., and E. L. Davis. 2010. Oral health of patients with intellectual disabilities: A systematic review. *Special Care in Dentistry* 30(3):110-117.

Anthony, M., J. M. Williams, and A. M. Avery. 2008. Health needs of migrant and seasonal farmworkers. *Journal of Community Health Nursing* 25(3):153-160.

APHA (American Public Health Association). 2008 (unpublished). *Community water fluoridation in the United States.* American Public Health Association.

Applebaum, E., T. N. Ruhlen, F. R. Kronenberg, C. Hayes, and E. S. Peters. 2009. Oral cancer knowledge, attitudes and practices: A survey of dentists and primary care physicians in Massachusetts. *Journal of the American Dental Association* 140(4):461-467.

Applewhite, H. L. 1969. Dental education as it relates to the community. *American Journal of Public Health and the Nation's Health* 59(10):1882-1886.

Armour, B. S., M. Swanson, H. B. Waldman, and S. P. Perlman. 2008. A profile of state-level differences in the oral health of people with and without disabilities, in the U.S., in 2004. *Public Health Reports* 123(1):67-75.

Arnold, C. L., T. C. Davis, H. J. Berkel, R. H. Jackson, I. Nandy, and S. London. 2001. Smoking status, reading level, and knowledge of tobacco effects among low-income pregnant women. *Preventive Medicine* 32(4):313-320.

Atchison, K. A., M. W. Gironda, D. Messadi, and C. Der-Martirosian. 2010. Screening for oral health literacy in an urban dental clinic. *Journal of Public Health Dentistry* 70(4):269-275.

Azarpazhooh, A., and P. A. Main. 2008. Fluoride varnish in the prevention of dental caries in children and adolescents: A systematic review. *Journal of the Canadian Dental Association* 74(1):73-79.

Bahekar, A. A., S. Singh, S. Saha, J. Molnar, and R. Arora. 2007. The prevalence and incidence of coronary heart disease is significantly increased in periodontitis: A meta-analysis. *American Heart Journal* 154(5):830-837.

Baker, D. W. 2006. The meaning and the measure of health literacy. *Journal of General Internal Medicine* 21(8):878-883.

Barth, J., and P. Lannen. 2010. Efficacy of communication skills training courses in oncology: A systematic review and meta-analysis. *Annals of Oncology*. Published electronically October 5, 2010. DOI: 10.1093/annonc/mdq441.

Bawden, J. W. 1998. Fluoride varnish: A useful new tool for public health dentistry. *Journal of Public Health Dentistry* 58(4):266-269.

Beck, J. D., D. J. Couper, K. L. Falkner, S. P. Graham, S. G. Grossi, J. C. Gunsolley, T. Madden, G. Maupome, S. Offenbacher, and D. D. Stewart. 2008. The periodontitis and vascular events (pave) pilot study: Adverse events. *Journal of Periodontology* 79(1):90-96.

Beltran-Aguilar, E. D., J. W. Goldstein, and S. A. Lockwood. 2000. Fluoride varnishes: A review of their clinical use, cariostatic mechanism, efficacy and safety. *Journal of the American Dental Association* 131(5):589-596.

Bergström, J. 2003. Tobacco smoking and risk for periodontal disease. Journal of Clinical *Periodontology* 30(2):107-113.

Berkowitz, R. J. 2006. Mutans streptococci: Acquisition and transmission. *Pediatric Dentistry* 28(2):106-109.

Betancourt, J. R., and A. R. Green. 2010. Commentary: Linking cultural competence training to improved health outcomes: Perspectives from the field. *Academic Medicine* 85(4): 583-585.

Blaizot, A., J. N. Vergnes, S. Nuwwareh, J. Amar, and M. Sixou. 2009. Periodontal diseases and cardiovascular events: Meta-analysis of observational studies. *International Dental Journal* 59(4):197-209.

Bray, R. M., L. L. Hourani, K. L. R. Olmsted, M. Witt, J. M. Brown, M. R. Pemberton, M. E. Marsden, B. Marriott, S. Scheffler, R. Vandermaas-Peeler, B. Weimer, S. Calvin, M. Bradshaw, K. Close, and D. Hayden. 2006. *2005 Department of Defense survey of health related behaviors among active duty military personnel*. Research Triangle Park, NC: RTI International.

Burt, B. A., S. A. Eklund, K. J. Morgan, F. E. Larkin, K. E. Guire, L. O. Brown, and J. A. Weintraub. 1988. The effects of sugars intake and frequency of ingestion on dental caries increment in a three-year longitudinal study. *Journal of Dental Research* 67(11):1422-1429.

Cannick, G. F., A. M. Horowitz, D. R. Garr, S. G. Reed, B. W. Neville, T. A. Day, R. F. Woolson, and D. T. Lackland. 2007. Use of the OSCE to evaluate brief communication skills training for dental students. *Journal of Dental Education* 71(9):1203-1209.

Carey, J. A., A. Madill, and M. Manogue. 2010. Communications skills in dental education: A systematic research review. *European Journal of Dental Education* 14(2):69-78.

Casamassimo, P. S., S. Thikkurissy, B. L. Edelstein, and E. Maiorini. 2009. Beyond the DMFT: The human and economic cost of early childhood caries. *Journal of the American Dental Association* 140(6):650-657.

Caspary, G., D. M. Krol, S. Boulter, M. A. Keels, and G. Romano-Clarke. 2008. Perceptions of oral health training and attitudes toward performing oral health screenings among graduating pediatric residents. *Pediatrics* 122(2):e465-e471.

CDA (California Dental Association). 2010. *Oral health during pregnancy and early childhood: Evidence-based guidelines for health professionals.* Sacramento, CA: California Dental Association.

CDC (Centers for Disease Control and Prevention). 1999a. Achievements in public health, 1900-1999: Fluoridation of drinking water to prevent dental caries. *Morbidity and Mortality Weekly Report* 48(41):933-940.

CDC. 1999b. Ten great public health achievements—United States, 1900-1999. *Morbidity and Mortality Weekly Report* 48(12):241-243.

CDC. 1999c. Water fluoridation and costs of Medicaid treatment for dental decay—Louisiana, 1995-1996. *Morbidity and Mortality Weekly Report* 48(34):753-757.

CDC. 2001. Recommendations for using fluoride to prevent and control dental caries in the United States. *MMWR Recommendations and Reports* 50(RR14):1-42.

CDC. 2010a. *CDC honors 65 years of community water fluoridation.* http://www.cdc.gov/fluoridation/65_years.htm (accessed September 16, 2010).

CDC. 2010b. *Community water fluoridation: 2008 water fluoridation statistics.* http://www.cdc.gov/fluoridation/statistics/2008stats.htm (accessed September 16, 2010).

Chávarry, N., M. V. Vettore, C. Sansone, and A. Sheiham. 2009. The relationship between diabetes mellitus and destructive periodontal disease: A meta-analysis. *Oral health & preventive dentistry* 7(2):107-127.

Chevarley, F. M. 2010. *Percentage of persons unable to get or delayed in getting needed medical care, dental care, or prescription medicines: United States, 2007.* Statistical brief #282. Rockville, MD: Agency for Healthcare Research and Quality.

CODA (Commission on Dental Accreditation). 2010. *Accreditation standards for dental education programs.* Chicago, IL: American Dental Assocation, Commission on Dental Accreditation.

Cohen, L. A., A. J. Bonito, C. Eicheldinger, R. J. Manski, M. D. Macek, R. R. Edwards, and N. Khanna. 2011. Comparison of patient visits to emergency departments, physician offices, and dental offices for dental problems and injuries. *Journal of Public Health Dentistry* 71(1):13-22.

Coogin, M. M., J. Greenspan, and S. J. Challacombe. 2005. Oral lesions in infection with human immunodeficiency virus. *Bulletin of the World Health Organization* 83(9):700-706.

Cromartie, J., and P. Nelson. 2009. *Baby boom migration and its impact on rural America.* Washington, DC: U.S. Department of Agriculture.

Cruz, G. D., R. Z. Le Geros, J. S. Ostroff, J. L. Hay, H. Kenigsberg, and D. M. Franklin. 2002. Oral cancer knowledge, risk factors and characteristics of subjects in a large oral cancer screening program. *Journal of the American Dental Association* 133(8):1064-1071.

Davis, E. E., A. S. Deinard, and E. W. H. Maïga. 2010. Doctor, my tooth hurts: The costs of incomplete dental care in the emergency room. *Journal of Public Health Dentistry* 70(3):205-210.

Deery, C., M. Heanue, S. Deacon, P. Robinson, A. Walmsley, H. Worthington, W. Shaw, and A. Glenny. 2004. The effectiveness of manual versus powered toothbrushes for dental health: A systematic review. *Journal of Dentistry* 32(3):197-211.

Dennison, J., L. Straffon, and F. More. 1990. Evaluating tooth eruption on sealant efficacy. *Journal of the American Dental Association* 121(5):610-614.

Detman, L. A., B. H. Cottrell, and M. F. Denis-Luque. 2010. Exploring dental care misconceptions and barriers in pregnancy. *Birth* 37(4):318-324.

DeVoe, J. E., G. E. Fryer, R. Phillips, and L. Green. 2003. Receipt of preventive care among adults: Insurance status and usual source of care. *American Journal of Public Health* 93(5):786-791.

DeWalt, D. A., and A. Hink. 2009. Health literacy and child health outcomes: A systematic review of the literature. *Pediatrics* 124(Supp. 3):S265-S274.

DeWalt, D. A., N. D. Berkman, S. Sheridan, K. N. Lohr, and M. P. Pignone. 2004. Literacy and health outcomes. *Journal of General Internal Medicine* 19(12):1228-1239.

DeWalt, D., R. Malone, M. Bryant, M. Kosnar, K. Corr, R. Rothman, C. Sueta, and M. Pignone. 2006. A heart failure self-management program for patients of all literacy levels: A randomized, controlled trial. *BMC Health Services Research* 6(1):30.

DeWalt, D. A., L. F. Callahan, V. H. Hawk, K. A. Broucksou, A. Hink, R. Rudd, and C. Brach. 2010. *Health literacy universal precautions toolkit*. Rockville, MD: Agency for Healthcare Research and Quality.

Dietrich, T., C. Culler, R. Garcia, and M. M. Henshaw. 2008. Racial and ethnic disparities in children's oral health: The National Survey of Children's Health. *Journal of the American Dental Association* 139(11):1507-1517.

Dolan, T. A., C. W. Peek, A. E. Stuck, and J. C. Beck. 1998. Functional health and dental service use among older adults. *Journal of Gerontology: Series A Biological Sciences and Medical Sciences* 53A(6):M413-M418.

Dolan, T. A., K. Atchison, and T. N. Huynh. 2005. Access to dental care among older adults in the United States. *Journal of Dental Education* 69(9):961-974.

Douglass, J. M., Y. Li, and N. Tinanoff. 2008. Association of *mutans streptococci* between caregivers and their children. *Pediatric Dentistry* 30(5):375-387.

D'Souza, G., A. R. Kreimer, R. Viscidi, M. Pawlita, C. Fakhry, W. M. Koch, W. H. Westra, and M. L. Gillison. 2007. Case–control study of human papillomavirus and oropharyngeal cancer. *New England Journal of Medicine* 356(19):1944-1956.

Dunning, J. M. 1986. *Principles of dental public health*. 4th ed. Cambridge, MA: Harvard University Press.

Dye, B. 2010. *Healthy People 2020: Current status and future direction*. Presentation at meeting of the Committee on an Oral Health Initiative, Washington, DC. March 31, 2010.

Dye, B., and G. Thornton-Evans. 2010. Trends in oral health by poverty status as measured by *Healthy People 2010* objectives. *Public Health Reports* 125(6):817-830.

Dye, B. A., S. Tan, V. Smith, B. G. Lewis, L. K. Barker, G. Thornton-Evans, P. I. Eke, E. D. Beltran-Aguilar, A. M. Horowitz, and L. Chien-Hsun. 2007. *Trends in oral health status: United States, 1988-1994 and 1999-2004*. Hyattsville, MD: National Center for Health Statistics.

Dye, B. A., O. Arevalo, and C. M. Vargas. 2010. Trends in paediatric dental caries by poverty status in the United States, 1988–1994 and 1999–2004. *International Journal of Paediatric Dentistry* 20(2):132-143.

Eberhardt, M. S., D. D. Ingram, D. M. Makuc, E. R. Pamuk, V. M. Freid, S. B. Harper, C. A. Schoenborn, and H. Xia. 2001. *Urban and rural health chartbook: Health, United States, 2001*. Hyattsville, MD: National Center for Health Statistics.

Edelstein, B. L., and C. H. Chinn. 2009. Update on disparities in oral health and access to dental care for America's children. *Academic Pediatrics* 9(6):415-419.

Ehlen, L. A., T. A. Marshall, F. Qian, J. S. Wefel, and J. J. Warren. 2008. Acidic beverages increase the risk of in vitro tooth erosion. *Nutrition Research* 28(5):299-303.

Eichler, K., S. Wieser, and U. Brügger. 2009. The costs of limited health literacy: A systematic review. *International Journal of Public Health* 54(5):313-324.

Eiser, A. R., and G. Ellis. 2007. Viewpoint: Cultural competence and the african american experience with health care: The case for specific content in cross-cultural education. *Academic Medicine* 82(2):176-183.

Eke, P., G. Thornton-Evans, L. Wei, W. Borgnakke, and B. Dye. 2010. Accuracy of NHANES periodontal examination protocols. *Journal of Dental Research* 89(11):1208-1213.

Featherstone, J. D. B. 2004. The continuum of dental caries—evidence for a dynamic disease process. *Journal of Dental Research* 83(Special Issue C):C39-C42.

Feldman, C., M. Giniger, M. Sanders, R. Saporito, H. Zohn, and S. Perlman. 1997. Special Olympics, special smiles: Assessing the feasibility of epidemiologic data collection. *Journal of the American Dental Association* 128(12):1687-1696.

Finlayson, T. L., K. Siefert, A. I. Ismail, and W. Sohn. 2007. Maternal self-efficacy and 1–5-year-old children's brushing habits. *Community Dentistry and Oral Epidemiology* 35(4):272-281.

Fisher-Owens, S. A., S. A. Gansky, L. J. Platt, J. A. Weintraub, M. J. Soobader, M. D. Bramlett, and P. W. Newacheck. 2007. Influences on children's oral health: A conceptual model. *Pediatrics* 120(3):e510-e520.

Fogacci, M. F., M. V. Vettore, and A. T. Thomé Leão. 2011. The effect of periodontal therapy on preterm low birth weight: A meta-analysis. *Obstetrics and Gynecology* 117(1):153-165

Forrest, J. L., A. M. Horowitz, and Y. Shmuely. 2000. Caries preventive knowledge and practices among dental hygienists. *Journal of Dental Hygiene* 74(3):183-195.

Forrest, J. L., A. M. Horowitz, and Y. Shmuely. 2001. Dental hygienists' knowledge, opinions, and practices related to oral and pharyngeal cancer risk assessment. *Journal of Dental Hygiene* 75(4):271-281.

Freeman, R., and A. Ismail. 2009. Assessing patients' health behaviours: Essential steps for motivating patients to adopt and maintain behaviours conducive to oral health. *Monographs in Oral Science* 21:113-127.

Freudenthal, J. J., and D. M. Bowen. 2010. Motivational interviewing to decrease parental risk-related behaviors for early childhood caries. *Journal of Dental Hygiene* 84(1):29-34.

Gaffield, M. L., B. J. Colley, D. M. Malvitz, and R. Romaguera. 2001. Oral health during pregnancy: An analysis of information collected by the Pregnancy Risk Assessment Monitoring System. *Journal of the American Dental Association* 132(7):1009-1016.

Gelskey, S. C. 1999. Cigarette smoking and periodontitis: Methodology to assess the strength of evidence in support of a causal association. *Community Dentistry and Oral Epidemiology* 27(1):16-24.

Gift, H. C., S. T. Reisine, and D. C. Larach. 1992. The social impact of dental problems and visits. *American Journal of Public Health* 82(12):1663-1668.

Gift, H. C., S. T. Reisine, and D. C. Larach. 1993. Erratum: The social impact of dental problems and visits. *American Journal of Public Health* 83(6):816.

Gift, H. C., S. B. Corbin, and R. E. Nowjack-Raymer. 1994. Public knowledge of prevention of dental disease. *Public Health Reports* 109(3):397-404.

Glanz, K. 2010, March 31. *Behavioral science and public health interventions.* Presentation at meeting of the Committee on an Oral Health Initiative, Washington, DC. March 31, 2010.

Glanz, K., and D. B. Bishop. 2010. The role of behavioral science theory in development and implementation of public health interventions. *Annual Review of Public Health* 31:399-418.

Glassman, P., and P. Subar. 2008. Improving and maintaining oral health for people with special needs. *Dental Clinics of North America* 52(2):447-461.

Glassman, P., T. Henderson, M. Helgeson, C. Meyerowitz, R. Ingraham, R. Isman, D. Noel, R. Tellier, and K. Toto. 2005. Oral health for people with special needs: Consensus statement on implications and recommendations for the dental profession. *CDA Journal* 33(8):619-623.

Gong, D. A., J. Y. Lee, R. G. Rozier, B. T. Pahel, J. A. Richman, and W. F. Vann. 2007. Development and testing of the test of functional health literacy in dentistry (TOFHLID). *Journal of Public Health Dentistry* 67(2):105-112.

Gordon, J. S., J. A. Andrews, D. A. Albert, K. M. Crews, T. J. Payne, and H. H. Severson. 2010. Tobacco cessation via public dental clinics: Results of a randomized trial. *American Journal of Public Health* 100(7):1307-1312.

Grembowski, D., C. Spiekerman, and P. Milgrom. 2008. Linking mother and child access to dental care. *Pediatrics* 122(4):e805-e814.

Griffin, S. O., B. F. Gooch, S. A. Lockwood, and S. L. Tomar. 2001a. Quantifying the diffused benefit from water fluoridation in the United States. *Community Dentistry and Oral Epidemiology* 29(2):120-129.

Griffin, S. O., K. Jones, and S. L. Tomar. 2001b. An economic evaluation of community water fluoridation. *Journal of Public Health Dentistry* 61(2):78-86.

Griffin, S. O., E. Regnier, P. M. Griffin, and V. Huntley. 2007. Effectiveness of fluoride in preventing caries in adults. *Journal of Dental Research* 86(5):410-415.

Griffin, S. O., E. Oong, W. Kohn, B. Vidakovic, B. F. Gooch, J. Bader, J. Clarkson, M. R. Fontana, D. M. Meyer, R. G. Rozier, J. A. Weintraub, and D. T. Zero. 2008. The effectiveness of sealants in managing caries lesions. *Journal of Dental Research* 87(2):169-174.

Grindefjord, M., G. Dahllöf, B. Nilsson, and T. Modeer. 1996. Stepwise prediction of dental caries in children up to 3.5 years of age. *Caries Research* 30(4):256-266.

Gussy, M. G., E. B. Waters, E. M. Riggs, S. K. Lo, and N. M. Kilpatrick. 2008. Parental knowledge, beliefs and behaviours for oral health of toddlers residing in rural Victoria. *Australian Dental Journal* 53(1):52-60.

Haraszthy, V., J. Zambon, M. Trevisan, M. Zeid, and R. Genco. 2000. Identification of periodontal pathogens in atheromatous plaques. *Journal of Periodontology* 71(10):1554-1560.

Havercamp, S. M., D. Scandlin, and M. Roth. 2004. Health disparities among adults with developmental disabilities, adults with other disabilities, and adults not reporting disability in North Carolina. *Public Health Reports* 119(4):418-426.

Heller, K. E., B. A. Burt, and S. A. Eklund. 2001. Sugared soda consumption and dental caries in the United States. *Journal of Dental Research* 80(10):1949-1953.

Hewlett, E. R., P. L. Davidson, T. T. Nakazono, S. E. Baumeister, D. C. Carreon, and J. R. Freed. 2007. Effect of school environment on dental students' perceptions of cultural competency curricula and preparedness to care for diverse populations. *Journal of Dental Education* 71(6):810-818.

HHS (Department of Health and Human Services). 2000a. *Healthy People 2010: Understanding and improving health.* 2nd ed. Washington, DC: U.S. Government Printing Office.

HHS. 2000b. *Oral health in America: A report of the surgeon general.* Rockville, MD: U.S. Department of Health and Human Services.

HHS. 2006. *Midcourse review: Healthy People 2010.* Washington, DC: U.S. Department of Health and Human Services.

HHS. 2011. *Proposed HHS recommendation for fluoride concentration in drinking water for prevention of dental caries.* http://www.hhs.gov/news/press/2011pres/01/pre_pub_frn_fluoride.html (accessed September 13, 2011).

Hobson, W. L., M. L. Knochel, C. L. Byington, P. C. Young, C. J. Hoff, and K. F. Buchi. 2007. Bottled, filtered, and tap water use in Latino and non-Latino children. *Archives of Pediatrics and Adolescent Medicine* 161(5):457-461.

Horowitz, A. M., P. Nourjah, and H. C. Gift. 1995. U.S. adult knowledge of risk factors and signs of oral cancers: 1990. *Journal of the American Dental Association* 126(1):39-45.

Horowitz, A. M., H.S. Moon, H. S. Goodman, and J. A. Yellowitz. 1998. Maryland adults' knowledge of oral cancer and having oral cancer examinations. *Journal of Public Health Dentistry* 58(4):281-287.

Horowitz, A. M., M. T. Canto, and W. L. Child. 2002. Maryland adults' perspectives on oral cancer prevention and early detection. *Journal of the American Dental Association* 133(8):1058-1063.

Horowitz, H. S. 1996. The effectiveness of community water fluoridation in the United States. *Journal of Public Health Dentistry* 56(5):253-258.

Howard, D., J. Gazmararian, and R. Parker. 2005. The impact of low health literacy on the medical costs of Medicare managed care enrollees. *American Journal of Medicine* 118(4):371-377.

Huebner, C. E., P. Milgrom, D. Conrad, and R. S. Y. Lee. 2009. Providing dental care to pregnant patients: A survey of Oregon general dentists. *Journal of the American Dental Association* 140(2):211-222.

Hughes, D. 2010. Oral health during pregnancy and early childhood: Barriers to care and how to address them. *Journal of the California Dental Association* 38(9):655-660.

Hung, H. C., W. Willett, A. Ascherio, B. A. Rosner, E. Rimm, and K. J. Joshipura. 2003. Tooth loss and dietary intake. *Journal of the American Dental Association* 134(9):1185-1192.

Hwang, S. S., V. C. Smith, M. C. McCormick, and W. D. Barfield. 2010. Racial/ethnic disparities in maternal oral health experiences in 10 states, Pregnancy Risk Assessment Monitoring System, 2004-2006. *Maternal and Child Health Journal.* Article first published online: 21 July 2010, DOI: 10.1007/s10995-010-0643-2.

Hyman, J. J., B. C. Reid, S. W. Mongeau, and A. K. York. 2006. The military oral health care system as a model for eliminating disparities in oral health. *Journal of the American Dental Association* 137(3):372-378.

IHS (Indian Health Service). 2002. *An oral health survey of American Indian and Alaska Native dental patients: Findings, regional differences, and national comparisons.* Rockville, MD: Indian Health Service, Division of Dental Services.

IOM (Institute of Medicine). 1997. *Dietary reference intakes.* Washington, DC: National Academy Press.

IOM. 2000. *Promoting health: Intervention strategies from social and behavioral research.* Washington, DC: National Academy Press.

IOM. 2003. *Unequal treatment: Confronting racial and ethnic disparities in healthcare.* Washington, DC: The National Academies Press.

IOM. 2004. *Health literacy: A prescription to end confusion.* Washington, DC: The National Academies Press.

IOM. 2005. *Preventing childhood obesity: Health in the balance.* Washington, DC: The National Academies Press.

IOM. 2008. *Retooling for an aging America.* Washington, DC: The National Academies Press.

IOM. 2009. *Adolescent health services: Missing opportunities.* Washington, DC: The National Academies Press.

Ismail, A. I., and W. Sohn. 1999. A systematic review of clinical diagnostic criteria of early childhood caries. *Journal of Public Health Dentistry* 59(3):171-191.

Isong, I. A., K. E. Zuckerman, S. R. Rao, K. A. Kuhlthau, J. P. Winickoff, and J. M. Perrin. 2010. Association between parents' and children's use of oral health services. *Pediatrics* 125(3):502-508.

Jablonski, R. A., C. L. Munro, M. J. Grap, C. M. Schubert, M. Ligon, and P. Spigelmyer. 2009. Mouth care in nursing homes: Knowledge, beliefs, and practices of nursing assistants. *Geriatric Nursing* 30(2):99-107.

Jackson, J. 2007. Nursing home fined $100,000 for death. *Petaluma Argus-Courier,* July 11, 2007.

Janket, S. J., A. E. Baird, S. K. Chuang, and J. A. Jones. 2003. Meta-analysis of periodontal disease and risk of coronary heart disease and stroke. *Oral Surgery, Oral Medicine, Oral Pathology, Oral Radiology, and Endodontics* 95(5):559-569.

JCNDE (Joint Commission on National Dental Examinations). 2011. *National board dental examinations*. http://www.ada.org/2289.aspx (accessed February 25, 2011).

Jeffcoat, M. K., J. C. Hauth, N. C. Geurs, M. S. Reddy, S. P. Cliver, P. M. Hodgkins, and R. L. Goldenberg. 2003. Periodontal disease and preterm birth: Results of a pilot intervention study. *Journal of Periodontology* 74(8):1214-1218.

Jones, D. B., W. J. Niendorff, and E. B. Broderick. 2000. A review of the oral health of American Indian and Alaska Native elders. *Journal of Public Health Dentistry* 60(Supp. 1):256-260.

Jones, M., J. Y. Lee, and R. G. Rozier. 2007. Oral health literacy among adult patients seeking dental care. *Journal of the American Dental Association* 138(9):1199-1208.

Joshipura, K. J., and C. Ritchie. 2005. Can the relation between tooth loss and chronic disease be explained by socio-economic status? *European Journal of Epidemiology* 20(3):203-204.

Kaiser Family Foundation. 2011. *Medicaid benefits: Dental services (October 2008)*. http://medicaidbenefits.kff.org/service.jsp?gr=off&nt=on&so=0&tg=0&yr=4&cat=6&sv=6 (accessed January 9, 2011).

Kelly, S. E., C. J. Binkley, W. P. Neace, and B. S. Gale. 2005. Barriers to care-seeking for children's oral health among low-income caregivers. *American Journal of Public Health* 95(8):1345-1351.

Kitchens, D. H. 2005. The economics of pit and fissure sealants in preventive dentistry: A review. *Journal of Contemporary Dental Practice* 6(3):95-103.

Kitchens, M., and B. M. Owens. 2007. Effect of carbonated beverages, coffee, sports and high energy drinks, and bottled water on the *in vitro* erosion characteristics of dental enamel. *Journal of Clinical Pediatric Dentistry* 31(3):153-159.

Kiyak, H. A., and M. Reichmuth. 2005. Barriers to and enablers of older adults' use of dental services. *Journal of Dental Education* 69(9):975-986.

Koh, H. 2010. A 2020 vision for Healthy People. *New England Journal of Medicine* 362(18): 1653-1656.

Kumar, J. V., O. Adekugbe, and T. A. Melnik. 2010. Geographic variation in Medicaid claims for dental procedures in New York state: Role of fluoridation under contemporary conditions. *Public Health Reports* 125(5):647-654.

Kuthy, R. A., M. S. Strayer, and R. J. Caswell. 1996. Determinants of dental user groups among an elderly, low-income population. *Health Services Research* 30(6):809-825.

Kutner, M., E. Greenberg, Y. Jin, and C. Paulsen. 2006. *The health literacy of America's adults: Results from the 2003 National Assessment of Adult Literacy*. Washington, DC: National Center for Health Statistics.

Lai, D. T. C., K. Cahill, Y. Qin, and J. L. Tang. 2010. Motivational interviewing for smoking cessation. Cochrane Database of Systematic Reviews(3): CD006936.

Lebby, K. D., F. Tan, and C. P. Brown. 2010. Maternal factors and disparities associated with oral clefts. *Ethnicity and Disease* 20(1 Supp. 1):146-149.

Lee, J. Y., T. J. Bouwens, M. F. Savage, and W. F. Vann, Jr. 2006. Examining the cost-effectiveness of early dental visits. *Pediatric Dentistry* 28(2):102-105.

Lee, J. Y., R. G. Rozier, S. Y. D. Lee, D. Bender, and R. E. Ruiz. 2007. Development of a word recognition instrument to test health literacy in dentistry: The REALD-30—a brief communication. *Journal of Public Health Dentistry* 67(2):94-98.

Lee, R. S.-Y., P. Milgrom, C. E. Huebner, and D. A. Conrad. 2010. Dentists' perceptions of barriers to providing dental care to pregnant women. *Women's Health Issues* 20(5):359-365.

Levinson, W., and D. Roter. 1993. The effects of two continuing medical education programs on communication skills of practicing primary care physicians. *Journal of General Internal Medicine* 8(6):318-324.

Lewis, C., and J. Stout. 2010. Toothache in U.S. children. *Archives of Pediatrics and Adolescent Medicine* 164(11):1059-1063.

Lewis, C. W., D. C. Grossman, P. K. Domoto, and R. A. Deyo. 2000. The role of the pediatrician in the oral health of children: A national survey. *Pediatrics* 106(6):e84.

Lewis, C., W. Mouradian, R. Slayton, and A. Williams. 2007. Dental insurance and its impact on preventative dental care visits for U.S. children. *Journal of the American Dental Association* 138(3):369-380.

Li, Y., and P. W. Caufield. 1995. The fidelity of initial acquisition of *mutans streptococci* by infants from their mothers. *Journal of Dental Research* 74(2):681-685.

Löe, H. 1993. Periodontal disease. The sixth complication of diabetes mellitus. *Diabetes Care* 16(1):329-334.

Lopez, N. J., P. C. Smith, and J. Guitierrez. 2002. Periodontal therapy may reduce the risk of preterm low birth weight in women with periodontal disease: A randomized control trial. *Journal of Periodontology* 73(8):911-924.

Lopez, N. J., I. Da Silva, J. Ipinza, and J. Guitierrez. 2005. Periodontal therapy reduces the rate of preterm low birth weight in women with pregnancy-associated gingivitis. *Journal of Periodontology* 76(Supp. 11):2144-2153.

López Pérez, R., S. A. Borges Yáñez, G. Jiménez García, and G. Maupomé. 2002. Oral hygiene, gingivitis, and periodontitis in persons with Down syndrome. *Special Care in Dentistry* 22(6):214-220.

Macones, G. A., S. Parry, D. B. Nelson, J. F. Strauss, J. Ludmir, A. W. Cohen, D. M. Stamilio, D. Appleby, B. Clothier, M. D. Sammel, and M. Jeffcoat. 2010. Treatment of localized periodontal disease in pregnancy does not reduce the occurrence of preterm birth: Results from the periodontal infections and prematurity study (pips). *American Journal of Obstetrics and Gynecology* 202(2):147.e141-147.e148.

Mancuso, C. A., and M. Rincon. 2006. Impact of health literacy on longitudinal asthma outcomes. *Journal of General Internal Medicine* 21(8):813-817.

Manski, R. J., and E. Brown. 2007. *Dental use, expenses, private dental coverage, and changes, 1996 and 2004.* Rockville, MD: Agency for Healthcare Research and Quality.

Manski, R. J., and E. J. Brown. 2010. *Dental coverage of adults ages 21-64, United States, 1997 and 2007.* Rockville, MD: Agency for Healthcare Research and Quality.

Manski, R. J., and L. S. Magder. 1998. Demographic and socioeconomic predictors of dental care utilization. *Journal of the American Dental Association* 129(2):195-200.

Manski, R. J., J. Moeller, J. Schimmel, P. A. St. Clair, H. Chen, L. Magder, and J. V. Pepper. 2010. Dental care coverage and retirement. *Journal of Public Health Dentistry* 70(1):1-12.

Marinho, V. C. 2009. Cochrane reviews of randomized trials of fluoride therapies for preventing dental caries. *European Archives of Paediatric Dentistry* 10(3):183-191.

Marinho, V. C., J. P. Higgins, S. Logan, and A. Sheiham. 2002. Fluoride varnishes for preventing dental caries in children and adolescents. *Cochrane Database of Systematic Reviews*(3): CD002279.

Marinho, V. C., J. P. Higgins, S. Logan, and A. Sheiham. 2003a. Topical fluoride (toothpastes, mouthrinses, gels or varnishes) for preventing dental caries in children and adolescents. *Cochrane Database of Systematic Reviews*(4): CD002782.

Marinho, V. C. C., J. P. T. Higgins, S. Logan, and A. Sheiham. 2003b. Fluoride toothpastes for preventing dental caries in children and adolescents. *Cochrane Database of Systematic Reviews*(1): CD002278.

Marsh, P. D. 2003. Are dental diseases examples of ecological catastrophes? *Microbiology* 149(2):279-294.

Marsh, P. D. 2006. Dental plaque as a biofilm and a microbial community—implications for health and disease. *BMC Oral Health* 6(Supp. 1):S14.

Marshall, T. A., B. Broffitt, J. Eichenberger-Gilmore, J. J. Warren, M. A. Cunningham, and S. M. Levy. 2005. The roles of meal, snack, and daily total food and beverage exposures on caries experience in young children. *Journal of Public Health Dentistry* 65(3):166-173.

Marur, S., G. D'Souza, W. H. Westra, and A. A. Forastiere. 2010. HPV-associated head and neck cancer: A virus-related cancer epidemic. *Lancet Oncology* 11(8):781-789.

McLeroy, K. R., D. Bibeau, A. Steckler, and K. Glanz. 1988. An ecological perspective on health promotion programs. *Health Education Quarterly* 15(4):351-377.

Merchant, A. T., W. Pitiphat, M. Franz, and K. J. Joshipura. 2006. Whole-grain and fiber intakes and periodontitis risk in men. *The American Journal of Clinical Nutrition* 83(6):1395-1400.

Michalowicz, B. S., J. S. Hodges, A. J. DiAngelis, V. R. Lupo, M. J. Novak, J. E. Ferguson, W. Buchanan, J. Bofill, P. N. Papapanou, D. A. Mitchell, S. Matseoane, and P. A. Tschida. 2006. Treatment of periodontal disease and the risk of preterm birth. *New England Journal of Medicine* 355(18):1885-1894.

Michalowicz, B. S., A. J. DiAngelis, M. J. Novak, W. Buchanan, P. N. Papapanou, D. A. Mitchell, A. E. Curran, V. R. Lupo, J. E. Ferguson, J. Bofill, S. Matseoane, A. S. Deinard, Jr., and T. B. Rogers. 2008. Examining the safety of dental treatment in pregnant women. *Journal of the American Dental Association* 139(6):685-695.

Miller, E., J. Y. Lee, D. A. DeWalt, and W. F. Vann, Jr. 2010. Impact of caregiver literacy on children's oral health outcomes. *Pediatrics* 126(1):107-114.

Miller, W. R. 1983. Motivational interviewing with problem drinkers. *Behavioural and Cognitive Psychotherapy* 11(02):147-172.

Miskell, P. 2005. *How Crest made business history.* http://hbswk.hbs.edu/archive/4574.html (accessed December 23, 2010).

Mobley, C., T. A. Marshall, P. Milgrom, and S. E. Coldwell. 2009. The contribution of dietary factors to dental caries and disparities in caries. *Academic Pediatrics* 9(6):410.

Morgan, M. A., J. Crall, R. L. Goldenberg, and J. Schulkin. 2009. Oral health during pregnancy. *Journal of Maternal-Fetal and Neonatal Medicine* 22(9):733-739.

Mork, J., A. K. Lie, E. Glattre, S. Clark, G. Hallmans, E. Jellum, P. Koskela, B. Møller, E. Pukkala, J. T. Schiller, Z. Wang, L. Youngman, M. Lehtinen, and J. Dillner. 2001. Human papillomavirus infection as a risk factor for squamous-cell carcinoma of the head and neck. *New England Journal of Medicine* 344(15):1125-1131.

Moynihan, P., and P. Petersen. 2004. Diet, nutrition and the prevention of dental diseases. *Public Health Nutrition* 7(1a):201-226.

Naar-King, S., J. T. Parsons, D. A. Murphy, X. Chen, D. R. Harris, and M. E. Belzer. 2009. Improving health outcomes for youth living with the human immunodeficiency virus: A multisite randomized trial of a motivational intervention targeting multiple risk behaviors. *Archives of Pediatrics and Adolescent Medicine* 163(12):1092-1098.

Nabi, G., J. Cody, G. Ellis, P. Herbison, and J. Hay-Smith. 2006. Anticholinergic drugs versus placebo for overactive bladder syndrome in adults. *Cochrane Database of Systematic Reviews*(4): CD003781.

Napier, G. L., and C. M. Kodner. 2008. Health risks and benefits of bottled water. *Primary Care* 35(4):789-802.

National Health and Medical Research Council. 2007. *A systematic review of the efficacy and safety of fluoridation.* Canberra, ACT, Australia: National Health and Medical Research Council.

NCHS (National Center for Health Statistics). 2011. *Health indicators warehouse: Community water fluoridation.* http://www.healthindicators.gov/Indicators/Communitywater fluoridation_1265/Profile/Data (accessed July 18, 2011).

Neuhauser, L. 2010. *Communicating with patients: A survey of dental team members—preliminary results*. Presentation at meeting of the Committee on an Oral Health Initiative, Washington, DC. June 28, 2010.

New York State Department of Health. 2006. *Oral health care during pregnancy and early childhood: Practice guidelines*. Albany, NY: New York State Department of Health.

Newbrun, E. 2010. What we know and do not know about fluoride. *Journal of Public Health Dentistry* 70(3):227-233.

Newnham, J. P., I. A. Newnham, C. M. Ball, M. Wright, C. E. Pennell, J. Swain, and D. A. Doherty. 2009. Treatment of periodontal disease during pregnancy: A randomized controlled trial. *Obstetrics and Gynecology* 114(6):1239-1248.

NIDCR (National Institute of Dental and Craniofacial Research). 2005. The invisible barrier: Literacy and its relationship with oral health. *Journal of Public Health Dentistry* 65(3):174-192.

NIDCR. 2010. *Prevalence (number of cases) of cleft lip and cleft palate*. http://www.nidcr.nih.gov/DataStatistics/FindDataByTopic/CraniofacialBirthDefects/PrevalenceCleft+LipCleftPalate.htm (accessed December 27, 2010).

NIDCR. 2011a. *Periodontal disease in adults (age 20 to 64)*. http://www.nidcr.nih.gov/DataStatistics/FindDataByTopic/GumDisease/PeriodontaldiseaseAdults20to64 (accessed February 14, 2011).

NIDCR. 2011b. *Periodontal disease in seniors (age 65 and over)*. http://www.nidcr.nih.gov/DataStatistics/FindDataByTopic/GumDisease/PeriodontaldiseaseSeniors65over (accessed February 14, 2011).

Nishida, M., S. G. Grossi, R. G. Dunford, A. W. Ho, M. Trevisan, and R. J. Genco. 2000a. Calcium and the risk for periodontal disease. *Journal of Periodontology* 71(7):1057-1066.

Nishida, M., S. G. Grossi, R. G. Dunford, A. W. Ho, M. Trevisan, and R. J. Genco. 2000b. Dietary Vitamin C and the risk for periodontal disease. *Journal of Periodontology* 71(8):1215-1223.

Nomura, L. H., J. L. D. Bastos, and M. A. Peres. 2004. Dental pain prevalence and association with dental caries and socioeconomic status in schoolchildren, southern brazil, 2002. *Brazilian Oral Research* 18:134-140.

Norris, L. J. 2007. *Testimony of the Public Justice Center on May 2, 2007 to the Subcommittee on Domestic Policy Committee on Oversight and Government Reform, U.S. House of Representatives (110th Congress), on the story of Deamonte Driver and ensuring oral health for children enrolled in Medicaid*.

Novak, K. F., A. W. Whitehead, J. M. Close, and A. L. Kaplan. 2004. Students' perceived importance of diversity exposure and training in dental education. *Journal of Dental Education* 68(3):355-360.

NRC (National Research Council). 1989. *Diet and health: Implications for reducing chronic disease risk*. Washington, DC: National Academy Press.

O'Connell, J. M., D. Brunson, T. Anselmo, and P. W. Sullivan. 2005. Costs and savings associated with community water fluoridation programs in Colorado. *Preventing Chronic Disease* 2(Special Issue):1-13.

Offenbacher, S., D. Lin, R. Strauss, R. McKaig, J. Irving, S. P. Barros, K. Moss, D. A. Barrow, A. Hefti, and J. D. Beck. 2006. Effects of periodontal therapy during pregnancy on periodontal status, biological parameters, and pregnancy outcomes: A pilot study. *Journal of Periodontology* 77(12):2011-2024.

Offenbacher, S., J. D. Beck, H. L. Jared, S. M. Maurriello, L. C. Mendoza, D. J. Couper, D. D. Stewart, A. P. Murtha, D. L. Cochran, D. J. Dudley, M. S. Reddy, N. C. Geurs, and J. C. Hauth. 2009. Effects of periodontal therapy on rate of preterm delivery: A randomized controlled trial. *Obstetrics and Gynecology* 114(3):551-559.

OMH (Office of Minority Health). 2001. *National standards for culturally and linguistically appropriate services in health care.* Washington, DC: U.S. Department of Health and Human Services.

Otto, M. 2007. For want of a dentist. *Washington Post*, February 28, P. B01.

Owens, P. L., B. D. Kerker, E. Zigler, and S. M. Horwitz. 2006. Vision and oral health needs of individuals with intellectual disability. *Mental Retardation and Developmental Disabilities Research Reviews* 12(1):28-40.

Paraskevas, S., J. D. Huizinga, and B. G. Loos. 2008. A systematic review and meta analyses on C reactive protein in relation to periodontitis. *Journal of Clinical Periodontology* 35(4):277-290.

Parnell, C., H. Whelton, and D. O'Mullane. 2009. Water fluoridation. *European Archives of Paediatric Dentistry* 10(3):141-148.

Patton, L. L., R. Agans, J. R. Elter, and J. H. Southerland. 2004. Oral cancer knowledge and examination experiences among North Carolina adults. *Journal of Public Health Dentistry* 64(3):173-180.

Pavia, M., C. Pileggi, C. G. A. Nobile, and I. F. Angelillo. 2006. Association between fruit and vegetable consumption and oral cancer: A meta-analysis of observational studies. *American Journal of Clinical Nutrition* 83(5):1126-1134.

Pew Center on the States. 2010. *The cost of delay: State dental policies fail one in five children.* Washington, DC: Pew Center on the States.

Pignone, M., D. A. DeWalt, S. Sheridan, N. Berkman, and K. N. Lohr. 2005. Interventions to improve health outcomes for patients with low literacy. *Journal of General Internal Medicine* 20(2):185-192.

Pihlstrom, B. L., B. S. Michalowicz, and N. W. Johnson. 2005. Periodontal diseases. *Lancet* 366(9499):1809-1820.

Pilcher, E. S., L. T. Charles, and C. J. Lancaster. 2008. Development and assessment of a cultural competency curriculum. *Journal of Dental Education* 72(9):1020-1028.

Polyzos, N. P., I. P. Polyzos, D. Mauri, S. Tzioras, M. Tsappi, I. Cortinovis, and G. Casazza. 2009. Effect of periodontal disease treatment during pregnancy on preterm birth incidence: A metaanalysis of randomized trials. *American Journal of Obstetrics and Gynecology* 200(3):225-232.

Polyzos, N. P., I. P. Polyzos, A. Zavos, A. Valachis, D. Mauri, E. G. Papanikolaou, S. Tzioras, D. Weber, and I. E. Messinis. 2010. Obstetric outcomes after treatment of periodontal disease during pregnancy: Systematic review and meta-analysis. *BMJ* 341. Published online December 29, 2010. DOI: 10.1136/bmj.c7017.

Probst, J., S. Laditka, J.-Y. Wang, and A. Johnson. 2007. Effects of residence and race on burden of travel for care: Cross-sectional analysis of the 2001 U.S National Household Travel Survey. *BMC Health Services Research* 7(1):40.

Quijano, A., A. J. Shah, A. I. Schwarcz, E. Lalla, and R. J. Ostfeld. 2010. Knowledge and orientations of internal medicine trainees toward periodontal disease. *Journal of Periodontology* 81(3):359-363.

Quiñonez, R. B., M. A. Keels, W. F. Vann, Jr., F. T. McIver, K. Heller, and J. K. Whitt. 2000. Early childhood caries: Analysis of psychosocial and biological factors in a high-risk population. *Caries Research* 35(5):376-383.

Quiñonez, R. B., S. M. Downs, D. Shugars, J. Christensen, and W. F. Vann, Jr. 2005. Assessing cost-effectiveness of sealant placement in children. *Journal of Public Health Dentistry* 65(2):82-89.

Ramos-Gomez, F. J., J. A. Weintraub, S. A. Gansky, C. I. Hoover, and J. D. Featherstone. 2002. Bacterial, behavioral and environmental factors associated with early childhood caries. *Journal of Clinical Pediatric Dentistry* 26(2):165-173.

Reid, B. C., R. Chenette, and M. D. Macek. 2003. Prevalence and predictors of untreated caries and oral pain among Special Olympic athletes. *Special Care in Dentistry* 23(4):139-142.

Rethman, M. P., W. Carpenter, E. E. W. Cohen, J. Epstein, C. A. Evans, C. M. Flaitz, F. J. Graham, P. P. Hujoel, J. R. Kalmar, W. M. Koch, P. M. Lambert, M. W. Lingen, B. W. Oettmeier, Jr., L. L. Patton, D. Perkins, B. C. Reid, J. J. Sciubba, S. L. Tomar, A. D. Wyatt, Jr., K. Aravamudhan, J. Frantsve-Hawley, J. L. Cleveland, and D. M. Meyer. 2010. Evidence-based clinical recommendations regarding screening for oral squamous cell carcinomas. *Journal of the American Dental Association* 141(5):509-520.

Richman, J. A., J. Y. Lee, R. G. Rozier, D. A. Gong, B. T. Pahel, and W. F. Vann, Jr.. 2007. Evaluation of a word recognition instrument to test health literacy in dentistry: The REALD-99. *Journal of Public Health Dentistry* 67(2):99-104.

Robinson, P., S. A. Deacon, C. Deery, M. Heanue, A. D. Walmsley, H. V. Worthington, A. M. Glenny, and B. C. Shaw. 2005. Manual versus powered toothbrushing for oral health. *Cochrane Database of Systematic Reviews*(1):CD002281.

Rollnick, S., and W. R. Miller. 1995. What is motivational interviewing? *Behavioural and Cognitive Psychotherapy* 23(4):325-334.

Rothman, K., and A. Keller. 1972. The effect of joint exposure to alcohol and tobacco on risk of cancer of the mouth and pharynx. *Journal of Chronic Diseases* 25(12):711-716.

Rothman, R. L., D. A. DeWalt, R. Malone, B. Bryant, A. Shintani, B. Crigler, M. Weinberger, and M. Pignone. 2004. Influence of patient literacy on the effectiveness of a primary care-based diabetes disease management program. *Journal of the American Medical Association* 292(14):1711-1716.

Rubak, S., A. Sandbæk, T. Lauritzen, and B. Christensen. 2005. Motivational interviewing: A systematic review and meta-analysis. *The British Journal of General Practice* 55(513):305-312.

Ruddy, G. 2007. *Health centers' role in addressing the oral health needs of the medically underserved.* Washington, DC: National Association of Community Health Centers.

Russell, S. L., and L. J. Mayberry. 2008. Pregnancy and oral health: A review and recommendations to reduce gaps in practice and research. *MCN The American Journal of Maternal/ Child Nursing* 33(1):32-37.

Sabbahi, D. A., H. P. Lawrence, H. Limeback, and I. Rootman. 2009. Development and evaluation of an oral health literacy instrument for adults. *Community Dentistry and Oral Epidemiology* 37(5):451-462.

Sadatmansouri, S., N. Sedighpoor, and M. Aghaloo. 2006. Effects of periodontal treatment phase I on birth term and birth weight. *Journal of the Indian Society of Pedodontics and Preventive Dentistry* 24(1):23-26.

Sakai, V. T., T. M. Oliveira, T. C. Silva, A. B. S. Moretti, D. Geller-Palti, V. A. Biella, and M. A. A. M. Machado. 2008. Knowledge and attitude of parents or caretakers regarding transmissibility of caries disease. *Journal of Applied Oral Science* 16(2):150-154.

Sanders, L. M., S. Federico, P. Klass, M. A. Abrams, and B. Dreyer. 2009. Literacy and child health: A systematic review. *Archives of Pediatrics and Adolescent Medicine* 163(2): 131-140.

Satur, J. G., M. G. Gussy, M. V. Morgan, H. Calache, and C. Wright. 2010. Review of the evidence for oral health promotion effectiveness. *Health Education Journal* 69(3):257-266.

Scannapieco, F. A., and A. W. Ho. 2001. Potential associations between chronic respiratory disease and periodontal disease: Analysis of National Health and Nutrition Examination Survey III. *Journal of Periodontology* 72(1):50-56.

Scannapieco, F. A., R. B. Bush, and S. Paju. 2003a. Associations between periodontal disease and risk for atherosclerosis, cardiovascular disease, and stroke. A systematic review. *Annals of Periodontology* 8(1):38-53.

Scannapieco, F. A., R. B. Bush, and S. Paju.. 2003b. Periodontal disease as a risk factor for adverse pregnancy outcomes. A systematic review. *Annals of Periodontology* 8(1):70-78.

Scherzer, T., J. C. Barker, H. Pollick, and J. A. Weintraub. 2010. Water consumption beliefs and practices in a rural Latino community: Implications for fluoridation. *Journal of Public Health Dentistry* 70(4):337-343.

Schwartzberg, J. G., A. Cowett, J. VanGeest, and M. S. Wolf. 2007. Communication techniques for patients with low health literacy: A survey of physicians, nurses, and pharmacists. *American Journal of Health Behavior* 31(Supp. 1):S96-S104.

Scott, T. L., J. A. Gazmararian, M. V. Williams, and D. W. Baker. 2002. Health literacy and preventive health care use among Medicare enrollees in a managed care organization. *Medical Care* 40(5):395.

Seirawan, H., J. Schneiderman, V. Greene, and R. Mulligan. 2008. Interdisciplinary approach to oral health for persons with developmental disabilities. *Special Care in Dentistry* 28(2):43-52.

Selden, C. R., M. Zorn, S. Ratzan, and R. M. Parker. 2000. *Current bibliographies in medicine: Health literacy.* Besthesda, MD: National Library of Medicine.

Seppä, L., T. Leppänen, and H. Hausen. 1995. Fluoride varnish versus acidulated phosphate fluoride gel: A 3-year clinical trial. *Caries Research* 29(5):327-330.

Shaw, L., M. Shaw, and T. Foster. 1989. Correlation of manual dexterity and comprehension with oral hygiene and periodontal status in mentally handicapped adults. *Community Dentistry and Oral Epidemiology* 17(4):187-189.

Shaw, R., and M. Robinson. 2010. The increasing clinical relevance of human papillomavirus type 16 (HPV-16) infection in oropharyngeal cancer. *British Journal of Oral and Maxillofacial Surgery.*

Silk, H., A. B. Douglass, J. M. Douglass, and L. Silk. 2008. Oral health during pregnancy. *American Family Physician* 77(8):1139-1144.

Silva, R. M. D. 2004. Characterization of *Streptococcus constellatus* strains recovered from a brain abscess and periodontal pockets in an immunocompromised patient. *Journal of Periodontology* 75(12):1720-1723.

Simpson, T. C., I. Needleman, S. H. Wild, D. R. Moles, and E. J. Mills. 2010. Treatment of periodontal disease for glycaemic control in people with diabetes. *Cochrane Database of Systematic Reviews*(5):CD004714.

Siriphant, P., T. F. Drury, A. M. Horowitz, and R. M. Harris. 2001. Oral cancer knowledge and opinions among Maryland nurse practitioners. *Journal of Public Health Dentistry* 61(3):138-144.

Skelton, J., T. A. Smith, W. T. Betz, L. J. Heaton, and T. T. Lillich. 2002. Improving the oral health knowledge of osteopathic medical students. *Journal of Dental Education* 66(11):1289-1296.

Skillman, S. M., M. P. Doescher, W. E. Mouradian, and D. K. Brunson. 2010. The challenge to delivering oral health services in rural America. *Journal of Public Health Dentistry* 70(Supp. 1):S49-S57.

Slavkin, H. C. 1997. First encounters: Transmission of infectious oral diseases from mother to child. *Journal of the American Dental Association* 128(6):773-778.

Slavkin, H. C., and B. J. Baum. 2000. Relationship of dental and oral pathology to systemic illness. *Journal of the American Medical Association* 284(10):1215-1217.

Sondik, E. J., D. T. Huang, R. J. Klein, and D. Satcher. 2010. Progress toward the *Healthy People 2010* goals and objectives. *Annual Review of Public Health* 31(1):271-281.

Sriraman, N. K., P. A. Patrick, K. Hutton, and K. S. Edwards. 2009. Children's drinking water: Parental preferences and implications for fluoride exposure. *Pediatric Dentistry* 31(4):310-315.

Stanton, M. W., and M. K. Rutherford. 2003. *Dental care: Improving access and quality.* Rockville, MD: Agency for Healthcare Research and Quality.

Steinberg, B. J., L. Minsk, J. I. Gluch, and S. K. Giorgio. 2008. Women's oral health issues. In *Women's health in clinical practice.* Totowa, NJ: Humana Press. Pp. 273-293.

Stiefel, D. J. 2002. Oral health and dental care access challenges. *Special Care in Dentistry* 22(3):26S-39S.

Sturgis, E. M., and P. M. Cinciripini. 2007. Trends in head and neck cancer incidence in relation to smoking prevalence. *Cancer* 110(7):1429-1435.

Sudore, R., and D. Schillinger. 2009. Interventions to improve care for patients with limited health literacy. *Journal of Clinical Outcomes Management* 16(1):20-29.

Sundin, B., L. Granath, and D. Birkhed. 1992. Variation of posterior approximal caries incidence with consumption of sweets with regard to other caries related factors in 15–18 year olds. *Community Dentistry and Oral Epidemiology* 20(2):76-80.

Suzuki, J., and A. Delisle. 1984. Pulmonary actinomycosis of periodontal origin. *Journal of Periodontology* 55(10):581-584.

Tarannum, F., and M. Faizuddin. 2007. Effect of periodontal therapy on pregnancy outcome in women affected by periodontitis. *Journal of Periodontology* 78(11):2095-2103.

Task Force on Community Preventive Services. 2002. Recommendations on selected interventions to prevent dental caries, oral and pharyngeal cancers, and sports-related craniofacial injuries. *American Journal of Preventive Medicine* 23(Supp. 1):16-20.

Taylor, G. W. 2001. Bidirectional interrelationships between diabetes and periodontal diseases: An epidemiologic perspective. *Annals of Periodontology* 6(1):99-112.

Teeuw, W. J., V. E. A. Gerdes, and B. G. Loos. 2010. Effect of periodontal treatment on glycemic control of diabetic patients: A systematic review and meta-analysis. *Diabetes Care* 33(2):421-427.

Tiller, S., K. Wilson, and J. Gallagher. 2001. Oral health status and dental service use of adults with learning disabilities living in residential institutions and in the community. *Community Dental Health* 18(3):167-171.

Tomar, S. L., and A. F. Reeves. 2009. Changes in the oral health of U.S. children and adolescents and dental public health infrastructure since the release of the Healthy People 2010 objectives. *Academic Pediatrics* 9(6):388-395.

Traebert, J., J. De Lacerda, T. Fischer, and Y. Jinbo. 2005. Dental caries and orofacial pain trends in 12-year-old school children between 1997 and 2003. *Oral health & preventive dentistry* 3(4):243.

Truman, B. I., B. F. Gooch, I. Sulemana, H. C. Gift, A. M. Horowitz, C. A. Evans, Jr., S. O. Griffin, and V. G. Carande-Kulis. 2002. Reviews of evidence on interventions to prevent dental caries, oral and pharyngeal cancers, and sports-related craniofacial injuries. *American Journal of Preventive Medicine* 23(Supp. 1):21-54.

Turner, T., W. L. Cull, B. Bayldon, P. Klass, L. M. Sanders, M. P. Frintner, M. A. Abrams, and B. Dreyer. 2009. Pediatricians and health literacy: Descriptive results from a national survey. *Pediatrics* 124(Supp. 3):S299-S305.

Twetman, S. 2009. Caries prevention with fluoride toothpaste in children: An update. *European Archives of Paediatric Dentistry* 10(3):162-167.

Uher, R., A. Farmer, N. Henigsberg, M. Rietschel, O. Mors, W. Maier, D. Kozel, J. Hauser, D. Souery, A. Placentino, J. Strohmaier, N. Perroud, A. Zobel, A. Rajewska-Rager, M. Z. Dernovsek, E. R. Larsen, P. Kalember, C. Giovannini, M. Barreto, P. McGuffin, and K. J. Aitchison. 2009. Adverse reactions to antidepressants. *British Journal of Psychiatry* 195(3):202-210.

Uppal, A., S. Uppal, A. Pinto, M. Dutta, S. Shrivatsa, V. Dandolu, and M. Mupparapu. 2010. The effectiveness of periodontal disease treatment during pregnancy in reducing the risk of experiencing preterm birth and low birth weight: A meta-analysis. *Journal of the American Dental Association* 141(12):1423-1434.

USDA (U.S. Department of Agriculture). 2009. *Rural population and migration.* http://www. ers.usda.gov/Briefing/Population/ (accessed January 7, 2011).

USMLE (U.S. Medical Licensing Examination). 2010. *2011 step 2 clinical skills: Content description and general information.* Philadelphia, PA: Federation of State Medical Boards of the United States and National Board of Medical Examiners.

Vargas, C. M., and C. R. Ronzio. 2006. Disparities in early childhood caries. *BMC Oral Health* 6(Supp. 1):S3-S7.

Vargas, C., J. Crall, and D. Schneider. 1998. Sociodemographic distribution of pediatric dental caries: NHANES III, 1988-1994. *Journal of the American Dental Association* 129(9):1229.

Vargas, C. M., E. A. Kramarow, and J. A. Yellowitz. 2001. *The oral health of older Americans.* Hyattsville, MD: National Center for Health Statistics.

Vargas, C. M., B. A. Dye, and K. L. Hayes. 2002. Oral health status of rural adults in the United States. *Journal of the American Dental Association* 133(12):1672-1681.

Vargas, C. M., B. A. Dye, and K. L. Hayes. 2003a. Oral health care utilization by U.S. rural residents, National Health Interview Survey 1999. *Journal of Public Health Dentistry* 63(3):150-157.

Vargas, C. M., C. R. Ronzio, and K. L. Hayes. 2003b. Oral health status of children and adolescents by rural residence, United States. *Journal of Rural Health* 19(3):260-268.

Vargas, C. M., J. A. Yellowitz, and K. L. Hayes. 2003c. Oral health status of older rural adults in the United States. *Journal of the American Dental Association* 134(4):479-486.

Vergnes, J. N., and M. Sixou. 2007. Preterm low birth weight and maternal periodontal status: A meta-analysis. *American Journal of Obstetrics and Gynecology* 196(2):135.e1-135.e7.

Vernon, J. A., A. Trujillo, S. Rosenbaum, and B. DeBuono. 2007. *Low health literacy: Implications for national health policy.* http://www.gwumc.edu/sphhs/departments/healthpolicy/dhp_publications/pub_uploads/dhpPublication_3AC9A1C2-5056-9D20-3D4BC6786 DD46B1B.pdf (accessed January 24, 2011).

Wagner, J. A., and D. Redford-Badwal. 2008. Dental students' beliefs about culture in patient care: Self-reported knowledge and importance. *Journal of Dental Education* 72(5):571-576.

Wagner, J., S. Arteaga, J. D'Ambrosio, C. E. Hodge, E. Ioannidou, C. A. Pfeiffer, L. Yong, and S. Reisine. 2007. A patient-instructor program to promote dental students' communication skills with diverse patients. *Journal of Dental Education* 71(12):1554-1560.

Wagner, J., S. Arteaga, J. D'Ambrosio, C. Hodge, E. Ioannidou, C. A. Pfeiffer, and S. Reisine. 2008. Dental students' attitudes toward treating diverse patients: Effects of a cross-cultural patient-instructor program. *Journal of Dental Education* 72(10):1128-1134.

Walsh, T., H. V. Worthington, A. M. Glenny, P. Appelbe, V. C. Marinho, and X. Shi. 2010. Fluoride toothpastes of different concentrations for preventing dental caries in children and adolescents. *Cochrane Database of Systematic Reviews*(1): CD007868.

Weinberger, A. H., E. L. Reutenauer, P. I. Jatlow, S. S. O'Malley, M. N. Potenza, and T. P. George. 2010. A double-blind, placebo-controlled, randomized clinical trial of oral selegiline hydrochloride for smoking cessation in nicotine-dependent cigarette smokers. *Drug and Alcohol Dependence* 107(2-3):188-195.

Weinstein, P., R. Harrison, and T. Benton. 2006. Motivating mothers to prevent caries: Confirming the beneficial effect of counseling. *Journal of the American Dental Association* 137(6):789-793.

Weintraub, J. A. 1989. The effectiveness of pit and fissure sealants. *Journal of Public Health Dentistry* 49(5):317–330.

Weintraub, J. A. 2001. Pit and fissure sealants in high-caries-risk individuals. *Journal of Dental Education* 65(10):1084-1090.

Weintraub, J. A. 2007. Family matters: Influence of biology and behavior on oral health. *New York State Dental Journal* 73(2):14-19.

Weintraub, J. A., S. C. Stearns, B. A. Burt, E. Beltran, and S. A. Eklund. 1993. A retrospective analysis of the cost-effectiveness of dental sealants in a children's health center. *Social Science and Medicine* 36(11):1483-1493.

Weintraub, J. A., S. C. Stearns, R. G. Rozier, and C. C. Huang. 2001. Treatment outcomes and costs of dental sealants among children enrolled in Medicaid. *American Journal of Public Health* 91(11):1877-1881.

Weintraub, J. A., F. Ramos-Gomez, B. Jue, S. Shain, C. I. Hoover, J. D. B. Featherstone, and S. A. Gansky. 2006. Fluoride varnish efficacy in preventing early childhood caries. *Journal of Dental Research* 85(2):172-176.

Weintraub, J. A., P. Prakash, S. G. Shain, M. Laccabue, and S. A. Gansky. 2010. Mothers' caries increases odds of children's caries. *Journal of Dental Research* 89(9):954-958.

Weiss, B. D. 2007. *Health literacy and patient safety: Help patients understand.* Chicago, IL: American Medical Association Foundation.

Weiss, B. D., and R. Palmer. 2004. Relationship between health care costs and very low literacy skills in a medically needy and indigent Medicaid population. *Journal of the American Board of Family Medicine* 17(1):44-46.

Weissman, A. M. 1997. Bottled water use in an immigrant community: A public health issue? *American Journal of Public Health* 87(8):1379-1380.

WHO (World Health Organization). 2010a. *Oral health.* http://www.who.int/topics/oral_health/en/ (accessed December 3, 2010).

WHO. 2010b. *Oral health: Risks to oral health and intervention.* http://www.who.int/oral_health/action/risks/en/index.html (accessed September 15, 2010).

WHO. 2010c. *Oral health: Tobacco.* http://www.who.int/oral_health/action/risks/en/index2.html (accessed September 15, 2010).

WHO. 2010d. *Oral health: Fluorides.* http://www.who.int/oral_health/action/risks/en/index1.html (accessed September 15, 2010).

WHO. 2010e. *Oral health: What is the burden of oral disease?* http://www.who.int/oral_health/disease_burden/global/en/index.html (accessed December 27, 2010).

Wilcox, A. J., R. T. Lie, K. Solvoll, J. Taylor, D. R. McConnaughey, F. Åbyholm, H. Vindenes, S. E. Vollset, and C. A. Drevon. 2007. Folic acid supplements and risk of facial clefts: National population based case-control study. *British Medical Journal* 334(7591):464-467.

Williams, M. V., D. W. Baker, E. G. Honig, T. M. Lee, and A. Nowlan. 1998. Inadequate literacy is a barrier to asthma knowledge and self-care. *Chest* 114(4):1008-1015.

Williams, M. V., T. Davis, R. M. Parker, and B. D. Weiss. 2002. The role of health literacy in patient-physician communication. *Family Medicine* 34(5):383-389.

Wolf, M. S., J. A. Gazmararian, and D. W. Baker. 2005. Health literacy and functional health status among older adults. *Archives of Internal Medicine* 165(17):1946-1952.

Wyszynski, D. F., D. L. Duffy, and T. H. Beaty. 1997. Maternal cigarette smoking and oral clefts: A meta-analysis. *Cleft Palate-Craniofacial Journal* 34(3):206-210.

Yellowitz, J. A., A. M. Horowitz, T. F. Drury, and H. S. Goodman. 2000. Survey of U.S. Dentists' knowledge of opinions about oral pharyngeal cancer. *Journal of the American Dental Association* 131(5):653-661.

Yeung, C. A. 2008. A systematic review of the efficacy and safety of fluoridation. *Evidence-Based Dentistry* 9(2):39-43.

Yuen, H. K., B. J. Wolf, D. Bandyopadhyay, K. M. Magruder, A. W. Selassie, and C. F. Salinas. 2010. Factors that limit access to dental care for adults with spinal cord injury. *Special Care in Dentistry* 30(4):151-156.

3

The Oral Health Care System

While the connections between oral health and overall health and well-being have been long established, oral health care and general health care are provided in almost entirely separate systems. Oral health is separated from overall health in terms of education and training, financing, workforce, service delivery, accreditation, and licensure. In the United States, medical and dental education and practice have been separated since the establishment of the first dental school in Baltimore in 1840 (University of Maryland, 2010). The financing of oral health care is characterized by a similar divide. For example, private health plans typically do not cover oral health care, and the benefits package for Medicare excludes oral health care almost entirely. These separations contribute to obstacles that impede the coordination of care for patients.

This chapter provides an overview of the oral health care system in America today—where services are provided, how those services are paid for, who delivers the services, how the workforce is educated and trained to provide these services, and how the workforce is regulated. The role of the U.S. Department of Health and Human Services (HHS) in oral health education and training, as well as in supporting the delivery of oral health care services, will be addressed in Chapter 4 of this report. Detailed examination of the role HHS plays in overseeing safety net providers such as Federally Qualified Health Centers (FQHCs[1]) was charged to the concurrent Institute of Medicine (IOM) Committee on Oral Health Access to

---

[1] A Federally Qualified Health Center (FQHC) is any health center that receives a grant established by section 330 of the Public Health Service Act (42 U.S.C. §254b).

Services. Therefore, this committee limited its examination of the safety net in this current report.

SITES OF ORAL HEALTH CARE

The current oral health care system is composed of two basic parts—the private delivery system and the safety net—and there is little integration of either sector with wider health care services. The two systems function almost completely separately; they use different financing systems, serve different clientele, and provide care in different settings. In the private delivery system, care is usually provided in small, private dental offices and financed primarily through employer-based or privately purchased dental plans and out-of-pocket payments. This model of care has remained relatively unchanged throughout the history of dentistry. The safety net, in contrast, is made up of a diverse and fragmented group of providers who are financed primarily through Medicaid and the Children's Health Insurance Program (CHIP), other government programs, private grants, as well as out-of-pocket payments.

In addition, some oral health care, especially for young children, has begun to be supplied by nondental providers in settings such as physicians' offices, which is discussed later in this chapter. This section gives a brief overview of the basic settings of oral health care by dental professionals—namely, dentists, dental hygienists, and dental assistants. The professionals themselves will be discussed later in this chapter.

The Private Practice Model

The structure of private practice provides dentists with considerable autonomy in their practice decisions (Wendling, 2010). Private practices tend to be located in areas that have the population to support them; thus, there are more practices located in urban areas than in rural, and more practices in high-income than in low-income areas (ADA, 2009b; Solomon, 2007; Wall and Brown, 2007). About 92 percent of professionally active dentists work in the private practice model (ADA, 2009d) (see Box 3-1 for definitions of types of dentists). Among all active private practice dentists (whose primary occupation was private practice), about 84 percent are independent dentists, 13 percent are employed dentists, and 3 percent are independent contractors (ADA, 2009d). About 60 percent of private practice dentists are solo dentists (Wendling, 2010). In addition, 80 percent of all active private practitioners and 83 percent of new active private practitioners are in general practice, while the remainder work in one of many specialty areas (see Table 3-1).

Dentists in the private practice setting see a variety of patients. The

BOX 3-1
Types of Dentists

A *professionally active dentist* is primarily or secondarily occupied in a private practice, dental school faculty/staff, armed forces, or other federal service (e.g., Veterans Administration, U.S. Public Health Service); or is a state or local government employee, hospital staff dentist, graduate student/intern/resident, or other health/dental organization staff member.

An *active private practitioner* is someone whose primary and/or secondary occupation is private practice.

A *new dentist* is anyone who has graduated from dental school within the last 10 years.

An *independent dentist* is a dentist running a sole proprietorship or one who is involved in a partnership.

A *solo dentist* is an independent dentist working alone in the practice he or she owns.

A *nonowner dentist* does not share in ownership of the practice.

An *employed dentist* works on a salary, commission, percentage, or associate basis.

An *independent contractor* contracts with owner(s) for use of space and equipment.

A *nonsolo dentist* works with at least one other dentist and can be an independent or nonowner dentist.

NOTE: Each of these types can be either general or specialty practitioners.
SOURCES: ADA, 2009b,d.

patients of independent general practitioners are spread relatively evenly across the age spectrum and equally divided by gender (ADA, 2009b). About two-thirds (63 percent) of their patients have private insurance; only about 7 percent receive publicly supported dental coverage, and the remaining 30 percent are not covered by any dental insurance (ADA, 2009b). Similarly, independent dentists' billings primarily are from private insurance and direct patient payments (44 percent and 39 percent, respectively) (ADA, 2009c). Nearly two-thirds of independent dentists (63 percent) and slightly more than half of new independent dentists (58 percent) do not have any patients in their practices covered by public sources (ADA, 2009b). However, in 2006, Bailit and colleagues estimated that 60 to 70 percent of underserved individuals who get care do so in the private care system (Bailit et al., 2006). While there is some disagreement as to whether dentists who care for patients with public coverage are considered part of

TABLE 3-1
Percentage Distribution of Active Private Practitioners by Practice,
Research, or Administration Area, 2007

Practice, Research, or Administration Area	All Active Private Practitioners	New Active Private Practitioners
General practice	80.1	83.3
Orthodontics and dentofacial orthopedics	5.7	4.7
Oral and maxillofacial surgery	3.7	1.9
Periodontics	2.8	1.7
Pediatric dentistry	3.0	4.4
Endodontics	2.6	2.6
Prosthodontics	1.6	0.8
Public health dentistry	0.3	0.4
Oral and maxillofacial pathology	0.1	0.1
Oral and maxillofacial radiology	0.0	0.0
Missing specialty area	0.1	0.1

SOURCE: ADA, 2009d.

the safety net, opportunities to expand care for vulnerable and underserved populations in private settings cannot be overlooked.

The Oral Health Safety Net

Some segments of the American population, namely socioeconomically disadvantaged groups, have difficulty accessing the private dental system due to geographic, financial, or other access barriers and must rely on the dental safety net (if they are seeking care) (Bailit et al., 2006; Brown, 2005; Wendling, 2010). While the term *safety net* may give the impression of an organized group of providers, the dental safety net comprises a group of unrelated entities that both individually and collectively have very limited capacity (Bailit et al., 2006; Edelstein, 2010a). One estimate of the current capacity of the safety net suggests that 7 to 8 million people may be served in these settings annually, and approximately another 2.5 million could be served with improved efficiency (Bailit et al., 2006). However, the safety net as it exists simply does not have the capacity to serve all of the people in need of care, which is estimated to be as high as 80 to 100 million individuals (Bailit et al., 2006; HHS, 2000). While there is a perception that the care provided in safety net settings is somehow inferior to the care provided in the private practice setting, there are no data to support this assumption. In fact, there are very little data regarding the quality of oral health care provided in any setting (see later in this chapter for more on quality assessment in the oral health care system).

Common types of safety net providers include FQHCs, FQHC look-alikes,[2] non-FQHC community health centers, dental schools, school-based clinics, state and local health departments, and community hospitals. Each type of provider offers some type of oral health care, but the extent of the services provided and the number of patients served varies widely and the safety net cannot care for everyone who needs it (Bailit et al., 2006; Edelstein, 2010a). Private sector efforts to supplement the safety net include the organization of single-day events to provide free dental care. In 2003, the ADA established the annual Give Kids a Smile Day; in 2011, the ADA estimated the event would involve about 45,000 volunteers providing care to nearly 400,000 children (ADA, 2011a). Another example includes the Missions of Mercy, which are often organized by state dental societies or private foundations. At these events, thousands of individuals have waited in lines for hours to receive care (Dickinson, 2010). These types of single-day events provide temporary relief to the access problem for some people, but they do not provide a regular source of care for people in need.

PAYING FOR ORAL HEALTH CARE

Multiple challenges exist in the financing of oral health care in the United States, including state budget crises, the relative lack of dental coverage, a payment system (like in general health care) that rewards treatment procedures rather than health promotion and disease prevention, and the high cost of dental services. Expenditures for dental services in the United States in 2009 were $102.2 billion, less than 5 percent of total spending on health care, a proportion that has remained fairly constant for the last two decades (CMS, 2011c).

Demand for dental care may vary with the economic climate of the country (Guay, 2005; Wendling, 2010). For example, the recent recession was identified as a key factor contributing to 2009 having the slowest rate of growth in health spending (4 percent) in the last 50 years (Martin et al., 2011). Notably, expenditures on dental services had a negative rate of

---

[2] FQHC look-alikes must meet all of the statutory requirements of FQHCs, but they do not receive grant funding under section 330 and are eligible for many, but not all, of the benefits extended to FQHCs.

growth (–0.1 percent) in 2009, down from a positive rate of growth of 5.1 percent in 2008.

Typical sources of health care insurance—Medicare, Medicaid, CHIP, and employers of all sizes—often do not include dental coverage, especially for adults. Employment status of adults ages 51–64 is a strong predictor of dental coverage (Manski et al., 2010c), and "routine dental care" is specifically excluded from the traditional Medicare benefits package. High-income older adults are more likely to have dental coverage than are other older adults (Manski et al., 2010c). In any case, individuals with dental coverage often incur high out-of-pocket costs for oral health care (Bailit and Beazoglou, 2008). Estimates regarding the severity of uninsurance for dental care include the following:

- In 2000, the surgeon general's report estimated that 108 million people (about 35 percent of the population) lacked dental coverage (HHS, 2000).
- A recent estimate based on enrollment in private dental plans found 130 million U.S. adults and children lack dental coverage (NADP, 2009).
- In 2004, 34 percent of adults ages 21–64 and about 70 percent of adults ages 65 and older lacked dental coverage (Manski and Brown, 2007).
- Nearly 25 percent of people who have private health insurance lack dental coverage (Bloom and Cohen, 2010).

Overall, rates of uninsurance for oral health care are almost three times the rates of uninsurance for medical care—34.6 percent (Manski and Brown, 2007) versus 14.7 percent (CDC, 2009).

Financing of oral health care greatly influences where and whether individuals receive care. For example, the national Medical Expenditure Panel Survey (MEPS) data show that in 2004, 57 percent of individuals with private dental coverage had at least one dental visit, compared to 32 percent of those with public dental coverage and 27 percent of uninsured individuals (Manski and Brown, 2007). At the individual level, insurance coverage and socioeconomic factors play a significant role in access to oral health care (Flores and Tomany-Korman, 2008; GAO, 2008; Isong et al., 2010; Liu et al., 2007). Financing also has an effect on providers' practice patterns, in part due to the low reimbursement rates of public insurers. Previous studies have shown that like in medicine, dentists' practice patterns are associated with financial incentives (Atchison and Schoen, 1990; Naegele et al., 2010; Porter et al., 1999). The following sections give a general overview of how care is financed in the United States.

Private Sources

As shown in Table 3-2, dental care is financed primarily through private sources, including individual out-of-pocket payments and private dental plans.

In 2008, dental services accounted for 22 percent of all out-of-pocket health care expenditures, ranking second only to prescription drug expenditures (see Figure 3-1).

Employers can add a separate oral health product to their overall coverage package, but often they do not. In 2006, 56 percent of all employers offered health insurance, but only 35 percent offered dental insurance (Manski and Cooper, 2010). The availability of dental coverage through one's employer is associated with the size of the establishment; that is, the larger the number of employees overall, the higher the incidence of stand-alone dental plans available to employees (Barsky, 2004; Ford, 2009). Higher-paid workers are also more likely to have access to and participate in stand-alone dental plans (Barsky, 2004; Ford, 2009). Employees are more likely to be offered access to medical insurance than dental insurance, and a higher percentage of employees will take advantage of available dental benefits as compared with the percentage of employees who take advantage of available medical benefits (BLS, 2010b).

TABLE 3-2
National Health Expenditures by Type of Expenditure and Source of Funds, 2009

Type of Expenditure	Total Spending (billions)	Percentage from Out-of-Pocket Payments (%)	Percentage from Private Insurance (%)	Percentage from Public Insurance (%)
Dental services	102.2	41.6	48.9	9.1
Physician and clinical services	505.9	9.5	47.0	33.5
Home health care	68.3	8.8	7.4	80.2
Nursing and continuing care	137.0	29.1	7.7	56.2
Prescription drugs	249.9	21.2	43.4	33.9
Hospital care	759.1	3.2	35.0	53.2

NOTES: Public insurance includes Medicare, Medicaid, CHIP, the Department of Defense, and the Department of Veterans' Affairs. Totals do not reach 100% as some expenditures were attributed to "Other Third Party Payers and Programs."
SOURCE: CMS, 2011b.

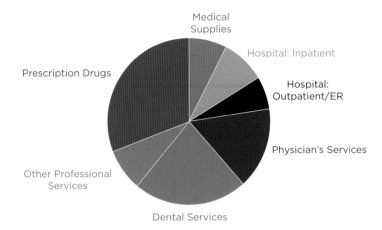

FIGURE 3-1
Out-of-pocket health care expenditures, 2008.
SOURCE: BLS, 2010a.

Public Sources

Of the $102.2 billion in dental expenditures, nearly 91 percent came from private funds (e.g., private insurance and out-of-pocket payments), and only 9 percent came from public funds (e.g., state and federal funds) (CMS, 2011b). In comparison, public funds account for about one-third of physician and clinical services (see Table 3-2). However, the reported national expenditure levels likely undercount the total public funds spent on improving oral health, because that total represents only the costs associated with direct services delivered by dentists (to the exclusion of the broader definition of *oral health*) and does not account for care provided in settings such as hospitals and nursing homes. While a much lower percentage of funds for dental services come from public sources as compared to the funding of many other services, the government may, in fact, have a very important role to play for those who cannot afford to pay for care.

Public sources are an important source of coverage for many vulnerable and underserved populations, but a recent report from the U.S. Government Accountability Office (GAO) found that finding providers to care for Medicaid populations "remains a challenge" (GAO, 2010). Low reimbursement by public programs is often cited as a disincentive for providers' to participate in publicly funded programs (Damiano et al., 1990; GAO, 2000; Lang and Weintraub, 1986; McKnight-Hanes et al., 1992; Venezie et al., 1997). Studies have shown, though, that in order to significantly increase participation rates, increased reimbursement is necessary but often requires additional efforts such as decreasing the administrative burdens of participation; changing provider perceptions of participating; and fostering relationships among state Medicaid staff, the state dental association, and local dentists (Borchgrevink et al., 2008; GAO, 2000; Greenberg et al., 2008; Wysen et al., 2004).

Medicaid and CHIP

Dental coverage is required for all Medicaid-enrolled children under age 21 (CMS, 2011a). This is a comprehensive benefit, including preventive, diagnostic, and treatment services. According to data from the Kaiser Family Foundation, Medicaid provides health care coverage to nearly 30 million children while CHIP covers an additional 6 million (KFF, 2011). Further, they note that together, Medicaid and CHIP provide health care coverage for one-third of children and over half (59 percent) of low-income children. However, exact documentation of these numbers may be challenging due to how enrollees are counted (e.g., at a point in time versus at any time in a given period).

Regarding the Early and Periodic Screening, Diagnosis and Treatment (EPSDT) Program, by law,[3] states must cover any Medicaid-covered service that would reasonably be considered medically necessary to prevent, correct, or ameliorate children's physical (including oral) and mental conditions. In contrast, Medicaid dental benefits are not required for adults, and even among those states that offer dental coverage for adult Medicaid recipients, the benefits are often limited to emergency care (ASTDD, 2011c). In FY2008, Medicaid spending on dental services accounted for 1.3 percent of all Medicaid payments (CMS, 2010b).

CHIP is a federally funded grant program that provides resources to states to expand health coverage to uninsured, low-income children. Millions of children have received coverage for medical care, and a portion of those have also been covered for dental care (Brach et al., 2003). The Children's Health Insurance Program Reauthorization Act (CHIPRA)[4] enacted in February 2009 requires all states to provide dental coverage to children (but not including their parents) covered under CHIP.

Medicare

As increasing numbers of baby boomers become eligible for Medicare, considerable attention is being paid to how these aging adults will pay for

---

[3] 42 U.S.C. §1396d(r)(3).
[4] *Children's Health Insurance Program Reauthorization Act of 2009*, Public Law 3, 111th Cong., 1st sess. (February 4, 2009).

and obtain oral health care (Ferguson et al., 2010; Manski et al., 2010a,b,c; Moeller et al., 2010). In the year 2000, almost 77 percent of dental care for older adults was paid by out-of-pocket expenditures, and 0.4 percent was covered by Medicaid (Brown and Manski, 2004). Medicare explicitly excludes coverage for routine dental care, specifically "for services in connection with the care, treatment, filling, removal, or replacement of teeth or structures directly supporting the teeth."[5]

In the initial Medicare program, "routine" physical checkups and routine foot care were excluded; comparatively, all dental services were excluded, not just "routine" dental services (CMS, 2010a). In 1980, Congress made an exception for "inpatient hospital services when the dental procedure itself made hospitalization necessary" (CMS, 2010a). Box 3-2 delineates the extent of the exclusion of oral health care from the Medicare program.

Federal Systems of Care

In addition to the public programs noted above, the federal government both directly provides and pays for the oral health care of several distinct segments of the U.S. population. This includes care provided both in public and private settings through the various branches of the military, the Bureau of Prisons, the Department of Homeland Security, and the Veterans Administration. The role of the federal government in providing care is discussed more fully in Chapter 4.

Impact of Health Care Reform

Between now and 2014, several provisions of the Patient Protection and Affordable Care Act (ACA)[6] will affect dental coverage. For example, provisions address coverage of oral health services for children and the expansion of Medicaid eligibility. Table 4-4 in Chapter 4 highlights some of the key provisions that will affect dental coverage.

THE DENTAL WORKFORCE

Traditionally, a combination of dentists, dental hygienists, and dental assistants directly provide oral health care. Dental laboratory technicians create bridges, dentures, and other dental prosthetics. In addition, new and evolving types of dental professionals (e.g., dental therapists) are being pro-

---

[5] *Social Security Act*, §1862(a)(12).

[6] *Patient Protection and Affordable Care Act*, Public Law 148, 111th Cong., 2nd sess. (March 23, 2010).

BOX 3-2
Exclusions (and Exceptions) to
Dental Coverage Under Medicare

Services Excluded Under Part B

A primary service (regardless of cause or complexity) provided for the care, treatment, removal, or replacement of teeth or structures directly supporting teeth (e.g., preparation of the mouth for dentures, removal of diseased teeth in an infected jaw).

A secondary service that is related to the teeth or structures directly supporting the teeth unless it is incident to and an integral part of a covered primary service that is necessary to treat a nondental condition (e.g., tumor removal) and it is performed at the same time as the covered primary service and by the same physician/dentist. In those cases in which these requirements are met and the secondary services are covered, Medicare does not make payment for the cost of dental appliances, such as dentures, even though the covered service resulted in the need for the teeth to be replaced, the cost of preparing the mouth for dentures, or the cost of directly repairing teeth or structures directly supporting teeth (e.g., alveolar process).

Exceptions to Services Excluded

Exceptions include the extraction of teeth to prepare the jaw for radiation treatment of neoplastic disease, as well as an oral or dental examination performed on an inpatient basis as part of comprehensive workup prior to renal transplant surgery or performed in a rural health clinic/FQHC prior to a heart valve replacement.

SOURCE: CMS, 2010a.

---

posed and, in some instances, used to provide some oral health care. The extent to which all of these professionals interact can vary greatly.

The surgeon general's 2000 report expressed concerns about

> a declining dentist-to population ratio, an inequitable distribution of oral health care professionals, a low number of underrepresented minorities applying to dental school, the effects of the costs of dental education and graduation debt on decisions to pursue a career in dentistry, the type and location of practice upon graduation, current and expected shortages in personnel for dental school faculties and oral health research, and an evolving curriculum with an ever-expanding knowledge base. (HHS, 2000)

Unfortunately, these concerns continue today.

The following section will focus on the traditional dental workforce in terms of its demographic profile, basic education and training, and racial and ethnic diversity, as well as the role of new and emerging members of the dental team. Later sections in this chapter will describe the roles and skills of other types of health care professionals (e.g., nurses, physicians) in the provision of oral health care.

Basic Demographics

The adequacy of the current supply of oral health professionals, both in terms of its numbers and skills, is difficult to assess for a variety of reasons related to changes in employment status, differing measures (e.g., licensed vs. active professionals), the holding of more than one position per worker, part-time employment, and the presence of multiple job titles. Predicting the need for specific types of practitioners is always difficult because many factors can affect the need and demand for oral health care (Brown, 2005; Guthrie et al., 2009). For example, improvements in oral health of the population might limit future demand for restorative care.

While it is debatable whether the number of professionals is adequate, it is more certain that the oral health workforce is not well distributed, with distinct areas showing significant needs (Hart-Hester and Thomas, 2003; Mertz and Grumbach, 2001; Saman et al., 2010). Even with a sufficient supply, geographic maldistribution could still persist (Wall and Brown, 2007). For example, even with financial incentives such as loan repayment, dentists willing to locate in rural areas might be unable to sustain a practice in these locations (Allison and Manski, 2007). More attention may be needed to where students are recruited from, as 57 percent of graduates report plans to return to work in their home states after graduation (Okwuje et al., 2010).

Job growth during the next decade is projected to be above average for all the dental professions, particularly for dental hygienists and dental assistants (see Table 3-3). In fact, dental hygienists rank twelfth on the list of the fastest-growing occupations (of all occupations) and fifth among occupations directly related to health care (see Table 3-4). Dental assistants rank fourteenth on the list of the fastest-growing occupations and sixth among occupations directly related to health care.

Dentists

Estimates of the number of dentists in the workforce vary significantly, likely due to how they are counted. As shown in Table 3-3, the Bureau of Labor Statistics (BLS) estimates that dentists held approximately 141,900 jobs in 2008, 85 percent of which were in general dentistry. However, in 2007, the American Dental Association (ADA) estimated that there were 181,725 professionally active dentists; 79 percent were general dentists

TABLE 3-3
Employment of Dental Occupations, 2008 and Projected 2018

Occupation	Number of Jobs		Percent Increase in Growth (%)
	2008	2018	
Dentists	141,900	164,000	16
General dentists	120,200	138,600	15
Dental hygienists	174,100	237,000	36
Dental assistants	295,300	400,900	36
Dental laboratory technicians	46,000	52,400	14

[a]The Bureau of Labor Statistics calculates replacement needs based on estimates of job openings due to retirement or other reasons for permanently leaving an occupation.

[b]Total job openings represent new positions due to both growth and replacement needs. Totals may not add precisely due to rounding.

SOURCES: BLS, 2010d,e,f,g.

(ADA, 2009d). The dentist-to-population ratio has remained relatively constant for nearly 20 years (about 60 dentists per 100,000 population) and is expected to decline in the coming decades (Wendling, 2010).

Among independent dentists in private practice, 43 percent are age 55 or older (ADA, 2009b). Like many other health care professions, concerns arise about replacement needs as these individuals retire. While most dentists are male, the proportion of female dentists is on the rise owing to the increased proportion of female dentists among younger dentists (see Figure 3-2). However, while dentistry is becoming increasingly gender diverse, the racial and ethnic profile of dentists has shown little change (see later in this section for a discussion of the racial and ethnic diversity of dental professions). Dentists' income can vary depending on the type of employment, ranging from an average total net income of about $114,000 for new employed dentists to over $350,000 for independent specialists (ADA, 2009c).

As discussed previously, professionally active dentists overwhelmingly work in the private practice setting (92 percent). Among the remaining dentists, occupations include[7]

---

[7] Does not total 100 percent due to rounding.

- Dental school faculty/staff member (1.7 percent),
- Armed forces (0.9 percent),
- Graduate student/intern/resident (1.3 percent),
- Hospital staff dentist (0.4 percent),
- State or local government employee (0.8 percent),
- Other federal service (0.8 percent), and
- Other health/dental organization staff (1.0 percent) (ADA, 2009d).

Among 2009 dental school graduates, 48 percent planned to enter private practice immediately, while 30 percent planned to go on to advanced education (e.g., residency), 11 percent planned to go into some form of government service, and less that one-half of 1 percent planned to enter teaching, research, or administration; the remainder were "other/undecided" (Okwuje et al., 2010).

TABLE 3-4
Top 15 Fastest-Growing Occupations, 2008 and Projected 2018

Occupation	Percent Change, 2008–2018
Biomedical engineers	72.0
Network systems and data communications analysts	53.4
Home health aides	50.0
Personal and home care aides	46.0
Financial examiners	41.2
Medical scientists, except epidemiologists	40.4
Physician assistants	39.0
Skin care specialists	37.9
Biochemists and biophysicists	37.4
Athletic trainers	37.0
Physical therapist aides	36.3
Dental hygienists	36.1
Veterinary technologists and technicians	35.8
Dental assistants	35.8
Computer software engineers, applications	34.0

SOURCE: BLS, 2010c.

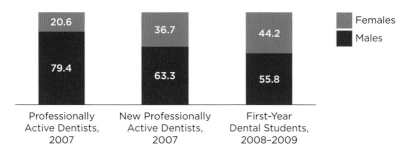

FIGURE 3-2
Percentage distribution of dentists by gender.
SOURCES: ADA, 2009d, 2010a.

Dental Hygienists

The dental hygiene profession began almost a century ago when a dentist trained his assistant to assist in preventive dental services (University of Bridgeport, 1998). Since then, dental hygiene has evolved to a licensed health care profession; dental hygienists, in concert with dentists, provide "preventive, educational, and therapeutic services supporting total health for the control of oral diseases and the promotion of oral health" (ADHA, 2010). In private dental practice, dental hygienists' work is generally billed under the dentist's provider number.

Dental hygienists are virtually all female (99 percent) (ADHA, 2009b). This is not changing dramatically: in 2008, only 2.8 percent of graduates of dental hygiene programs were male (ADA, 2009a). The mean age of dental hygienists is about 44 years of age (ADHA, 2009b), which, like dentists, may lend to concerns about the numbers nearing retirement. Dental hygienists are primarily employed in private dental practices but may also work in educational institutions and in public health settings such as school-based clinics, prisons, long-term care, and other institutional care facilities (ADHA, 2009b). In 2008, dental hygienists held about 174,100 jobs, with a median annual wage of about $66,500 (BLS, 2010e).[8] Nearly 30 percent of dental hygienists do not receive any benefits (ADHA, 2009b).

In spite of BLS projections for a 36 percent growth in the employment of dental hygienists between 2008 and 2018 (see Table 3-4), the dental hygiene workforce may also be experiencing challenges due to geographic maldistribution. For example, a 2009 survey of dental hygienists showed that 68 percent of respondents reported finding employment was somewhat or very difficult in their geographic area (up from 31 percent in 2007), and

---

[8] Because dental hygienists may hold more than one job, this is an overestimate of the number of practicing dental hygienists.

of these, 80 percent felt that there were too many hygienists living in the area (ADHA, 2009a,b).

Dental Assistants

Dental assistants primarily work in a clinical capacity, but other roles include administrative positions, practice management, and education (McDonough, 2007). Most dental assistants work in private practices and as assistants to general dentists, but many dental assistants work in specialty practices. Across the country, there are different job titles and categories for dental assistants in different states (ADAA/DANB Alliance, 2005). The BLS estimates that dental assistants held 295,000 jobs in 2008, with a median annual wage of about $32,000 (BLS, 2010d). Like dental hygienists, dental assistants are nearly all female (McDonough, 2007). Expanded function dental assistants (EFDAs) may perform some limited restorative functions under the supervision of a dentist (Skillman et al., 2010). Both the U.S. Army Dental Command and the Indian Health Service have programs to train and employ EFDAs (IHS, 2011; Luciano et al., 2006). While the title of EFDA is commonly used to describe all dental assistants who can perform extended duties, there are many other titles given to dental assistants with expanded duties (e.g., expanded duties dental assistant, advanced dental assistant, registered restorative assistant in extended functions), and many states permit dental assistants to perform specific extended functions (e.g., coronal polishing, administration or monitoring of sedation, pit and fissure sealants) (DANB, 2007). In fact, some states permit certified dental assistants to act at the level of an EFDA, even though titles such as *certified dental assistant* or *registered dental assistant* are used (DANB, 2007). As stated by the Dental Assistant National Board, "without a single, nationally-accepted set of guidelines that govern the practice of dental assisting in the country, it is difficult to execute a concise overview" of the profession (DANB, 2007).

Dental Laboratory Technicians

In 2008, dental laboratory technicians (or "dental technicians") held about 46,000 jobs in 2008 with a median annual wage of about $34,000 (BLS, 2010g). Dental technicians work in a variety of settings, including dentists' offices, their own private businesses, or small privately owned offices. Among all students enrolled during the 2008–2009 academic year, 40 percent were age 23 and younger and slightly more than half were female (ADA, 2009a).

Education and Training

Prior to the 20th century, dental and allied dental education occurred through apprenticeships and training in proprietary schools (Haden et al., 2001). The education of dental professionals evolved and formalized over time to take place in a variety of locations, including dental schools, 4-year colleges and universities, community colleges, and technical schools. The ADA's Commission on Dental Accreditation (CODA) accredits predoctoral dental education programs; programs for dental hygienists, dental assistants, and dental laboratory technicians; and advanced dental educational programs (i.e., residencies) (Department of Education, 2010). While the number of programs is increasing, faculty recruitment, especially for dental schools and dental hygiene programs, is a persistent problem; this is often due to low salary (ADHA, 2006; Chmar et al., 2008; Walker et al., 2008). In addition, several efforts have emphasized the need to revise the way that dental students are educated and trained, including the need to provide care in a more patient-centered fashion, as well as for students to gain more clinical experiences in the community setting (Cohen et al., 1985; Formicola et al., 1999, 2006; HHS, 2010; IOM, 1995; Lamster et al., 2008). More effort is also needed to improve the health literacy and cultural competency of students.

The sections below provide some highlights as to the overall education and training of the dental professions. Chapter 4 provides more information on the role of HHS in education and training.

Dentists

U.S. dental schools typically offer a 4-year curriculum; students take 2 years of predominantly basic science classes followed by 2 years of predominantly clinical experience, after which they are awarded either a Doctor of Dental Medicine (DMD), or a Doctor of Dental Surgery (DDS). The number of dental schools in the United States is increasing, and more dentists are being produced. In 2009, there were 57 dental schools, of which 37 were public, 16 were private, and 4 were private, state-related institutions (ADA, 2010a). At that time, 8 new dental schools were in various stages of development (Guthrie et al., 2009). About 4,800 dentists graduate each year (ADA, 2010a). In 1999, there were 55 dental schools that graduated about 4,100 dentists annually (ADA, 2010a.)

The cost of dental education is a barrier to entry, especially for low-income and underrepresented minority students (IOM, 2004; Sullivan Commission, 2004; Walker et al., 2008). In 2008–2009, the average annual tuition for dental schools was $27,961 for state residents and $41,561 for nonresidents, similar to the tuition for medical students (AAMC, 2011;

ADA, 2010a); the difference is significant considering that many states do not have a single dental school. As this problem exists for several professions, the Western Interstate Commission for Higher Education created the Professional Student Exchange Program in which students from certain states may receive assistance to attend health professional schools (including dental schools) in other states (WICHE, 2011). There is also great variation between public and private institutions.

In 2009, average dental education debt was $164,000, and 77 percent of graduates had at least $100,000 in debt (Okwuje et al., 2010). Comparatively, the average educational debt for medical school graduates in 2009 was approximately $156,000, and 79 percent of graduates had at least $100,000 in debt (AMA, 2011). Debt among dental graduates varies widely; those with higher levels of debt are more likely to enter private practice immediately upon graduation and less likely to pursue advanced education as compared to those with no debt (Okwuje et al., 2010).

Dentists have the option of postgraduate education that provides further training in general dentistry or one of the nine recognized specialty areas. In 2008–2009, there were 723 specialty and postdoctoral general dentistry programs in the United States, including dental residencies and fellowship programs (ADA, 2010b). Currently, about 30 percent of graduating dental students plan to pursue postgraduate training (Okwuje et al., 2010). In the 2008–2009 academic year, there were nearly more than 44,500 applications[9] for residency programs slots and about 3,000 first-year enrollees (ADA, 2010b).

Dental Hygienists

In the 2008–2009 academic year, there were 301 dental hygiene education programs accredited by CODA (ADA, 2009a). Most of these programs award associate degrees (82 percent), but others award baccalaureate degrees, diplomas, and certificates (ADA, 2009a). In 2008, there were about 6,700 dental hygiene graduates. In the early years of the profession, dental hygiene education programs were often colocated with dental education programs in schools of dentistry (Haden et al., 2001). Today, about two-thirds of dental hygiene education programs are located in community, junior, and technical colleges (ADHA, 2006), which may decrease the amount of interaction between dentists and dental hygienists during their training, and therefore not prepare them to work as a team. Annual tuition can vary widely. For example, community colleges have an average annual tuition of $3,154, while the average annual tuition for programs colocated with dentals schools is $12,659 (ADA, 2009a). While the educational admissions

---

[9] This reflects the number of applications and not the unique number of applicants.

requirements for dental hygiene education programs vary widely, more than 80 percent of first-year students have completed at least 2 years of college (ADA, 2009a). Faculty in dental hygiene education programs are mostly dental hygienists (76 percent), and 21 percent are dentists (ADA, 2009a).

Dental Assistants

Dental assistants are trained on the job or in formal education programs. Education programs in dental assisting may be located in postsecondary institutions that are accredited by CODA, postsecondary institutions that are not accredited, high schools, vocational programs, and technical schools (ADAA/DANB Alliance, 2005). Dental assistants may also be trained on the job by their employers. Considering the numerous alternate pathways to working in dental assisting and the variability in state licensure and certification practices, as described previously, it is difficult to generalize a description of the workforce as a whole or to assess the impact of the various training alternatives (ADAA/DANB Alliance, 2005; Neumann, 2004). Little is known about the wide variety of programs that are not accredited by CODA.

In 2008–2009, CODA accredited 273 dental assisting programs, almost all of which (87 percent) were in public institutions (ADA, 2009a). Average cost for tuition and fees in a CODA-accredited dental assisting program in the 2008–2009 academic year for in-district students was $6,791 (ADA, 2009a). Among students enrolled in CODA-accredited dental assisting programs in the 2008–2009 academic year, 63 percent were age 23 and under, and less than 5 percent were male. In 2008, there were 6,110 graduates from CODA-accredited programs (ADA, 2009a).

Virtually all CODA-accredited programs require a high school diploma (or even higher level of education) for admission (ADA, 2009a). Most CODA-accredited programs are 1 year in length leading to a certificate or diploma. However, a few have a 2-year curriculum resulting in an associate degree. About 14 percent of faculty in CODA-accredited programs are dentists, 70 percent are dental assistants, and 28 percent are dental hygienists (ADA, 2009a).[10]

Dental Laboratory Technicians

There are no formal education or training requirements for dental technicians, and most learn required skills through on-the-job training; however, some formal programs exist in universities, community and junior

---

[10] Some faculty members reported more than one discipline, so these numbers do not total 100 percent.

colleges, vocational schools, and the military (BLS, 2010g). In the 2008–2009 academic year, there were 20 CODA-accredited programs (ADA, 2009a). Virtually all faculty (91 percent) are dental laboratory technicians (ADA, 2009a). Most accredited programs last 2 years, and 13 confer an associate's degree. In the 5-year period from 2004–2009, applications to these programs decreased by nearly 13 percent (ADA, 2009a). Average total tuition and fees range from $7,838 for in-district students to $18,214 for out-of-state students (ADA, 2009a). In 2008, there were 234 total graduates from accredited dental laboratory technology programs (ADA, 2009a).

Racial and Ethnic Diversity

The racial and ethnic profile of the dental workforce is not representative of the overall population (see Table 3-5). While diversity among the dental professions students has increased in the previous decade (see Table 3-6), the numbers still are not significantly different. Evidence shows that a diverse health professions workforce (including race and ethnicity, gender, and geographic distribution) leads to improved access for underserved populations, greater patient satisfaction, and better communication (HRSA, 2006; IOM, 2004). Health care professionals from underrepresented minority (URM) populations, in part due to patient preference, often account for a disproportionate amount of the services provided to underserved populations (including both URM and low-income populations) (Brown et al., 2000; HRSA, 2006; IOM, 2003; Mitchell and Lassiter, 2006). For example, a 1996 survey by the ADA revealed that nearly 77 percent of white den-

TABLE 3-5
Dental Professions by Percentage of Race and Hispanic Ethnicity, 2000

	General Population	Dentists	Dental Hygienists	Dental Assistants
White[a]	75.1	82.8	90.9	75.8
Black or African American[a]	12.3	3.3	2.3	5.6
Asian[a]	3.6	8.8	2.0	3.6
Hispanic or Latino Origin	12.5	3.6	3.7	12.6

[a]Category excludes Hispanic origin.
SOURCES: U.S. Census Bureau, 2000, 2002.

TABLE 3-6
Percentage of Dental Professions School and Program Enrollment
by Race and Hispanic Ethnicity, 2000–2001 and 2008–2009

	Enrolled Dental Students		Enrolled Dental Hygiene Students		Enrolled Dental Assistant Students[a]	
	2000–2001	2008–2009	2000–2001	2008–2009	2000–2001	2008–2009
White	63.4	59.9	82.3	78.6	68.4	60.2
Black	4.8	5.8	4.2	4.4	12.5	15.1
Asian	24.8	23.4	4.6	7.0	2.9	4.8
Hispanic	5.3	6.2	5.7	7.3	9.7	11.1

[a]Includes only dental assistant students enrolled in CODA-approved programs.
Racial and ethnic diversity of entire dental assistant workforce may be different.
SOURCES: ADA, 2002, 2009a, 2010a.

tists' patients were white, while 62 percent of African American dentists' patients were African American and 27 percent were white (ADA, 1998). More recently, among dental students graduating in 2008, 80 percent of African American students and 75 percent of Hispanic students expected at least one-quarter of their patients would be from underserved racial and ethnic populations; nearly 37 percent of the African American students and 27 percent of the Hispanic students expected at least half their practice would come from these populations (Okwuje et al., 2009). In comparison, only 43.5 percent of white students expected at least one-quarter of their patients to come from underserved racial and ethnic populations, and only 6.5 percent expected at least half of their practice to be comprised from these populations (Okwuje et al., 2009). It is important to note that the recruitment of low-income students (regardless of race or ethnicity) may also be important in the future care of URM patients (Andersen et al., 2010).

Several factors complicate recruitment of underrepresented minorities into dentistry including lack of exposure to and knowledge of the dental profession, minimal opportunities for mentorship from dental professionals, and competition from other health professions for underrepresented minority students who are academically qualified (Haden et al., 2003).

Bridge and Pipeline Programs

Bridge and pipeline programs are two strategies used to attract and retain underrepresented minority, lower-income, and rural students to health care professions. Bridge programs primarily focus on elementary school students through high school graduates while pipeline programs focus on undergraduate and preprofessional students. Both programs have a long history in health professions (e.g., dentistry, medicine, nursing, pharmacy) (Awé and Bauman, 2010; Brooks et al., 2002; Brunson et al., 2010; Cantor et al., 1998; Formicola et al., 2010; Grumbach and Chen, 2006; Hesser et al., 1996; Kim et al., 2009; Lewis, 1996; Rackley et al., 2003; Thomson et al., 2010).

Pipeline interventions for improving racial and ethnic diversity in the health professions in general have shown promise (HHS, 2009). In 2001, the Robert Wood Johnson Foundation, in collaboration with the California Endowment and the W.K. Kellogg Foundation, created the initiative *Pipeline, Profession, and Practice: Community-Based Dental Education*,[11] which ended in July 2010. This project provided much insight into strategies for successful implementation (Lavizzo-Mourey, 2010; Leviton, 2009). Overall, dental pipeline programs show promise, but gains to date have been small and individual programs have had variable results regarding the ultimate enrollment and retention of students, dependent upon the program's characteristics (Andersen et al., 2005; Markel et al., 2008; Price et al., 2007; Thind et al., 2008; Veal et al., 2004). Moreover, it has yet to be determined whether these programs will have a long-term effect on increasing diversity in dentistry. Evidence suggests that pipeline programs require a sustained commitment by participating schools and sufficient resources to maintain momentum (Brunson et al., 2010; Thind et al., 2009).

One example of an effort to increase the diversity of the dental workforce is the ADA Career Guidance and Diversity Committee, which sponsors the Student Ambassador Program. In this program, ambassadors reach out to high school and college students regarding careers in dentistry (ADA, 2011b). Strategies include increasing collaborations between dental schools and college prehealth advisors, providing shadowing opportunities, and linking to existing career guidance programs.

New and Emerging Members of the Dental Team

Many health care professions have become embroiled over the creation of new types of practitioners as well as over the expansion of scope of practice for existing practitioners. Within the dental professions, efforts to define or expand scopes of practice for dental professionals have been plagued by a decades-long, contentious history (Dunning, 1958; Edelstein, 2010b; Fales, 1958; Hammons and Jamison, 1967, 1968; Hammons et al., 1971; Nash, 2009; Nash and Willard, 2010). Early experiments to have dental

---

[11] For information on participating schools, funding levels, activities, accomplishments, and community partners, see the RWJF project website at: http://www.dentalpipeline.org.

hygiene students perform discrete restorative procedures indicated that the quality of the care provided by these students was equal to that of dental students, but follow-up studies were not performed amidst the concerns of organized dentistry for patient safety (Dunning, 1958; Garcia et al., 2010; Lobene and Kerr, 1979; Sisty et al., 1978). Dental therapists and dental nurses have been used internationally for decades (Ambrose et al., 1976; Gallagher and Wright, 2003; GAO, 2010; Nash and Nagel, 2005b; Nash et al., 2008; Pew Center on the States and National Academy for State Health Policy, 2009; Sun et al., 2010). In particular, New Zealand and Australia have used these dental professionals since the early 20th century. Suggestions to perform a demonstration of the New Zealand school dental nurse in the United States occurred as early as 1947 (Dunning, 1958), but they were not acted upon, again due to the concerns of dentists for patient safety.

The use of dental therapists to provide basic educational, preventive, and restorative services in the United States has been especially contentious. Recently, the Indian Health Service (IHS) has used dental therapists to perform specific functions in order to address oral health access difficulties for American Indian communities (Bolin, 2008; Fiset, 2005; Nash and Nagel, 2005a,b; Wetterhall et al., 2010). In 2003, the Alaska Native Tribal Health Consortium first sent several Alaskan students to New Zealand to train as dental therapists, and the consortium is currently working with the University of Washington to train these students in Alaska (DENTEX, 2010; Nash and Nagel, 2005b). The first assessment of dental therapists in the United States indicated there was no significant difference between treatment provided by dental therapists and treatment provided by dentists (Bolin, 2008). A more recent evaluation indicates that the care provided by dental therapists in the United States is both effective and acceptable to patients (Wetterhall et al., 2010). Further, residents of communities served by dental therapists report that access to care has improved. It is important to note the narrow scope of this evaluation in that the authors examined the implementation of the dental therapist model in just five practice sites. In addition, they noted: "We undertook this challenging effort knowing that there are few, if any, widely accepted, evidence-based standards for assessing dental practice performance. Further, for the logical comparison group—that is, dentists in private practice—there are virtually no data for any of the outcomes that we undertook to observe and measure" (Wetterhall et al., 2010).

Aside from the dental therapist, several other workforce models have been recently proposed to either introduce new types of professionals or expand the scope of work of existing professionals. For example, in 2009, the Minnesota legislature approved the certification of a master's level "advanced dental therapist"[12] to work in remote consultation with a dentist and provide some restorative procedures (GAO, 2010). The Community Dental Health Coordinator (CDHC), developed by the ADA, would provide oral health education and some limited preventive services under the supervision of a dentist (GAO, 2010; Pew Center on the States and National Academy for State Health Policy, 2009). The registered dental hygienist in alternative practice (RDHAP) started as a pilot project in the 1970s; the RDHAP is licensed (only in California) to provide care directly to patients but must have a documented relationship with a dentist for referral, consultation, and emergencies (Mertz and Glassman, 2011).

All of these new and emerging members of the dental team (and several others) have been targeted to reach populations that for a variety of reasons (e.g., transportation, geographic location, dental coverage issues) have difficulty accessing care. While there are differences, all depend on the practitioner being part of a larger health care team (Garcia et al., 2010). Many of these models remain controversial, with some arguing for their ability to increase access, and others voicing concerns for patient safety and the quality of care provided by these practitioners (ADA, 2007; AGD, 2008; Edelstein, 2010b; GDA, 2010; Pew Center on the States and National Academy for State Health Policy, 2009).

Lessons from Other Health Care Professions

Concerns have been raised in other fields when new types of practitioners were being developed or when existing professionals sought to extend their scopes of practice (Carson-Smith and Minarik, 2007; Daly, 2006; Huijbregts, 2007; RCHWS, 2003; Wing et al., 2004). While nurse practitioners and physician assistants are largely seen as well-accepted members of the health care team, their development was also resisted, and extension of their scopes of practice remains a sensitive issue. Professional tensions typically center around the quality of care provided by individuals with less training, but in many cases, evidence has not supported this. Advanced practice nurses are often involved in high-risk procedures such as childbirth and the administration of anesthesia, yet the evidence base continues to grow that the quality of their care is similar to that of physicians. For example, studies on certified nurse midwives have shown good maternal outcomes and cost savings in comparison with obstetricians (MacDorman and Singh, 1998; Oakley et al., 1996; Rosenblatt et al., 1997). Certified registered nurse anesthetists (CRNAs), like many nonphysician health care professionals, are an important source of care in rural populations: CRNAs are the sole providers of anesthesia in more than two-thirds of

---

[12] 2009 Minn. Laws Ch. 95, Art. 3.

all rural hospitals (AANA, 2011). In 2001, CMS ruled that states could opt out of requirements for physician supervision of CRNAs, a decision that was opposed by anesthesiologists due to concerns for quality of care (Dulisse and Cromwell, 2010). However, a study of the time period from 1996 until 2005 revealed that there was an increase in the number of procedures performed by CRNAs, but there was no concomittant increase in adverse events (Dulisse and Cromwell, 2010). These examples provide some evidence on the ability to use nonphysician health care professionals to provide quality care in some situations.

Conclusions

While dentists continue to raise concerns for the quality of care provided by individuals (apart from dentists) who might perform restorative care, there is a lack of evidence documenting poorer quality of the services performed by these individuals or poorer outcomes resulting from their care. There are many studies of the safety and quality of dental therapists and dental nurses around the world, but these models occur in different systems of care delivery and financing. Evaluations in the United States to date have been limited, and it is nearly impossible to compare their quality to that of existing dental professionals, since little evidence exists on the quality of care provided by traditional dental practitioners (see a discussion of quality of care later in this chapter). The committee considered the concerns raised by dentists, the unresolved needs of certain segments of the population (e.g., vulnerable and underserved populations), international evidence, and the experiences seen in developing new roles and responsibilities among other health care professions. In addition, the committee recognizes that there is little evidence to indicate which route would be best—developing new types of providers or expanding the scope of existing dental professionals. Due to the variety of challenges, the committee concludes that the exploration of new workforce models (including both new types of dental professionals as well as expansion of the role of existing professionals) is one part of a complex solution to improving oral health care. There may, in fact, be roles for different models depending on the needs of the population and sites of care. Without further research and evaluation, with monitoring for any concerns about the quality of care, better workforce models cannot be developed. Regardless of state laws, many factors will influence the ultimate success of new workforce models, including the support of dentists, the support of state Medicaid agencies, and a viable mechanism for paying the new types of practitioners (Nolan et al., 2003).

THE NONDENTAL ORAL HEALTH WORKFORCE

As oral health has increasingly become recognized as integral to overall health, nondental health care professionals have become increasingly involved in the prevention, diagnosis, and treatment of oral diseases. Studies show that training primary care clinicians in oral health leads to their increased ability to recognize oral disease and may help to increase their referrals to dentists (Dela Cruz et al., 2004; Mouradian et al., 2003; Pierce et al., 2002). In addition, practice changes resulting from this training can lead to increased access to preventive services and decreased dental disease (Chu et al., 2007; Douglass et al., 2009b; Kressin et al., 2009; Rozier et al., 2010). As discussed in Chapter 2, all types of health care professionals need improvements in their oral health literacy skills. In order to do so, educational programs will need to adapt curricula not only to teach basic oral health knowledge but also to impart a greater understanding of the importance of oral health to their individual disciplines. This section considers the education, training, and potential role of several nondental health care professions in the oral health care of the nation. At the end of the section, the role of nondental health care professionals as a whole in the delivery of preventive services for oral health is discussed.

Physicians

The need for physicians to learn about oral health has been recognized for nearly a century (Gies, 1926). Today, many physicians still do not receive education or training in oral health either during medical school, during residency training, or in continuing education programs (Krol, 2010; Mouradian et al., 2003). In addition, the breadth and depth of existing education and training efforts is highly variable (Douglass et al., 2009a; Ferullo et al., 2011). Even though many physicians recognize the importance of oral health (including their own role), they often do not feel prepared to provide oral health care. (See a discussion in Chapter 2 regarding health care professionals' knowledge of oral health.) Dentists also express some hesitation about involving physicians in oral health care; while a large majority of directors of advanced general dentistry residencies supported physician inclusion of routine dental assessments (87.1 percent) and prevention counseling (83.3 percent) in well-child care, less than a third (31.2 percent) supported physicians applying fluoride varnish (Raybould et al., 2009).

Medical Schools

Very few medical schools include curriculum on oral health, despite the presence of oral health topics on medical licensing exams (Ferullo et al., 2011; Krol, 2004; Mouradian et al., 2005; USMLE, 2010a,b). A recent survey indicated that almost 70 percent of medical schools include 4 hours or less of oral health in their curriculum; this includes the more than 10 percent of schools that have no oral health curriculum hours at all (Ferullo et al., 2011). The most frequently covered oral health topics include oral cancer, oral anatomy, and oral health and overall health; fewer than 50 percent of schools that teach oral health cover the risks of dental caries (Ferullo et al., 2011).

In 2004, the Josiah Macy, Jr. Foundation funded a 3-year grant to examine dental education, *New Models of Dental Education* (Formicola et al., 2005; Machen, 2008). As part of the project, three panels were convened to discuss different aspects of oral health education and each produced a report (Johnson et al., 2008; Lamster et al., 2008; Mouradian et al., 2008). One panel produced the report, *Curriculum and Clinical Training in Oral Health for Physicians and Dentists*, which emphasized the role for physicians in the identification and referral of patients with oral health needs (Mouradian et al., 2008). Subsequently, the American Association of Medical Colleges published learning objectives for oral health (AAMC, 2008). Courses that have incorporated these objectives have significantly increased students knowledge of oral health topics, even in a short time period (Silk et al., 2009). One medical school at the forefront of oral health education, the University of Washington Medical School, created and has started to implement a comprehensive oral health curriculum for medical students; results show students have more confidence in identification of oral disease and attitudes toward oral health care improved (Mouradian, 2010; Mouradian et al., 2005, 2006).

Pediatricians

A 2000 national survey of pediatricians found that more than 90 percent believed they had an important role in the recognition of oral diseases and the provision of counseling regarding the prevention of caries, and three-quarters expressed interest in the application of fluoride varnish in their practices (Lewis et al., 2000). However, half reported no oral health training in either medical school or residency. A 2006 survey found that two-thirds of graduating pediatrics residents thought they should be performing oral health assessments on their patients, but only about one-third of pediatrics residents receive any oral health training during their residencies, and of those that do, two-thirds get less than 3 hours of training. (Caspary et al., 2008). Only about 14 percent had clinical observation time with a dentist.

The American Academy of Pediatrics (AAP), the professional society for general pediatrics, has developed explicit educational guidelines for oral health training in pediatric residency (AAP, 2011c). In addition, the pediatric board exam has questions about oral health (ABP, 2009). However, the residency review committee for pediatrics has not yet identified oral health as a required topic for pediatric residencies.

Family Medicine Physicians

Family medicine has taken a number of steps to incorporate oral health into residency curriculum. The Society of Teachers of Family Medicine Group on Oral Health published an oral health curriculum for family medicine in 2005 (it was updated in 2008), and the residency review committee for family medicine residencies added oral health as a requirement in 2006 (ACGME, 2007; Society of Teachers of Family Medicine Group on Oral Health, 2011). Yet, a recent survey showed only three-fourths of the residency directors knew of the oral health requirement, and only about two-thirds of the programs were actually including oral health content, with the most common training time being 2 hours per year (Douglass et al., 2009a).

Internal Medicine Physicians

Of the primary care specialties, internal medicine has done the least to incorporate oral health. Oral health education is not a requirement for internal medicine residencies, although the geriatrics subspecialty requires education in prevention of oral diseases, and the sleep medicine subspecialty requires residents to have experience receiving consults from oral maxillofacial surgeons (ACGME, 2008, 2009a,b). No specific curricula exist to educate internal medicine residents or physicians in oral health. In a survey of internal medicine trainees, 90 percent reported receiving no training on periodontal disease during medical school, and 23 percent said they never referred patients to dentists (Quijano et al., 2010).

Nurses

The nursing workforce is the largest workforce of health professionals in the nation, with 3.1 million registered nurses including over 141,000 nurse practitioners (NPs) (ANA, 2011a, 2011b). In a recent "call to action" to the nursing profession, Clemmens and Kerr (2008) noted that "oral health has not been a high nursing priority in the past" and urged the profession to "increase nursing's awareness, knowledge, and skill about the significance that oral health holds." However, as with other nondental health care professions, the training of nurses in oral health and hygiene is highly variable and often inadequate (Jablonski, 2010).

NPs in particular may have an important role to play in oral health care. A recent study found that "substantial parallels exist in the education and practice of dentists and [NPs] including basic, social, and some clinical science education, practice models, research synergies, and community service" (Spielman et al., 2005). NPs have been defined as primary care providers (IOM, 1996) and can see patients independently and perform histories and physicals, perform lab tests, and diagnose and treat both acute and chronic conditions. NPs emphasize health promotion and disease prevention and especially focus on the health of individuals in the context of their families and communities. NPs commonly practice in rural areas and health professional shortage areas, and the growth of the profession, in part, is due to their role in caring for underserved populations (Grumbach et al., 2003; Harper and Johnson, 1998). As such, they may serve as a front-line screening source for oral diseases. NPs have been shown to provide high-quality care, be cost-effective, have high levels of patient satisfaction with their care, and contribute to increased productivity (Budzi et al., 2010; Hooker et al., 2005; Mezey et al., 2005; Todd et al., 2004).

Criteria set by the National Task Force on Quality Nurse Practitioner Education (2008) do not delineate any specific competencies for oral health. In 2006, the Arizona School of Health Sciences and the Arizona School of Dentistry and Oral Health developed a set of proposed oral health competencies for nurse practitioners and physician assistants (PAs) (Danielsen et al., 2006). As shown in Table 3-7, a subsequent survey of NPs and PAs revealed that many do not feel prepared for some of these basic competencies.

In addition to NPs, there are more than 3 million direct-care workers (e.g., nurse aides) who work in places where dental professionals typically do not provide care (e.g., assisted living facilities, home health agencies) (PHI, 2010). These nursing personnel also have the opportunity to be involved in the detection of oral diseases. In nursing home settings, certified nursing assistants are responsible for the provision of oral hygiene care for

TABLE 3-7
Perceived Competence of Nurse Practitioners and Physician Assistants (Percent)

	Nurse Practitioners	Physician Assistants
Can perform an oral exam	43	53
Can recognize oral symptoms of systemic disease	22	34
Can discern "obvious pathology and conditions of the oral cavity"	40	63

SOURCE: Danielsen et al., 2006.

residents, but they are often unprepared for this task and make it a low priority (Chalmers, 1996; Coleman and Watson, 2006; Jablonski et al., 2009).

Pharmacists

As health care professionals in community settings, the role of the pharmacist has expanded over time from merely dispensing medications to being an important partner with other health care professionals. Pharmacists are often involved in health promotion and disease prevention activities such as public health education, health screenings, and the provision of vaccines. In 2008, pharmacists held almost 270,000 jobs; about 65 percent worked in retail settings, and 22 percent worked in hospitals (BLS, 2009a). The BLS notes a likely increase in the need for pharmacists to provide services in settings such as doctors' offices and nursing facilities as well as to increasingly offer patient care services, such as the administration of vaccines (BLS, 2009a).

Regarding oral health specifically, customers may approach pharmacists regarding the treatment of oral health conditions such as mouth ulcers, cold sores, and persistent pain (Cohen et al., 2009; Macleod et al., 2003; Sowter and Raynor, 1997; Weinberg and Maloney, 2007). Pharmacists can have an important role in the management and treatment of oral disease such as through education on selection and use of daily oral hygiene products as well as referrals to dentists as necessary. Pharmacists could also monitor the prescription of dietary fluoride supplements, especially as it might relate to the status of that community's water fluoridation. No formal assessment has been done to evaluate the extent and depth of education and instruction that pharmacy students receive regarding oral health.

Physician Assistants

As primary care providers, PAs also have great opportunities and responsibilities to be involved in oral health care (Berg and Coniglio, 2006; Danielsen et al., 2006). PAs work under the supervision of a physician, but they can often work apart from the physician's direct presence and can prescribe medications and bill for health care services. The BLS projects the PA profession to be the seventh fastest-growing occupation between 2008 and 2018 (see Table 3-4). In 2008, PAs held about 74,800 jobs; more than half of these jobs were located in physicians' offices, and about one-quarter were in hospitals (BLS, 2009b).

About half of PAs work in primary care (Brugna et al., 2007; Hooker and Berlin, 2002). Like NPs, PAs are an especially important source of care for rural communities, for low-income and minority populations, and in health professional shortage areas (Grumbach et al., 2003), and they have been shown to provide quality and cost-effective care (Ackermann and Kemle, 1998; Brugna et al., 2007; Jones and Cawley, 1994).

Very little is known about the extent of oral health education in the PA curricula. As in nurse practitioner programs, standards set by the Accreditation Review Commission on Education for the Physician Assistant (ARC-PA, 2010) do not delineate any specific competencies for oral health. In the previously mentioned survey performed by the Arizona School of Health Sciences and the Arizona School of Dentistry and Oral Health, many PAs feel unprepared for some basic oral health competencies (see Table 3-7). Interestingly, that survey showed that 10 percent of PAs did not think it was important for them to understand what the various dental specialties could do for their patients (compared to 2 percent of nurse practitioners) (Danielsen et al., 2006). A recent survey of PA program directors found "over 75 percent believed that dental disease prevention should be addressed in PA education, yet only 21 percent of programs actually did so" (Jacques et al., 2010). The number of curriculum hours dedicated to oral health ranged from 0 to 14 hours, with an average of 3.6 hours.

The Role of Nondental Health Care Professionals in Preventive Care

One solution for improving access to preventive care for oral health, especially for children, has been to expand the use of nondental health care professionals (Douglass et al., 2009b; Hallas and Shelley, 2009; Okunseri et al., 2009). Nondental health care professionals can incorporate oral health into their routine exams and wellness visits with basic risk assessments, oral exams, anticipatory guidance, and the provision of basic preventive services (Cantrell, 2008; Riter et al., 2008). The application of fluoride varnish is a prime example for the potential expanded role of nondental health care professionals. Fluoride varnish is increasingly being applied by nondental health care professionals and in community-based settings (AAP, 2011b; ASTDD, 2007). In spite of evidence on the effectiveness of fluoride varnish (see Chapter 2), it is not approved by the FDA for its use in the prevention of dental caries (ASTDD, 2007), which may deter some health care professionals from using it for this purpose.

In the past, nondental health care professionals could not be reimbursed for preventive care in oral health, but this is changing. As of 2010, 39 state Medicaid programs reimbursed primary medical care providers for preventive oral health services, 2 approved such reimbursement but did not have funding, and another 3 allowed reimbursement under certain circumstances (AAP, 2010). This is an increase from 2008, when only 25 states reimbursed physicians for these types of services, and 2009, when 34 states did so (Cantrell, 2008, 2009). In addition, some states also reimburse NPs and PAs for these services (Cantrell, 2008). The three types of services typically reimbursed include oral examination, screening, and risk assessment; anticipatory guidance and caregiver education; and application of fluoride varnish (Cantrell, 2009). In 2009, 25 states required the health care professionals undergo training before they could be reimbursed (Cantrell, 2009). Aside from lack of reimbursement, other barriers to engaging nondental health care professionals in preventive care (both for oral health as well as other health conditions) can include the lack of familiarity with oral health issues, lack of confidence in their skills, skepticism on the efficacy of preventive services, and inadequate time in the patient visit (Lewis et al., 2000; Rozier et al., 2003; Sanchez et al., 1997).

Several individual state-based initiatives have arisen to help improve nondental health care professionals' involvement in providing basic preventive services for oral health. One well-known example is North Carolina's Into the Mouths of Babes (IMB) which targets children up to age 3 (Rozier et al., 2003, 2010). IMB stemmed from earlier work in the 1990s where poor oral health was identified as one of the most serious problems for children and their families in the Appalachian region of the state. With support from the North Carolina Medicaid program, CMS, the Health Resources and Services Administration (HRSA), and the Centers for Disease Control and Prevention, lessons learned from that work led to the statewide demonstration of IMB in 2001. The project aims to improve practitioners' oral health knowledge, incorporate caregiver counseling and fluoride varnish application into primary care practices, and increase screenings and dental referrals for children with oral diseases or are at risk for diseases (Close et al., 2010). Reimbursement is provided for up to 6 visits for children up to age 3. Between 2001 and 2002, nearly 1,600 nondental health care professionals were trained (Rozier et al., 2003). About half of the participants were pediatricians or family physicians and another one-third were registered nurses; others included PAs, NPs, and a variety of other health care professionals. In 2006, almost one-third of all well-child visits for this age group included preventive care for oral health (Rozier et al., 2010). In 2009, the North Carolina Department of Health and Human Services reported a ten-fold increase in the number of preventive procedures since the inception of IMB (NC Department of Health and Human Services, 2009). Program successes have been attributed to a broad-based, collaborative coalition, support from the professions themselves, an active effort to improve awareness about oral diseases, and adequate resources (Rozier et al., 2003). A recent survey of participants in the program identified some of the barriers to success, including difficulty integrating the services into practices (reported by 42 percent), difficulty in applying fluoride varnish (29 percent), reluctance of other office personnel (26 percent), and difficulty in making dental referrals (21 percent) (Close et al., 2010). In order to better integrate the application of fluoride varnish into primary care setting, providers may need to look to the model of immunization as an example of successfully integrating the delivery of preventive services in these settings.

HHS has also actively supported programs that seek to improve the use of nondental health care professionals in oral health care. For example, *Bright Futures* was initiated by HRSA's Maternal and Child Health Bureau in 1990 to improve children's health in general through health promotion and disease prevention (AAP, 2011a). The project includes a collaboration of many different organizations and includes information, guidance, and training on oral health issues from pregnancy through adolescence. Currently, the American Academy of Pediatrics (AAP) is MCHB's lead collaborator; AAP has developed a new edition of the Bright Futures Guidelines, which focus on health promotion and disease prevention (MCHB, 2011). The website (www.brightfutures.org) includes online training modules for child health professionals in oral health management and risk assessment.

PUBLIC HEALTH WORKERS

Public health workers include many of the professions previously mentioned, including both dental and nondental health care professionals. The 1988 IOM report *The Future of Public Health* defined the mission of public health as "fulfilling society's interest in assuring conditions in which people can be healthy" (IOM, 1988). That committee went on to say:

> [Public health's] aim is to generate organized community effort to address the public interest in health by applying scientific and technical knowledge to prevent disease and promote health. The mission of public health is addressed by private organizations and individuals as well as by public agencies. But the governmental public health agency has a unique function: to see to it that vital elements are in place and that the mission is adequately addressed. (IOM, 1988)

As with other segments of the health care workforce, the public health workforce is difficult to enumerate due to the variety of professions involved, lack of a common taxonomy for job titles and duties, and a lack of a single comprehensive licensure or certification process for public health (HRSA, 2000). Both dental and nondental health care professionals may be involved in dental public health. Little is known about the extent of training in oral health among schools of public health, even though graduates may be involved in oral health issues during their careers. A 2001 survey of schools of public health showed that 60 percent of schools had no faculty with a degree in dentistry or dental hygiene (Tomar, 2006). In addition, only 15 percent of schools offered a Master of Public Health degree with a concentration in dental public health.

The predecessor to the present-day American Association of Public

Health Dentistry (AAPHD) was established in 1937 and represents a variety of public health professionals involved in oral health care (AAPHD, 2004). In 1948, the Association of State and Territorial Dental Directors was established to represent the directors and staff of state dental public health programs and is currently an affiliate of the Association of State and Territorial Health Officials (ASTDD, 2011a). In 1951, the American Dental Association (ADA) recognized dental public health as a specialty of dentistry (AAPHD, 2004). In 2005, estimates of the number of public health dentists ranged from 153 (the number of diplomats of the American Board of Public Health Dentistry) to 498 (the number of dentist members of the AAPHD) to 543 (the number of members in the ADA directory reporting a specialty of "dental public health") (Tomar, 2005). HHS supports dental public health residency programs (see Chapter 4). Public health dentists often work for governments at the federal, state, county, and local levels (Tomar, 2006). While public health is a key part of the practice of dental hygiene, little is known about public health workers with specialty in dental hygiene.

While HHS is a key leader in establishing the general public health infrastructure of the country, much dental public health activity takes place at the state and local levels. Dental public health workers often are involved in state- and locally funded activities (e.g., sealant programs, fluoridation programs) that aim to assure access to services. Most states have established an oral health plan, whether as a part of the state's direct dental public health activities, or as a part of a larger health plan (CDC, 2011). Such plans are usually developed and overseen by oral health directors or dental directors under the umbrella of state departments of (public) health. The range of services and activities provided under the auspices of state public health dentistry, vary considerably, however, and range from assessment (e.g., gathering oral health data through surveillance activities), to policy development (e.g., related to access), to assurance (e.g., providing clinical preventive and treatment services, supporting community-level water fluoridation) (ASTDD, 2011b).

Oral health data gathered through state and local public health dental programs allow state and federal agencies to identify trends in oral diseases (e.g., dental caries) and oral health professional shortage areas, and provide the basis for future planning. State-level dental public health programs provide both population and individual-level preventive, promotive, and restorative care. State public health dental programs, through county and city health departments, also provide fluoride varnish, mouth rinse, and fluoride tablets (ASTDD, 2011b).

INTERPROFESSIONAL TEAM CARE

In 2001, the ADA stated, "A formal dialogue among all health care professions should be established to develop a plan for greater cooperation and integration of knowledge in medical and dental predoctoral education, hospital settings, continuing education programs, and research facilities" (ADA, 2001). The importance of interaction between dentists and other health care professionals is a not new finding. In 1917, Sidney J. Rauh, Chairman of the Oral Hygiene Committee of the Ohio State Dental Society, noted,

> It has been found imperative that physicians and surgeons possess at least a theoretical knowledge of disease-breeding conditions met with in the teeth and jaws, but it is even more important for the dentist to appreciate the close relationship between his profession and that of the physician, surgeon, bacteriologist, chemist, and public health official. (Rauh, 1917)

Still, health care professionals are typically trained separately by discipline. As a result, professionals may gain little understanding of or appreciation for the expertise of other professionals or the skills needed to effectively participate on a team, including how and when to refer patients to each other and how to best communicate with each other. The value of interprofessional care, especially to care for patients with complex care needs, and the importance of interprofessional education and training have been increasingly acknowledged in recent years (Baum and Axtell, 2005; Blue et al., 2010; Buelow et al., 2008; Dodds et al., 2010; Dyer, 2003; Fulmer et al., 2005; Hall and Weaver, 2001; Howe and Sherman, 2006; Lerner et al., 2009; Misra et al., 2009; O'Leary et al., 2010; Wilder et al., 2008; Williams et al., 2006). In particular, evidence is growing that interprofessional care leads to better care coordination, communication, and, ultimately, better patient outcomes, improved satisfaction, and cost savings (Hammick et al., 2007; HHS, 2010; McKinnon and Jorgenson, 2009; Reeves et al., 2008, 2010; Snyder et al., 2010). The AAP policy statement on the role of pediatricians in prevention calls for collaboration between primary care pediatricians and local dentists in order to establish a dental home (AAP, 2008). The newly formed Center for Medicare and Medicaid Innovation has several projects looking at the effectiveness of team care (Carey, 2010). (See Chapter 4 for more on the center.) While more professionals are gaining experience in interprofessional training, little evidence exists to determine which methods are best for imparting the knowledge and skills necessary to work as a team member, how such training affects patterns of practice, or how it affects patient outcomes (Cooper et al., 2001; Hall and Weaver, 2001; Remington et al., 2006; Thistlethwaite and Moran, 2010).

For oral health care, two levels of team care may exist—first among dental professionals and second among various health care professionals. As will be discussed in Chapter 4, the federal government has a history of training dental professionals to work together more effectively. More research will be needed for understanding the dynamics of the dental team as new types of dental professionals emerge. In addition, little research exists on the interprofessional education and training of dental professionals and nondental professionals together in caring for mutual patients who have complex oral health needs (Haden et al., 2010; Hallas and Shelley, 2009; Wilder et al., 2008). In 2005, New York University created a unique partnership in which a college of nursing was located within the college of dentistry. As part of the interdisciplinary educational model, pediatric nurse practitioner students work alongside dental students to provide care in school clinics and Head Start programs (Garcia et al., 2010; Hallas and Shelley, 2009). This allows the pediatric nurse practitioner students to learn about caries risk assessment and how to apply fluoride varnish while the dental students can become more familiar with the role of the nurse in oral health.

In January 2010, the Advisory Committee on Training in Primary Care Medicine and Dentistry recommended that "training grants should provide funds to develop, implement, and evaluate training programs that promote interprofessional practice in the patient-centered medical-dental home model of care" (HHS, 2010). They also stated that "funding should support clinical sites that prepare trainees for interprofessional practice by educating medical, dental, physician assistant, and other trainees together on health care teams."

REGULATING THE ORAL HEALTH WORKFORCE

Regulation of the health care workforce in general occurs at several levels. The primary role of the federal government is to protect consumers and promote fair competition. The state has a legitimate interest in protecting the public as well, and each state develops their own scope of practice law for each health care profession that covers such things as who may enter a profession, what types of minimal competency requirements must be satisfied for licensure, and what services they may provide. Finally, the private sector is involved in the regulation of the health care workforce in that they often offer voluntary credentialing; sometimes these types of credentials are required for licensure. For professions and occupations without licensure requirements, credentialing may be one source of information for consumers. HHS has virtually no role in the regulation of health care professions, so this discussion is to provide an overview of the issues as they relate to the overall oral health care system.

The Role of the Federal Government

The Federal Trade Commission (FTC) is charged by Congress with preventing "unfair methods of competition in or affecting commerce, and unfair or deceptive acts or practices in or affecting commerce,"[13] including the enforcement of antitrust laws and other basic consumer protection laws. Both the FTC and the Department of Justice advocate against the acts of professions that limit or prevent competition for the delivery of health care services by another profession (e.g., scope of practice laws or licensure restrictions) without providing counterveiling consumer benefit (Chiarello, 2009). In recent years, the FTC has been involved in two notable cases directly related to oral health. Beginning in 2003, the FTC intervened when the South Carolina Board of Dentistry amended state practice acts to override legislation that expanded the scope of practice of hygienists to allow preventive services to be provided in school settings without the direct presence of a dentist (FTC, 2004, 2010). More recently, the FTC became involved in actions surrounding a 2009 state bill (HB 687) supported by the Louisiana Dental Association to make it illegal for *anyone* to provide school-based oral health care for a fee (FTC, 2009; Moller, 2010). In both cases, the FTC said that the actions restricted care to underserved populations without evidence of counterveiling benefit.

The Role of States

While the education, training, and testing of most health care professionals and the accreditation of educational programs have national standards, the scope of practice for individual professions is established at the state level, often resulting in wide variability among states. As was briefly discussed earlier in this chapter, professional battles and controversy over expanding a profession's scope of practice are not new to the health care professions or unique to oral health care (Carson-Smith and Minarik, 2007; Daly, 2006; Dulisse and Cromwell, 2010; Huijbregts, 2007; RCHWS, 2003; Wing et al., 2004). Several previous IOM reports have supported the idea of expanding scope of practice in alignment with professional competencies (IOM, 2008, 2010).

State health professions' licensing boards tend to have an overrepresentation of the profession they are regulating (Dower, 2009; IOM, 1989). This is especially relevant in the dental professions, since boards of dentistry regulate the dental hygiene profession. When one class of professionals is regulated by a different group of professionals, practice may be restricted and it is often difficult to effect change in scope of practice (FTC and

---

[13] 15 U.S.C. §45.

DOJ, 2004; Nolan et al., 2003). Variations in permissible practice among the states are broad, especially for dental hygienists and dental assistants (ADAA/DANB Alliance, 2005; HRSA, 2004). As in medicine where physicians are given significant latitude to delegate to other health professions, in dentistry, dentists are provided with autonomy to delegate at their professional discretion. While part of the purpose of restricting scope of practice is to protect consumers from unsafe or untrained providers, some data suggest that overly restrictive licensure laws in oral health are not tied to better health outcomes; in fact, stringent laws have been tied to increased consumer costs, (IOM, 1989; Kleiner and Kudrle, 2000; Shepard, 1978).

The Role of the Private Sector

Certification is a process by which a private organization imposes a certain level of standards, either through testing or some other method, in order to become "certified." Certification is often used as a measure of competence, especially in professions which do not have a formal licensure. The Dental Assisting National Board estimates that almost 12 percent of dental assistants in the United States are certified dental assistants (CDAs) by the Dental Assisting National Board (ADAA/DANB Alliance, 2005). As of 2011, 29 states recognize or require CDA certification to perform expanded duties, and a total of 38 states plus the District of Columbia recognize or require one or more of the components of the full CDA exam for particular expanded functions (e.g., Radiation Health and Safety Exam, Infection Control Exam) (DANB, 2011).

Dental technicians can voluntarily become certified dental technicians (CDTs) by the National Board for Certification in Dental Laboratory Technology, an independent board established by the National Association of Dental Laboratories (BLS, 2010g). Certification can occur in crowns and bridges, ceramics, partial dentures, complete dentures, and orthodontic appliances. Three states (Kentucky, South Carolina, and Texas) require dental laboratories to employ at least one CDT, and in Florida dental laboratories must register with the state, and at least one technician must meet requirements for continuing education (18 hours every 2 years) (BLS, 2010g).

ORAL HEALTH AND QUALITY MEASUREMENT

Despite the current interest in the quality of health care, little is known about the quality of oral health care provided in this country. Measurement and assessment of the quality of oral health care lag far behind similar work in the rest of health care (Stanton and Rutherford, 2003). For decades, significant research, resources, and expert opinion has focused on the quality and safety problems in health care, but oral health has largely been left out of these discussions. In 1998, then President Clinton's Advisory Commission on Consumer Protection and Quality in the Health Care Industry (1998) found that "[a] key element of improving health care quality is the nation's ability to measure the quality and provide easily understood, comparable information on the performance of the industry." The National Quality Forum, a consensus-based entity responsible for endorsing quality measures, was formed as a result of that commission's recommendations. In 2001, the IOM called for increasing national attention to the quality problems in American health care in *Crossing the Quality Chasm* (IOM, 2001). That report specifically highlighted the urgent need for more and better measures and other information about performance. It recommended that the field make that information widely and publicly available so the public and health professionals would have the necessary information to make informed health and health care decisions. In 2006, the IOM issued a related report, *Performance Measures: Accelerating Improvement,* that observed that measuring performance in health care is a critical step toward understanding and resolving health care quality problems (IOM, 2006). It also noted that "[t]here are many obstacles to rapid progress in improving the quality of health care, but none exceeds the fact that the nation still lacks a coherent, goal-oriented, consistent, and efficient system for assessing and reporting on the performance of the health care system." Further, the report warned that "[f]ailure to establish a well-functioning national performance measurement and reporting system would severely compromise our ability to achieve the essential quality improvements called for in the *Quality Chasm* report."

Efforts to develop, endorse, and implement a range of measures to understand the six aims of quality developed in the *Crossing the Quality Chasm* report (safety, timeliness, equity, effectiveness, efficiency, and patient-centeredness) are ongoing. The health care field has made some significant progress in the effort to measure health care quality (IOM, 2006). However, as the 2006 IOM report found, many significant gaps in health care quality measurement remain, particularly pertaining to measures of equity, efficiency, and patient centeredness. One ongoing significant challenge for health care quality measurement has been developing and implementing measures of significant outcomes relevant to patients. Cost metrics have also been challenging to develop and implement. Further creation of measures of outcomes and cost across the continuum of patient care or episode of care remain a challenge. The ACA directed the Centers for Medicare and Medicaid Services (CMS) to promote the development of these sorts of episode measures for health care, but that work is ongoing.

Arguably, none of this vast and expanding effort specifically includes attention to oral health care or measures of the quality (as defined by the six aims of quality) of oral health care. A quick review of measures currently endorsed by the National Quality Forum finds no measures related to oral health (NQF, 2010). Further, the most recent annual editions of the National Healthcare Quality Report and the National Healthcare Disparities Report only included information about access to dental services, and not about the state of quality in oral health care (AHRQ, 2010).

Current Oral Health Quality Measures

In oral health care, four types of quality measures are generally available: (1) measures of technical excellence, (2) patient satisfaction (as opposed to patient experience), (3) service use, and (4) structure and process measures (Bader, 2009a). The first type of measures, technical excellence in individual restorations, is not strongly associated with long-term outcomes or patient satisfaction (Bader, 2009a; Evans et al., 2005). The criteria for judgment of technical excellence tend to be subjective and therefore make standardization and comparison difficult. A second set of measures are measures of patient satisfaction. While many patient satisfaction instruments exist for oral health care, they tend to be short, are imprecise at determining the source of expressed dissatisfaction, and are also difficult to compare (Bader, 2009a). They also have not kept up with the movement in the broader health care field toward measuring a fuller range of patient experience.

Measures of service use, a third type of measures, may be used to answer specific access questions such as the proportion of a population that receives a dental service. These measures may also be used to evaluate adherence to evidence-based treatment guidelines; however, few guidelines exist, and the comparison of two practitioners is difficult because the service-use measures need to be risk- (and need-) adjusted for the possible differences in the patient populations being compared, but there are no well-accepted case mix adjustors in dentistry (Bader, 2009a).

The last group of measures in general use in private oral health care practice today includes some general structure and process measures (aside from service-use measures). Structural measures include evaluations of facilities, equipment, and personnel administration. While these are considered to reflect good practice and may have some basis in regulation (e.g., shielding around X-ray equipment), very little evidence supports their relative importance to specific treatment outcomes other than protection of patient health (Bader, 2009a). Process measures include assessment of such functions as infection control, imaging, diagnosis, and treatment planning. Again, very little evidence supports the importance of these measures to the outcomes of care, but they are assumed to reflect good practice (Bader, 2009a).

Overall, quality assessment in dentistry today is relatively weak and does not assess either the appropriateness or the effectiveness of care. The only clinical outcome measure is technical excellence, which focuses on the provider's intervention, not the patient's long-term outcome (Bader, 2009a). The only patient-oriented outcome measure is patient satisfaction, which is inherently flawed as a clinical evaluation tool. In addition, there is no single source of oversight or reporting on any measures that are currently in use.

Limitations to Expanding Quality Measurement in Oral Health Care

The construction of quality measures depends on robust, timely, accurate, and reliable data sources. In health care, for instance, those data sources in the past have largely depended on administrative claims data. There is great hope in the future for more and better health care clinical data for cost and quality measurement from electronic sources (DesRoches and Jha, 2009). There is significant activity under way in health care to increase the adoption of electronic health records and to promote the meaningful use of those electronic tools to enhance the collection of clinical data for performance measurement. All that work to gather clinical data electronically is an ongoing significant challenge in health care. It is, however, largely nascent in oral health care (Langabeer et al., 2008).

Quality measurement in oral health care will also depend on administrative claims sources, at least in part, and until there is broad adoption and meaningful use of electronic formats in oral health care. Unfortunately, oral health care has an additional technical challenge: the absence of a universally accepted and used diagnosis code among dentists (Bader, 2009a; Garcia et al., 2010). Several code sets are available for oral health, but they have not been put into general use. Oral diseases are included in the International Statistical Classification of Diseases and Related Health Problems (ICD) codes, which have been almost universally adopted in medicine. The ICD oral health codes have been criticized, however, because they are interspersed with medically oriented diseases, and they do not distinguish between primary and permanent teeth (Leake, 2002). The ADA has developed a comprehensive system of diagnosis codes, the Systematized Nomenclature of Dentistry (SNODENT), but it has yet to be released (Bader, 2009a). Several closed-panel delivery systems have also developed oral health code sets for use inside their systems, but they are not available to the general public (Bader, 2009a).

The development of new measures depends on evidence-based standards and guidelines from which to create metrics. Quality measurement in oral health is hampered by the absence of a strong evidence base for most oral health treatments and, therefore, a lack of evidence-based guidelines (Bader, 2009b). In fact, a significant percentage of Cochrane reviews in dentistry did not have enough evidence to answer the research question posed (Bader, 2009a,b). Dental research is challenged in part because with the typical small practice design, it can be difficult to obtain outcomes data due to the need to gather data from multiple practices as well as the variety of forms that are used to collect the same data. The practice design also makes it difficult to disseminate evidence when it exists; most dentists work alone, so information sharing is limited, and few have chairside access to journals or computers (Bader, 2009b).

Future Directions for Quality Measurement in Oral Health Care

Quality improvement in oral health is hampered by an insufficient evidence base for interventions, insufficient data sources, and a lack of quality measures. Based on and building from the logic of the extensive past work on quality and quality measurement by the IOM and many others in overall health care, HHS and others need to prioritize developing quality assessment in oral health. Oral health care needs better measures to understand the state of quality in oral health care, identify quality and disparities problems, and begin to develop appropriate solutions to address those problems. One of the first steps is promoting the development of measures of the quality of oral health care. Ideally, the effort to build oral health care measures could learn from and perhaps build upon the existing health care measurement enterprise.

In 2008, CMS called upon the ADA to take the lead in developing performance measures to assess the quality of dental care being provided to children across the country. The project, known as the Dental Quality Alliance (DQA), began with its first meeting in late 2010 and was scheduled to begin measures development in early 2011 (Rich, 2010). The mission of the DQA is "to advance performance measurement as a means to improve oral health, patient care, and safety through a consensus-building process" (Rich, 2010). The DQA will identify and develop evidence-based oral health care performance measures, advance the effectiveness and scientific basis of clinical performance measurement, and seek to foster greater professional accountability, transparency, and value in oral health care (Rich, 2010).

Beyond basic quality measurement, the development of better measures for the quality of oral health care is needed to perform comparative effectiveness research for many oral health interventions. For example, in 2009, the IOM produced a study that identified the 100 priority topics for comparative effectiveness research in all of health care. Two of the topics were related to oral health:

- ORAL-A: Compare the clinical and cost-effectiveness of surgical care and a medical model of prevention and care in managing periodontal disease to increase tooth longevity and reduce systemic secondary effects in other organ systems, and

- ORAL-B: Compare the effectiveness of the various delivery models (e.g., primary care, dental offices, schools, mobile vans) in preventing dental caries in children (IOM, 2009).

The committee concluded that much more needs to be done to improve the quality assessment and improvement efforts in oral health to answer some of the basic questions regarding improving oral health and oral health access.

KEY FINDINGS AND CONCLUSIONS

The committee noted the following key findings and conclusions:

Sites of Care

- Oral health is provided in two separate systems—private offices and the safety net—neither of which function adequately for vulnerable populations.

Financing Oral Health Care

- Out-of-pocket payments account for 44 percent of dental expenditures, and dental services account for 22 percent of all out-of-pocket health care expenditures.
- High out-of-pocket costs, lack of dental coverage, and limited financial means create barriers to receiving oral health care.
- Ideally, dental coverage would be included as part of health care coverage, but the cost of doing so makes this potential merger extraordinarily challenging.
- More research is needed on the economic and social impacts of increasing coverage (both in terms of numbers of individuals as well as the breadth of services).
- More research is needed on how different financing systems and the incentives therein might affect care delivery, including provider participation, cost-effectiveness, and efficiency.

Workforce

- Health care professionals from underrepresented minority groups often account for a disproportionate share of care for patients from those same populations.

- Although it is improving slowly, the racial and ethnic profile of the dental workforce does not reflect the population as a whole.
- Several models of new and emerging dental professionals have been developed, but little research exists on which type has the most promise to improve access or how they can best be integrated into the workforce and targeted to vulnerable populations.
- Interprofessional, team-based care has the potential to improve care-cooridination, patient outcomes, and produce cost savings, yet most health care professionals are not trained to work in either intra- or interdisciplinary teams.
- While the regulation of health care professions occurs at the state level, HHS has a role to play in the demonstration and testing of new workforce models.

Education and Training

- Many nondental health care professionals are well suited and willing to integrate oral health care into the primary care setting, but they are not trained to do so.
- Nondental health care professionals have a significant role to play in oral health promotion and disease prevention, especially for children. Key modalities include basic examinations and risk assessments, patient and caregiver counseling, and the application of topical fluorides.

Quality

- In general, dentists do not use a universally accepted diagnosis coding system.
- Oral health lags significantly behind the remainder of the health care system in developing quality measures, and as a result, little is known about the quality of oral health care.
- Much more needs to be done to improve the quality assessment, improvement, and reporting efforts in oral health in order to answer some of the basic questions regarding improving oral health and oral health access.

REFERENCES

AAMC (Association of American Medical Colleges). 2008. *Contemporary issues in medicine: Oral health education for medical and dental students.* Washington, DC: American Association of Medical Colleges.

AAMC. 2011. *Cost of a medical education.* https://www.aamc.org/students/considering/financing/ (accessed February 23, 2011).

AANA (American Association of Nurse Anesthetists). 2011. *AANA overview.* http://www.aana.com/aboutaana.aspx?id=100&linkidentifier=id&itemid=100 (accessed February 26, 2011).

AAP (American Academy of Pediatrics). 2008. Policy statement: Preventive oral health intervention for pediatricians. *Pediatrics* 122(6):1387-1394.

AAP. 2010. *Fluoride information by state.* http://www.aap.org/commpeds/dochs/oralhealth/fluoride.cfm (accessed February 25, 2011).

AAP. 2011a. *Bright futures: History.* http://brightfutures.aap.org/history.html (accessed February 26, 2011).

AAP. 2011b. *Oral health risk assessment: Training for pediatricians and other child health professionals.* http://www.aap.org/oralhealth/cme/page46.htm (accessed February 25, 2011).

AAP. 2011c. *Protecting all children's teeth: A pediatric oral health training program.* http://www.aap.org/oralhealth/pact/index.cfm (accessed January 6, 2011).

AAPHD (American Association of Public Health Dentistry). 2004. *History of the American Association of Public Health Dentistry.* http://www.aaphd.org/default.asp?page=history.htm (accessed February 22, 2011).

ABP (American Board of Pediatrics). 2009. *General pediatrics certification examination: Content outline.* Chapel Hill, NC: American Board of Pediatrics.

ACGME (Accreditation Council for Graduate Medical Education). 2007. *ACGME program requirements for graduate medical education in family medicine.* Chicago, IL: Accreditation Council for Graduate Medical Education.

ACGME. 2008. *ACGME program requirements for graduate medical education in sleep medicine.* Chicago, IL: Accreditation Council for Graduate Medical Education.

ACGME. 2009a. *ACGME program requirements for graduate medical education in geriatric medicine.* Chicago, IL: Accreditation Council for Graduate Medical Education.

ACGME. 2009b. *ACGME program requirements for graduate medical education in internal medicine.* Chicago, IL: Accreditation Council for Graduate Medical Education.

Ackermann, R. J., and K. A. Kemle. 1998. The effect of a physician assistant on the hospitalization of nursing home residents. *Journal of the American Geriatrics Society* 46(5):610-614.

ADA (American Dental Association). 1998. *1996 dentist profile survey.* Chilcago, IL: American Dental Association.

ADA. 2001. *Future of dentistry.* Chicago, IL: American Dental Association.

ADA. 2007. *American Indian and Alaska Native oral health access summit: Summary report.* Santa Ana Pueblo, NM: American Dental Association.

ADA. 2009a. *2008-09 survey of allied dental education.* Chicago, IL: American Dental Association.

ADA. 2009b. *2008 survey of dental practice: Characteristics of dentists in private practice and their patients.* Chicago, IL: American Dental Association.

ADA. 2009c. *2008 survey of dental practice: Income from the private practice of dentistry.* Chicago, IL: American Dental Association.

ADA. 2009d. *Distribution of dentists in the United States by region and state, 2007.* Chicago, IL: American Dental Association.

ADA. 2010a. *2008-09 survey of dental education: Academic programs, enrollment, and graduates—volume 1.* Chicago, IL: American Dental Association.

ADA. 2010b. *2008-2009 survey of advanced dental education.* Chicago, IL: American Dental Association.

ADA. 2011a. *Ninth GKAS Day a Success.* http://www.ada.org/news/5416.aspx (accessed February 21, 2011).

ADA. 2011b. *Students drive diversity initiatives.* http://www.ada.org/news/5408.aspx (accessed August 30, 2011).

ADAA (American Dental Assistants Association)/DANB (Dental Assisting National Board) Alliance. 2005. *Addressing a uniform national model for the dental assisting profession.* Chicago, IL: Dental Assisting National Board.

ADHA (American Dental Hygienists' Association). 2006. *Dental hygiene education program director survey.* Chicago, IL: American Dental Hygienists' Association.

ADHA. 2009a. *2009 dental hygiene job market & employment survey.* http://www.adha.org/downloads/Job_employment_survey_2009_exec_sum.pdf (accessed November 30, 2010).

ADHA. 2009b. *Survey of dental hygienists in the United States: 2007.* Chicago, IL: American Dental Hygienists' Association.

ADHA. 2010. *Frequently asked questions.* http://www.adha.org/faqs/index.html (accessed November 23, 2010).

AGD (Academy of General Dentistry). 2008. *White paper on increasing access to and utilization of oral health care services.* Chicago, IL: Academy of General Dentistry.

AHRQ (Agency for Healthcare Research and Quality). 2010. *National healthcare quality & disparities reports: NHQRDRnet.* http://nhqrnet.ahrq.gov/nhqrdr/jsp/nhqrdr.jsp (accessed November 29, 2010).

Allison, R. A., and R. J. Manski. 2007. The supply of dentists and access to care in rural Kansas. *Journal of Rural Health* 23(3):198-206.

AMA (American Medical Association). 2011. *Medical student debt.* http://www.ama-assn.org/ama/pub/about-ama/our-people/member-groups-sections/medical-student-section/advocacy-policy/medical-student-debt.shtml (accessed January 5, 2011).

Ambrose, E. R., A. B. Hord, and W. J. Simpson. 1976. *A quality evaluation of specific dental services provided by the Saskatchewan dental plan: Final report:* Regina, Saskatchewan: Saskatchewan Dental Plan.

ANA (American Nurses Association). 2011a. *More about RNs and advance practice RNs.* http://www.nursingworld.org/EspeciallyForYou/StudentNurses/RNsAPNs.aspx (accessed September 1, 2011).

ANA. 2011b. *Who we are.* http://nursingworld.org/FunctionalMenuCategories/AboutANA/WhoWeAre.aspx (accessed February 21, 2011).

Andersen, R. M., P. L. Davidson, K. A. Atchison, E. Hewlett, J. R. Freed, J. A. Friedman, A. Thind, J. J. Gutierrez, T. T. Nakazono, and D. C. Carreon. 2005. Pipeline, profession, and practice program: Evaluating change in dental education. *Journal of Dental Education* 69(2):239-248.

Andersen, R. M., D. C. Carreon, P. L. Davidson, T. T. Nakazono, S. Shahedi, and J. J. Gutierrez. 2010. Who will serve? Assessing recruitment of underrepresented minority and low-income dental students to increase access to dental care. *Journal of Dental Education* 74(6):579-592.

ARC-PA (Accreditation Review Commission on Education for the Physician Assistant). 2010. *Accreditation standards for physician assistant education,* 4th ed. Johns Creek, GA: Accreditation Review Commission on Education for the Physician Assistant.

ASTDD (Association of State and Territorial Dental Directors). 2007. *Fluoride varnish: An evidence-based approach.* http://www.astdd.org/docs/Sept2007FINALFlvarnishpaper.pdf (accessed February 26, 2011).

ASTDD. 2011a. *About ASTDD.* http://www.astdd.org/about-us/ (accessed March 12, 2011).

ASTDD. 2011b. *State & territorial dental public health activities: A collection of descriptive summaries.* http://www.astdd.org/state-activities/ (accessed August 1, 2011).

ASTDD. 2011c. *Synopses of state dental public health programs: Data for FY 2009-2010.* http://www.astdd.org/docs/State_Synopsis_Report_SUMMARY_2011.pdf (accessed August 1, 2011).

Atchison, K. A., and M. H. Schoen. 1990. A comparison of quality in a dual-choice dental plan: Capitation versus fee-for-service. *Journal of Public Health Dentistry* 50(3):186-193.

Awé, C., and J. Bauman. 2010. Theoretical and conceptual framework for a high school pathway to pharmacy program. *American Journal of Pharmaceutical Education* 74(8): Article 149.

Bader, J. D. 2009a. Challenges in quality assessment of dental care. *Journal of the American Dental Association* 140(12):1456-1464.

Bader, J. D. 2009b. Stumbling into the age of evidence. *Dental Clinics of North America* 53(1):15-22.

Bailit, H., and T. Beazoglou. 2008. Financing dental care: Trends in public and private expenditures for dental services. *Dental Clinics of North America* 52(2):281-295.

Bailit, H., T. Beazoglou, N. Demby, J. McFarland, P. Robinson, and R. Weaver. 2006. Dental safety net: Current capacity and potential for expansion. *Journal of the American Dental Association* 137(6):807-815.

Barsky, C. B. 2004. Incidence benefits measures in the national compensation survey. *Monthly Labor Review* 127(8):21-28.

Baum, K. D., and S. Axtell. 2005. Trends in north american medical education. *Keio Journal of Medicine* 54(1):22-28.

Berg, P., and D. Coniglio. 2006. Oral health in children: Overlooked and undertreated. *Journal of the American Academy of Physician Assistants* 19(4):40.

Bloom, B., and R. A. Cohen. 2010. *Dental insurance for persons under age 65 years with private health insurance: United States, 2008.* Hyattsville, MD: National Center for Health Statistics.

BLS (Bureau of Labor Statistics). 2009a. *Occupational outlook handbook, 2010-11 edition, pharmacists.* http://www.bls.gov/oco/ocos079.htm (accessed December 28, 2010).

BLS. 2009b. *Occupational outlook handbook, 2010-11 edition, physician assistants.* http://www.bls.gov/oco/ocos081.htm (accessed December 28, 2010).

BLS. 2010a. *Consumer out-of-pocket health care expenditures in 2008.* http://www.bls.gov/opub/ted/2010/ted_20100325_data.htm (accessed January 9, 2011).

BLS. 2010b. *Employee benefits survey: Health care benefits, March 2010.* http://www.bls.gov/ncs/ebs/benefits/2010/benefits_health.htm (accessed December 28, 2010).

BLS. 2010c. *Employment projections: Fastest growing occupations.* http://www.bls.gov/emp/ep_table_103.htm (accessed December 28, 2010).

BLS. 2010d. *Occupational outlook handbook 2010-11 edition, dental assistants.* http://www.bls.gov/oco/ocos163.htm (accessed December 28, 2010).

BLS. 2010e. *Occupational outlook handbook, 2010-11 edition, dental hygienists.* http://www.bls.gov/oco/ocos097.htm (accessed December 28, 2010).

BLS. 2010f. *Occupational outlook handbook, 2010-11 edition, dentists.* http://www.bls.gov/oco/ocos072.htm (accessed January 5, 2011).

BLS. 2010g. *Occupational outlook handbook, 2010-11 edition, medical, dental, and ophthalmic laboratory technicians.* http://www.bls.gov/oco/ocos238.htm (accessed January 6, 2011).

Blue, A., B. F. Brandt, and M. H. Schmitt. 2010. American interprofessional health collaborative: Historical roots and organizational beginnings. *Journal of Allied Health* 39(Supp. 1):204-209.

Bolin, K. A. 2008. Assessment of treatment provided by dental health aide therapists in Alaska. *Journal of the American Dental Association* 139(11):1530-1535.

Borchgrevink, A., A. Snyder, and S. Gehshan. 2008. *The effects of Medicaid reimbursement rates on access to dental care.* Washington, DC: National Academy for State Health Policy.

Brach, C., E. M. Lewit, K. VanLandeghem, J. Bronstein, A. W. Dick, K. S. Kimminau, B. LaClair, E. Shenkman, L. P. Shone, N. Swigonski, and P. G. Szilagyi. 2003. Who's enrolled in the state children's health insurance program (SCHIP)? An overview of findings from the child health insurance research initiative (CHIRI). *Pediatrics* 112(6 Supp. 2): e499-e507.

Brooks, E. S., T. C. Gravely, S. A. Hornback, L. C. Cunningham, A. L. McCann, and J. L. Long. 2002. Bridge to dentistry: One dental school's approach to improving its enrollment of underrepresented minorities. *Journal of the American College of Dentists* 69(1):23-30.

Brown, E., and R. J. Manski. 2004. *Dental services: Use, expenses, and sources of payment, 1996-2000.* Rockville, MD: Agency for Healthcare Research and Quality.

Brown, L. J. 2005. *Adequacy of current and future dental workforce: Theory and analysis.* Chicago, IL: American Dental Association.

Brown, L. J., K. S. Wagner, and B. Johns. 2000. Racial/ethnic variations of practicing dentists. *Journal of the American Dental Association* 131(12):1750-1754.

Brugna, R. A., J. F. Cawley, and M. D. Baker. 2007. Physician assistants in geriatric medicine. *Clinical Geriatrics* 15(10):22-29.

Brunson, W. D., D. L. Jackson, J. C. Sinkford, and R. W. Valachovic. 2010. Components of effective outreach and recruitment programs for underrepresented minority and low-income dental students. *Journal of Dental Education* 74(10 Supp.):S74-S86.

Budzi, D., S. Lurie, K. Singh, and R. Hooker. 2010. Veterans' perceptions of care by nurse practitioners, physician assistants, and physicians: A comparison from satisfaction surveys. *Journal of the American Academy of Nurse Practitioners* 22(3):170-176.

Buelow, J. R., C. Rathsack, D. Downs, K. Jorgensen, J. R. Karges, and D. Nelson. 2008. Building interdisciplinary teamwork among allied health students through live clinical case simulations. *Journal of Allied Health* 37(2):e109-e123.

Cantor, J. C., L. Bergeisen, and L. C. Baker. 1998. Effect of an intensive educational program for minority college students and recent graduates on the probability of acceptance to medical school. *Journal of the American Medical Association* 280(9):772-776.

Cantrell, C. 2008. *The role of physicians in children's oral health.* Portland, ME: National Association for State Health Policy.

Cantrell, C. 2009. *Engaging primary care medical providers in children's oral health.* Portland, ME: National Academy for State Health Policy.

Carey, M. A. 2010. *New Medicare/Medicaid projects aimed at cheaper, better care.* http://www.kaiserhealthnews.org/Stories/2010/November/17/cms-innovation-center-berwick.aspx (accessed January 9, 2011).

Carson-Smith, W. Y., and P. A. Minarik. 2007. Advanced practice nurses: A new skirmish in the continuing battle over scope of practice. *Clinical Nurse Specialist* 21(1):52-54.

Caspary, G., D. M. Krol, S. Boulter, M. A. Keels, and G. R.C. 2008. Perceptions of oral health training and attitudes toward performing oral health screenings among graduating pediatric residents. *Pediatrics* 122(2):e465-e471.

CDC (Centers for Disease Control and Prevention). 2009. *Lack of health insurance and type of coverage.* http://www.cdc.gov/nchs/data/nhis/earlyrelease/200906_01.pdf (accessed August 19, 2010).

CDC. 2011. *State oral health plans.* http://www.cdc.gov/OralHealth/state_programs/OH_plans/index.htm (accessed September 8, 2011).

Chalmers, J. M. 1996. Factors influencing nurses' aides' provision of oral care for nursing facility residents. *Special Care in Dentistry* 16(2):71-79.

Chiarello, G. P. 2009. *Regulating the professions: The intersection of competition and consumer protection policies.* Paper presented at the IOM workshop The U.S. Oral Health Workforce in the Coming Decade, Washington, DC.

Chmar, J. E., R. G. Weaver, and R. W. Valachovic. 2008. Dental school vacant budgeted faculty positions, academic years 2005-06 and 2006-07. *Journal of Dental Education* 72(3):370-385.

Chu, M., L. E. Sweis, A. H. Guay, and R. J. Manski. 2007. The dental care of U.S. children: Access, use and referrals by nondentist providers, 2003. *Journal of the American Dental Association* 138(10):1324-1331.

Clemmens, D. A., and A. R. Kerr. 2008. Improving oral health in women: Nurses' call to action. *MCN American Journal of Maternal/Child Nursing* 33(1):10-14.

Close, K., R. G. Rozier, L. P. Zeldin, and A. R. Gilbert. 2010. Barriers to the adoption and implementation of preventive dental services in primary medical care. *Pediatrics* 125(3):509-517.

CMS (Centers for Medicare and Medicaid Services). 2010a. *Medicare dental coverage: Overview*. http://www.cms.hhs.gov/MedicareDentalCoverage (accessed November 22, 2010).

CMS. 2010b. *MSIS tables: Details for 2008*. http://www.cms.gov/MedicaidDataSourcesGenInfo/MSIS/itemdetail.asp?filterType=dual, data2&filterValue=Medicaid Payments by Service Category&filterByDID=2&sortByDID=1&sortOrder=ascending&itemID=CMS1229918&intNumPerPage=10 (accessed February 23, 2011).

CMS. 2011a. *Medicaid dental coverage*. http://www.cms.gov/MedicaidDentalCoverage/ (accessed June 10, 2011).

CMS. 2011b. *National health expenditures accounts: Definitions, sources, and methods, 2009*. https://www.cms.gov/NationalHealthExpendData/downloads/dsm-09.pdf (accessed July 29, 2011).

CMS. 2011c. *National health expenditures by type of service and source of funds: CY 1960-2009*. http://www.cms.gov/NationalHealthExpendData/02_NationalHealthAccountsHistorical.asp (accessed June 14, 2011).

Cohen, D. W., P. P. Cormier, and J. L. Cohen. 1985. *Educating the dentist of the future: the Pennsylvania Experiment*. Philadelphia: University of Pennsylvania Press.

Cohen, L. A., A. J. Bonito, D. R. Akin, R. J. Manski, M. D. Macek, R. R. Edwards, and L. J. Cornelius. 2009. Role of pharmacists in consulting with the underserved regarding toothache pain. *Journal of the American Pharmacists Association: JAPhA* 49(1):38-42.

Coleman, P., and N. M. Watson. 2006. Oral care provided by certified nursing assistants in nursing homes. *Journal of the American Geriatrics Society* 54(1):138-143.

Cooper, H., C. Carlisle, T. Gibbs, and C. Watkins. 2001. Developing an evidence base for interdisciplinary learning: A systematic review. *Journal of Advanced Nursing* 35(2):228-237.

Daly, R. 2006. Physician coalition prepares for scope-of-practice battles. *Psychiatric News* 41(3):10.

Damiano, P. C., E. R. Brown, J. D. Johnson, and J. P. Scheetz. 1990. Factors affecting dentist participation in a state Medicaid program. *Journal of Dental Education* 54(11):638-643.

DANB (Dental Assisting National Board). 2007. *Dental assisting job titles in the U.S.* http://www.danb.org/PDFs/JobTitles.pdf (accessed February 23, 2011).

DANB. 2011. *2011 CDA exam application packet*. http://www.danb.org/PDFs/CDAApplication.pdf (accessed September 8, 2011).

Danielsen, R., J. Dillenberg, and C. Bay. 2006. Oral health competencies for physician assistants and nurse practitioners. *Journal of Physician Assistant Education* 17(4):12-16.

Dela Cruz, G. G., R. G. Rozier, and G. Slade. 2004. Dental screening and referral of young children by pediatric primary care providers. *Pediatrics* 114(5).

DENTEX. 2010. *Dental health aide training program*. http://depts.washington.edu/dentexak/mission.html (accessed September 19, 2011).

Department of Education. 2010. *College accreditation in the United States: Specialized accrediting agencies*. http://www2.ed.gov/admins/finaid/accred/accreditation_pg7.html#health (accessed December 22, 2010).

DesRoches, C. M., and A. Jha. 2009. *On the cusp of change: Health information technology in the United States, 2009.* Princeton, NJ: Robert Wood Johnson Foundation.

Dickinson, T. D. 2010. *The MOM experience: Pathways to collaboration and conversation.* Presentation at meeting of the Committee on Oral Health Access to Services, Washington, DC. March 4, 2010.

Dodds, J., W. Vann, J. Lee, A. Rosenberg, K. Rounds, M. Roth, M. Wells, E. Evens, and L. H. Margolis. 2010. The UNC-CH MCH leadership training consortium: Building the capacity to develop interdisciplinary MCH leaders. *Maternal and Child Health Journal* 14(4):642-648.

Douglass, A. B., M. Deutchman, J. Douglass, W. Gonsalves, R. Maier, H. Silk, J. Tysinger, and A. S. Wrightson. 2009a. Incorporation of a national oral health curriculum into family medicine residency programs. *Family Medicine* 41(3):159-160.

Douglass, A. B., J. M. Douglass, and D. M. Krol. 2009b. Educating pediatricians and family physicians in children's oral health. *Academic Pediatrics* 9(6):452-456.

Dower, C. 2009. Regulatory *challenges to improving oral health care in the U.S.* Presentation at the IOM workshop The U.S. Oral Health Workforce in the Coming Decade, Washington, DC. February 10, 2009.

Dulisse, B., and J. Cromwell. 2010. No harm found when nurse anesthetists work without supervision by physicians. *Health Affairs* 29(8):1469-1475.

Dunning, J. M. 1958. Extending the field for dental auxiliary personnel in the United States. *American Journal of Public Health* 48(8):1059-1064.

Dyer, J. A. 2003. Multidisciplinary, interdisciplinary, and transdisciplinary: Educational models and nursing education. *Nursing Education Perspectives* 24(4):186-188.

Edelstein, B. 2010a. The dental safety net, its workforce, and policy recommendations for its enhancement. *Journal of Public Health Dentistry* 70(Supp. 1):S32-S39.

Edelstein, B. 2010b. *Training new dental health providers in the U.S.* Battle Creek, MI: W.K. Kellogg Foundation.

Evans, A. W., R. M. A. Leeson, and A. Petrie. 2005. Correlation between a patient-centred outcome score and surgical skill in oral surgery. *British Journal of Oral and Maxillofacial Surgery* 43(6):505-510.

Fales, M. H. 1958. The potential role of the dental hygienist in public health programs. *American Journal of Public Health* 48(8):1054-1058.

Ferguson, D. A., B. J. Steinberg, and T. Schwien. 2010. Dental economics and the aging population. *Compendium of continuing education in dentistry* (Jamesburg, NJ : 1995) 31(6):418-420, 422, 424-425.

Ferullo, A., H. Silk, and J. A. Savageau. 2011. A national survey of oral health curriculum in all U.S. allopathic and osteopathic medical schools. *Academic Medicine* 86(2):252-825.

Fiset, L. 2005. *A report on quality assessment of primary care provided by dental therapists to Alaska natives.* Seattle, WA: University of Washington School of Dentistry.

Flores, G., and S. C. Tomany-Korman. 2008. The language spoken at home and disparities in medical and dental health, access to care, and use of services in U.S. children. *Pediatrics* 121(6):e1703-e1714.

Ford, J. L. 2009. *The new health participation and access data from the National Compensation Survey.* http://www.bls.gov/opub/cwc/cm20091022ar01p1.htm (accessed December 27, 2010).

Formicola, A. J., J. McIntosh, S. Marshall, D. Albert, D. Mitchell-Lewis, G. P. Zabos, and R. Garfield. 1999. Population-based primary care and dental education: A new role for dental schools. *Journal of Dental Education* 63(4):331-338.

Formicola, A J., H. Bailit, T. Beazoglou, and L. A. Tedesco. 2005. The Macy study: A framework for consensus. *Journal of Dental Education* 69(11): 1183-1185.

Formicola, A. J., R. Myers, J. F. Hasler, M. Peterson, W. Dodge, H. L. Bailit, T. Beazoglou, and L. A. Tedesco. 2006. Evolution of dental school clinics as patient care delivery centers. *Journal of Dental Education* 70(12):1271-1288.

Formicola, A. J., K. C. D'Abreu, and L. A. Tedesco. 2010. Underrepresented minority dental student recruitment and enrollment programs: An overview from the dental pipeline program. *Journal of Dental Education* 74(10 Supp.):S67-S73.

FTC (Federal Trade Commission). 2004. *Opinion and order of the commission: Docket no. 9311.* http://www.ftc.gov/os/adjpro/d9311/040728commissionopinion.pdf (accessed January 10, 2011).

FTC. 2009. *FTC staff comment before the Louisiana House of Representatives concerning Louisiana House Bill 687 on the practice of in-school dentistry.* http://www.ftc.gov/os/2009/05/V090009louisianahb687amendment.pdf (accessed September 8, 2011).

FTC. 2010. *Overview of FTC antitrust actions in health care services and products.* Washington, DC: Federal Trade Commission.

FTC and DOJ (Department of Justice). 2004. *Improving health care: A dose of competition.* Washington, DC: Federal Trade Commission and Department of Justice.

Fulmer, T., K. Hyer, E. Flaherty, M. Mezey, N. Whitelaw, M. Orry Jacobs, R. Luchi, J. C. Hansen, D. A. Evans, C. Cassel, E. Kotthoff-Burrell, R. Kane, and E. Pfeiffer. 2005. Geriatric interdisciplinary team training program: Evaluation results. *Journal of Aging and Health* 17(4):443-470.

Gallagher, J. L., and D. A. Wright. 2003. General dental practitioners' knowledge of and attitudes towards the employment of dental therapists in general practice. *British Dental Journal* 194(1):37-41.

GAO (Government Accountability Office). 2000. *Factors contributing to low use of dental services by low-income populations.* Washington, DC: U.S. General Accounting Office.

GAO. 2008. *Extent of dental disease in children has not decreased, and millions are estimated to have untreated tooth decay.* Washington, DC: U.S. Government Accountability Office.

GAO. 2010. *Efforts underway to improve children's access to dental services, but sustained attention needed to address ongoing concerns.* Washington, DC: U.S. Government Accountability Office.

Garcia, R. I., R. E. Inge, L. Niessen, and D. P. DePaola. 2010. Envisioning success: The future of the oral health care delivery system in the United States. *Journal of Public Health Dentistry* 70(Supp. 1):S58-S65.

GDA (Georgia Dental Association). 2010. *White paper on Georgia's oral health status, access to and utilization of oral health care services.* Atlanta, GA: Georgia Dental Association.

Gies, W. J. 1926. *Dental education in the United States and Canada.* New York: Carnegie Foundation for the Advancement of Teaching.

Greenberg, B. J. S., J. V. Kumar, and H. Stevenson. 2008. Dental case management: Increasing access to oral health care for families and children with low incomes. *Journal of the American Dental Association* 139(8):1114-1121.

Grumbach, K., and E. Chen. 2006. Effectiveness of University of California postbaccalaureate premedical programs in increasing medical school matriculation for minority and disadvantaged students. *Journal of the American Medical Association* 296(9):1079-1085.

Grumbach, K., L. G. Hart, E. Mertz, J. Coffman, and L. Palazzo. 2003. Who is caring for the underserved? A comparison of primary care physicians and nonphysician clinicians in California and Washington. *Annals of Family Medicine* 1(2):97-104.

Guay, A. H. 2005. Dental practice: Prices, production and profits. *Journal of the American Dental Association* 136(3):357-361.

Guthrie, D., R. W. Valachovic, and L. J. Brown. 2009. The impact of new dental schools on the dental workforce through 2022. *Journal of Dental Education* 73(12):1353-1360.

Haden, N. K., K. E. Morr, and R. W. Valachovic. 2001. Trends in allied dental education: An analysis of the past and a look to the future. *Journal of Dental Education* 65(5):480-495.

Haden, N. K., F. A. Catalanotto, C. J. Alexander, H. Bailit, A. Battrell, J. Broussard Jr., J. Buchanan, C. W. Douglass, C. E. Fox 3rd, P. Glassman, R. I. Lugo, M. George, C. Meyerowitz, E. R. Scott 2nd, N. Yaple, J. Bresch, Z. Gutman-Betts, G. G. Luke, M. Moss, J. C. Sinkford, R. G. Weaver, and R. W. Valachovic. 2003. Improving the oral health status of all Americans: Roles and responsibilities of academic dental institutions: The report of the ADEA President's Commission. *Journal of Dental Education* 67(5):563-583.

Haden, N. K., W. D. Hendricson, D. K. Kassebaum, R. R. Ranney, G. Weinstein, E. L. Anderson, and R. W. Valachovic. 2010. Curriculum change in dental education, 2003-09. *Journal of Dental Education* 74(5):539-557.

Hall, P., and L. Weaver. 2001. Interdisciplinary education and teamwork: A long and winding road. *Medical Education* 35(9):867-875.

Hallas, D., and D. Shelley. 2009. Role of pediatric nurse practitioners in oral health care. *Academic Pediatrics* 9(6):462-466.

Hammick, M., D. Freeth, I. Koppel, S. Reeves, and H. Barr. 2007. A best evidence systematic review of interprofessional education: BEME guide no. 9. *Medical Teacher* 29(8):735-751.

Hammons, P. E., and H. C. Jamison. 1967. Expanded functions for dental auxiliaries. *Journal of the American Dental Association* 75(3):658-672.

Hammons, P. E., and H. C. Jamison. 1968. New duties for dental auxiliaries—the Alabama experience. *American Journal of Public Health and the Nation's Health* 58(5):882-886.

Hammons, P. E., H. C. Jamison, and L. L. Wilson. 1971. Quality of service provided by dental therapists in an experimental program at the University of Alabama. *Journal of the American Dental Association* 82(5):1060-1066.

Harper, D. C., and J. Johnson. 1998. The new generation of nurse practitioners: Is more enough? *Health Affairs* 17(5):158-164.

Hart-Hester, S., and C. Thomas. 2003. Access to health care professionals in rural Mississippi. *Southern Medical Journal* 96(2):149-154.

Hesser, A., E. Pond, L. Lewis, and B. Abbot. 1996. Evaluation of a supplementary retention program for African-American baccalaureate nursing students. *Journal of Nursing Education* 35(7):304-309.

HHS (Department of Health and Human Services). 2000. *Oral health in America: A report of the surgeon general.* Rockville, MD: U.S. Department of Health and Human Services.

HHS. 2009. *Pipeline programs to improve racial and ethnic diversity in the health professions: An inventory of federal programs, assessment of evaluation approaches, and critical review of the research literature.* Rockville, MD: U.S. Department of Health and Human Services.

HHS. 2010. *Advisory committee on training in primary care medicine and dentistry: The redesign of primary care with implications for training.* Rockville, MD: U.S. Department of Health and Human Services.

Hooker, R. S., and L. E. Berlin. 2002. Trends in the supply of physician assistants and nurse practitioners in the United States. *Health Affairs* 21(5):174-181.

Hooker, R. S., D. J. Cipher, and E. Sekscenski. 2005. Patient satisfaction with physician assistant, nurse practitioner, and physician care: A national survey of Medicare beneficiaries. *Journal of Clinical Outcomes Management* 12(2):88-92.

Howe, J. L., and D. W. Sherman. 2006. Interdisciplinary educational approaches to promote team-based geriatrics and palliative care. *Gerontology and Geriatrics Education* 26(3):1-16.

HRSA (Health Resources and Services Administration). 2000. *The public health workforce: Enumeration 2000.* ftp://ftp.hrsa.gov//bhpr/nationalcenter/phworkforce2000.pdf (accessed February 22, 2011).

HRSA. 2004. *The professional practice environment of dental hygienists in the fifty states and the District of Columbia, 2001.* http://bhpr.hrsa.gov/healthworkforce/reports/hygienists/dh1.htm (accessed January 10, 2011).

HRSA. 2006. *The rationale for diversity in the health professions: A review of the evidence.* Rockville, MD: Department of Health and Human Services.

Huijbregts, P. A. 2007. Chiropractic legal challenges to the physical therapy scope of practice: Anybody else taking the ethical high ground? *Journal of Manual and Manipulative Therapy* 15(2):69-80.

IHS (Indian Health Service). 2011. Indian health manual, part 3, chapter 2, dental. http://www.ihs.gov/ihm/index.cfm?module=dsp_ihm_pc_p3c2 (accessed February 28, 2011).

IOM (Institute of Medicine). 1988. *The future of public health.* Washington, DC: National Academy Press.

IOM. 1989. *Allied health services: Avoiding crises.* Washington, DC: National Academy Press.

IOM. 1995. *Dental education at the crossroads: Challenges and change.* Washington, DC: National Academy Press.

IOM. 1996. *Primary care: America's health in a new era.* Washington, DC: National Academy Press.

IOM. 2001. *Crossing the quality chasm: A new health system for the 21st century.* Washington, DC: National Academy Press.

IOM. 2003. *Unequal treatment: Confronting racial and ethnic disparities in health care.* Washington, DC: The National Academies Press.

IOM. 2004. *In the nation's compelling interest: Ensuring diversity in the health-care workforce.* Washington, DC: The National Academies Press.

IOM. 2006. *Performance measures: Accelerating improvement.* Washington, DC: The National Academies Press.

IOM. 2008. *Retooling for an aging America.* Washington, DC: The National Academies Press.

IOM. 2009. *Initial national priorities for comparative effectiveness research.* Washington, DC: The National Academies Press.

IOM. 2010. *The future of nursing: Leading change, advancing health.* Washington, DC: The National Academies.

Isong, I. A., K. E. Zuckerman, S. R. Rao, K. A. Kuhlthau, J. P. Winickoff, and J. M. Perrin. 2010. Association between parents' and children's use of oral health services. *Pediatrics* 125(3):502-508.

Jablonski, R. 2010. *Nursing education and research (geriatrics).* Presentation at meeting of the Committee on an Oral Health Initiative, Washington, DC. June 28, 2010.

Jablonski, R. A., C. L. Munro, M. J. Grap, C. M. Schubert, M. Ligon, and P. Spigelmyer. 2009. Mouth care in nursing homes: Knowledge, beliefs, and practices of nursing assistants. *Geriatric Nursing* 30(2):99-107.

Jacques, P. F., C. Snow, M. Dowdle, N. Riley, K. Mao, and W. C. Gonsalves. 2010. Oral health curricula in physician assistant programs: A survey of physician assistant program directors. *Journal of Physician Assistant Education* 21(2):22-30.

Johnson, L., R. J. Genco, C. Damsky, N. K. Haden, S. Hart, T. C. Hart, C. F. Shuler, L. A. Tabak, and L. A. Tedesco. 2008. Genetics and its implications for clinical dental practice and education: Report of panel 3 of the Macy study. *Journal of Dental Education* 72(Supp. 2):86-94.

Jones, P. E., and J. F. Cawley. 1994. Physician assistants and health system reform: Clinical capabilities, practice activities, and potential roles. *Journal of the American Medical Association* 271(16):1266-1272.

KFF (Kaiser Family Foundation). 2011. *Health coverage of children: The role of Medicaid and CHIP.* http://www.kff.org/uninsured/upload/7698-05.pdf (accessed March 1, 2011).

Kim, M. J., K. Holm, P. Gerard, B. McElmurry, M. Foreman, S. Poslusny, and C. Dallas. 2009. Bridges to the doctorate: Mentored transition to successful completion of doctoral study for underrepresented minorities in nursing science. *Nursing Outlook* 57(3):166-171.

Kleiner, M. M., and R. T. Kudrle. 2000. Does regulation affect economic outcomes? The case of dentistry. *Journal of Law and Economics* 43(2):547-582.

Kressin, N., M. Nunn, H. Singh, M. Orner, L. Pbert, C. Hayes, C. Culler, S. Glicken, S. Palfrey, and P. Geltman. 2009. Pediatric clinicians can help reduce rates of early childhood caries: Effects of a practice-based intervention. *Medical Care* 47(11):1121-1128.

Krol, D. M. 2004. Educating pediatricians on children's oral health: Past, present, and future. *Pediatrics* 113(5):e487-e492.

Krol, D. M. 2010. Children's oral health and the role of the pediatrician. *Current Opinion in Pediatrics* 22(6):804-808.

Lamster, I. B., L. A. Tedesco, D. M. Fournier, J. M. Goodson, A. R. Gould, N. K. Haden, T. H. Howell, Jr., T. K. Schleyer, J. A. Ship, and D. T. W. Wong. 2008. New opportunities for dentistry in diagnosis and primary health care: Report of panel 1 of the Macy study. *Journal of Dental Education* 72(Supp. 2):66-72.

Lang, W. P., and J. A. Weintraub. 1986. Comparison of Medicaid and non-Medicaid dental providers. *Journal of Public Health Dentistry* 46(4):207-211.

Langabeer II, J. R., M. F. Walji, D. Taylor, and J. A. Valenza. 2008. Economic outcomes of a dental electronic patient record. *Journal of Dental Education* 72(10):1189-1200.

Lavizzo-Mourey, R. 2010. Foreword. *Journal of Dental Education* 74(Supp. 10):S7-S8.

Leake, J. 2002. Diagnostic codes in dentistry—Definition, utility and developments to date. *Journal-Canadian Dental Association* 68(7):403-407.

Lerner, S., D. Magrane, and E. Friedman. 2009. Teaching teamwork in medical education. *Mount Sinai Journal of Medicine* 76(4):318-329.

Leviton, L. C. 2009. Foreword. *Journal of Dental Education* 73(Supp. 2):S5-S7.

Lewis, C. L. 1996. A state university's model program to increase the number of its disadvantaged students who matriculate into health professions schools. *Academic Medicine* 71(10):1050-1057.

Lewis, C. W., D. C. Grossman, P. K. Domoto, and R. A. Deyo. 2000. The role of the pediatrician in the oral health of children: A national survey. *Pediatrics* 106(6):e84.

Liu, J., J. C. Probst, A. B. Martin, J.-Y. Wang, and C. F. Salinas. 2007. Disparities in dental insurance coverage and dental care among U.S. children: The National Survey of Children's Health. *Pediatrics* 119(Supp. 1):S12-S21.

Lobene, R. R., and A. Kerr. 1979. *The Forsyth experiment: An alternative system for dental care.* Cambridge, MA: Harvard University Press.

Luciano, W. J., L. G. Rothfuss, and A. S. v. Gonten. 2006. The expanded function dental assistant training program. Army Medical Department Journal January-March 2006:16-20.

MacDorman, M. F., and G. K. Singh. 1998. Midwifery care, social and medical risk factors, and birth outcomes in the USA. *Journal of Epidemiology and Community Health* 52(5):310-317.

Machen, J. B. 2008. Will we allow dentistry to be left behind? Principles underlying dental education and practice. *Journal of Dental Education* 72(2 Supp):10-13.

Macleod, I., G. Bell, and A. Lorimer. 2003. A role for pharmacists in cancer detection. *Pharmaceutical Journal* 270(7240):367.

Manski, R. J., and E. Brown. 2007. *Dental use, expenses, private dental coverage, and changes, 1996 and 2004.* Rockville, MD: Agency for Healthcare Research and Quality.

Manski, R. J., and P. F. Cooper. 2010. Characteristics of employers offering dental coverage in the United States. *Journal of the American Dental Association* 141(6):700-711.

Manski, R. J., J. Moeller, H. Chen, P. A. St. Clair, J. Schimmel, L. Magder, and J. V. Pepper. 2010a. Dental care expenditures and retirement. *Journal of Public Health Dentistry* 70(2):148-155.

Manski, R. J., J. Moeller, H. Chen, P. A. St. Clair, J. Schimmel, L. Magder, and J. V. Pepper. 2010b. Dental care utilization and retirement. *Journal of Public Health Dentistry* 70(1): 67-75.

Manski, R. J., J. Moeller, J. Schimmel, P. A. St. Clair, H. Chen, L. Magder, and J. V. Pepper. 2010c. Dental care coverage and retirement. *Journal of Public Health Dentistry* 70(1): 1-12.

Markel, G., M. Woolfolk, and M. R. Inglehart. 2008. Feeding the pipeline: Academic skills training for predental students. *Journal of Dental Education* 72(6):653-661.

Martin, A., D. Lassman, L. Whittle, A. Catlin, J. Benson, C. Cowan, B. Dickensheets, M. Hartman, P. McDonnell, O. Nuccio, and B. Washington. 2011. Recession contributes to slowest annual rate of increase in health spending in five decades. *Health Affairs* 30(1):11-20.

McDonough, D. 2007. *What's new in ADAA demographics*. http://findarticles.com/p/articles/mi_m0MKX/is_1_76/ai_n18645509/ (accessed March 9, 2011).

MCHB (Maternal and Child Health Bureau). 2011. *Bright Futures for Infants, Children, and Adolescents*. http://mchb.hrsa.gov/programs/training/brightfutures.htm (accessed March 1, 2011).

McKinnon, A., and D. Jorgenson. 2009. Pharmacist and physician collaborative prescribing: For medication renewals within a primary health centre. *Canadian Family Physician* 55(12):e86-e91.

McKnight-Hanes, C., D. R. Myers, and J. C. Dushku. 1992. Method of payment for children's dental services by practice type and geographic location. *Pediatric Dentistry* 14(5):338-341.

Mertz, E., and P. Glassman. 2011. Alternative practice dental hygiene in California: Past, present, and future. *CDA Journal* 39(1).

Mertz, E. A., and K. Grumbach. 2001. Identifying communities with low dentist supply in California. *Journal of Public Health Dentistry* 61(3):172-177.

Mezey, M., S. G. Burger, H. G. Bloom, A. Bonner, M. Bourbonniere, B. Bowers, J. B. Burl, E. Capezuti, D. Carter, J. Dimant, S. A. Jerro, S. C. Reinhard, and M. Ter Maat. 2005. Experts recommend strategies for strengthening the use of advanced practice nurses in nursing homes. *Journal of the American Geriatrics Society* 53(10):1790-1797.

Misra, S., R. H. Harvey, D. Stokols, K. H. Pine, J. Fuqua, S. M. Shokair, and J. M. Whiteley. 2009. Evaluating an interdisciplinary undergraduate training program in health promotion research. *American Journal of Preventive Medicine* 36(4):358-365.

Mitchell, D. A., and S. L. Lassiter. 2006. Addressing health care disparities and increasing workforce diversity: The next step for the dental, medical, and public health professions. *American Journal of Public Health* 96(12):2093-2097.

Moeller, J. F., H. Chen, and R. J. Manski. 2010. Investing in preventive dental care for the Medicare population: A preliminary analysis. *American Journal of Public Health* 100(11):2262-2269.

Moller, J. 2010. Mobile dental clinic rules endorsed by legislative committee. *Times-Picayune*, August 20. P. A02.

Mouradian, W. E. 2010. *Wanted . . . physicians who understand oral health*. Presentation at meeting of the Committee on an Oral Health Initiative, Washington, DC. June 28, 2010.

Mouradian, W. E., J. H. Berg, and M. J. Somerman. 2003. Addressing disparities through dental-medical collaborations, part 1. The role of cultural competency in health disparities: Training of primary care medical practitioners in children's oral health. *Journal of Dental Education* 67(8):860-868.

Mouradian, W. E., A. Reeves, S. Kim, R. Evans, D. Schaad, S. G. Marshall, and R. Slayton. 2005. An oral health curriculum for medical students at the University of Washington. *Academic Medicine* 80(5):434-442.

Mouradian, W. E., A. Reeves, S. Kim, C. Lewis, A. Keerbs, R. L. Slayton, D. Gupta, R. Oskouian, D. Schaad, and T. Kalet. 2006. A new oral health elective for medical students at the University of Washington. *Teaching and Learning in Medicine* 18(4):336-342.

Mouradian, W., C. N. Bertolami, L. Tedesco, C. Aschenbrener, S. J. Crandall, R. M. Epstein, M. Da Fonseca, N. K. Haden, A. Ruffin, J. J. Sciubba, S. Silverton, and R. P. Strauss. 2008. Curriculum and clinical training in oral health for physicians and dentists: Report of panel 2 of the Macy study. *Journal of Dental Education* 72(Supp. 2):73-85.

NADP (National Association of Dental Plans). 2009. *Dental benefits improve access to dental care.* http://www.nadp.org/Libraries/HCR_Documents/nadphcr-dentalbenefitsimprove accesstocare-3-28-09.sflb.ashx (accessed January 10, 2011).

Naegele, E. R., J. Cunha-Cruz, and P. Nadanovsky. 2010. Disparity between dental needs and dental treatment provided. *Journal of Dental Research* 89(9):975-979.

Nash, D. A. 2009. Adding dental therapists to the health care team to improve access to oral health care for children. *Academic Pediatrics* 9(6):446-451.

Nash, D. A., and R. J. Nagel. 2005a. A brief history and current status of a dental therapy initiative in the United States. *Journal of Dental Education* 69(8):857-859.

Nash, D. A., and R. J. Nagel. 2005b. Confronting oral health disparities among American Indian/Alaska Native children: The pediatric oral health therapist. *American Journal of Public Health* 95(8):1325-1329.

Nash, D. A., and W. R. Willard. 2010. On why the dental therapists' "movement" in the United States should focus on children—not adults. *Journal of Public Health Dentistry* 70(4):259-261.

Nash, D. A., J. W. Friedman, T. B. Kardos, R. L. Kardos, E. Schwarz, J. Satur, D. G. Berg, J. Nasruddin, E. G. Mumghamba, E. S. Davenport, and R. Nagel. 2008. Dental therapists: A global perspective. *International Dental Journal* 58(2):61-70.

National Task Force on Quality Nurse Practitioner Education. 2008. *Criteria for evaluation of nurse practitioner programs.* Washington, DC: National Organization of Nurse Practitioner Faculties.

NC Department of Health and Human Services. 2009. *2008-2009 annual report: North Carolina oral health section.* http://www.ncdhhs.gov/dph/oralhealth/library/includes/08-09%20OHS%20Annual%20Report.pdf (accessed February 26, 2011).

Neumann, L. M. 2004. Trends in dental and allied dental education. *Journal of the American Dental Association* 135(9):1253-1259.

Nolan, L., B. Kamoie, J. Harvey, L. Vaquerano, S. Blake, S. Chawla, J. Levi, and S. Rosenbaum. 2003. *The effects of state dental practice laws allowing alternative models of preventive oral health care delivery to low-income children.* Washington, DC: Center for Health Services Research and Policy, School of Public Health and Health Services, The George Washington University.

NQF (National Quality Forum). 2010. *NQF-endorsed standards.* http://www.qualityforum.org/Measures_List.aspx (accessed November 29, 2010).

Oakley, D., M. E. Murray, T. Murtland, R. Hayashi, H. F. Andersen, F. Mayes, and J. Rooks. 1996. Comparisons of outcomes of maternity care by obstetricians and certified nurse-midwives. *Obstetrics and Gynecology* 88(5):823-829.

Okunseri, C., A. Szabo, S. Jackson, N. M. Pajewski, and R. I. Garcia. 2009. Increased children's access to fluoride varnish treatment by involving medical care providers: Effect of a Medicaid policy change. *Health Services Research* 44(4):1144-1156.

Okwuje, I., E. Anderson, and R. W. Valachovic. 2009. Annual ADEA survey of dental school seniors: 2008 graduating class. *Journal of Dental Education* 73(8):1009-1032.

Okwuje, I., E. Anderson, and R. W. Valachovic. 2010. Annual ADEA survey of dental school seniors: 2009 graduating class. *Journal of Dental Education* 74(9):1024-1045.

O'Leary, K. J., D. B. Wayne, C. Haviley, M. E. Slade, J. Lee, and M. V. Williams. 2010. Improving teamwork: Impact of structured interdisciplinary rounds on a medical teaching unit. *Journal of General Internal Medicine* 25(8):826-832.

Pew Center on the States and National Academy for State Health Policy. 2009. *Help wanted: A policy maker's guide to new dental providers*. Washington, DC: Pew Center on the States, National Academy for State Health Policy.

PHI. 2010. *Facts 3: Who are direct care workers?* http://www.directcareclearinghouse.org/download/PHI%20FactSheet3_singles.pdf (accessed September 27, 2010).

Pierce, K. M., R. G. Rozier, and W. F. Vann. 2002. Accuracy of pediatric primary care providers' screening and referral for early childhood caries. *Pediatrics* 109(5):e82.

Porter, J., P. C. Coyte, J. Barnsley, and R. Croxford. 1999. The effects of fee bundling on dental utilization. *Health Services Research* 34(4):901-921.

President's Advisory Commission on Consumer Protection and Quality in the Health Care Industry. 1998. *Quality first: Better health care for all Americans*. http://www.hcquality commission.gov/final/ (accessed November 29, 2010).

Price, S. S., W. D. Brunson, D. A. Mitchell, C. J. Alexander, and D. L. Jackson. 2007. Increasing the enrollment of underrepresented minority dental students: Experiences from the dental pipeline program. *Journal of Dental Education* 71(3):339-347.

Quijano, A., A. J. Shah, A. I. Schwarcz, E. Lalla, and R. J. Ostfeld. 2010. Knowledge and orientations of internal medicine trainees toward periodontal disease. *Journal of Periodontology* 81(3):359-363.

Rackley, B., J. Wheat, C. Moore, R. Garner, and B. Harrell. 2003. The southern rural access program and Alabama's rural health leaders pipeline: A partnership to develop needed minority health care professionals. *Journal of Rural Health* 19(5):354-360.

Rauh, S. J. 1917. The present status of and necessity for mouth hygiene. *American Journal of Public Health* 7:631-636.

Raybould, T. P., A. S. Wrightson, C. S. Massey, T. A. Smith, and J. Skelton. 2009. Advanced general dentistry program directors' attitudes on physician involvement in pediatric oral health care. *Special Care in Dentistry* 29(6):232-236.

RCHWS (Regional Center for Health Workforce Studies). 2003. *Changes in the scope of practice and the supply of non-physician clinicians in Texas*. San Antonio, TX: Regional Center for Health Workforce Studies, Center for Health Economics and Policy, The University of Texas Health Science Center at San Antonio.

Reeves, S., M. Zwarenstein, J. Goldman, H. Barr, D. Freeth, M. Hammick, and I. Koppel. 2008. Interprofessional education: Effects on professional practice and health care outcomes. *Cochrane Database of Systematic Reviews*(1). Issue 1. Art. No.: CD002213. DOI: 10.1002/14651858.CD002213.pub2.

Reeves, S., M. Zwarenstein, J. Goldman, H. Barr, D. Freeth, I. Koppel, and M. Hammick. 2010. The effectiveness of interprofessional education: Key findings from a new systematic review. *Journal of Interprofessional Care* 24(3):230-241.

Remington, T. L., M. A. Foulk, and B. C. Williams. 2006. Evaluation of evidence for interprofessional education. *American Journal of Pharmaceutical Education* 70(3).

Rich, K. 2010. *Dental quality alliance*. http://www.medicaiddental.org/Docs/2010/Rich_Quality.pdf (accessed February 18, 2011).

Riter, D., R. Maier, and D. Grossman. 2008. Delivering preventive oral health services in pediatric primary care: A case study. *Health Affairs* 27(6):1728-1732.

Rosenblatt, R. A., S. A. Dobie, L. G. Hart, R. Schneeweiss, D. Gould, T. R. Raine, T. J. Benedetti, M. J. Pirani, and E. B. Perrin. 1997. Interspecialty differences in the obstetric care of low-risk women. *American Journal of Public Health* 87(3):344-351.

Rozier, R. G., B. K. Sutton, J. W. Bawden, K. Haupt, G. D. Slade, and R. S. King. 2003. Prevention of early childhood caries in north carolina medical practices: Implications for research and practice. *Journal of Dental Education* 67(8):876-885.

Rozier, R. G., S. C. Stearns, B. T. Pahel, R. B. Quinonez, and J. Park. 2010. How a North Carolina program boosted preventive oral health services for low-income children. *Health Affairs* 29(12):2278-2285.

Saman, D. M., O. Arevalo, and A. O. Johnson. 2010. The dental workforce in Kentucky: Current status and future needs. *Journal of Public Health Dentistry* 70(3):188-196.

Sanchez, O., N. Childers, L. Fox, and E. Bradley. 1997. Physicians' views on pediatric preventive dental care. *Pediatric Dentistry* 19(6):377-383.

Shepard, L. 1978. Licensing restrictions and the cost of dental care. *Journal of Law and Economics* 21(1):187-201.

Silk, H., S. O. G. Stille, R. Baldor, and E. Joseph. 2009. Implementation of STFM's "Smiles for Life" oral health curriculum in a medical school interclerkship. *Family Medicine* 41(7):487-491.

Sisty, N. L., W. G. Henderson, C. L. Paule, and J. F. Martin. 1978. Evaluation of student performance in the four-year study of expanded functions for dental hygienists at the University of Iowa. *Journal of the American Dental Association* 97(4):613-627.

Skillman, S. M., M. P. Doescher, W. E. Mouradian, and D. K. Brunson. 2010. The challenge to delivering oral health services in rural America. *Journal of Public Health Dentistry* 70(Supp. 1):S49-S57.

Snyder, M. E., A. J. Zillich, B. A. Primack, K. R. Rice, M. A. Somma McGivney, J. L. Pringle, and R. B. Smith. 2010. Exploring successful community pharmacist-physician collaborative working relationships using mixed methods. *Research in Social and Administrative Pharmacy* 6(4):307-321.

Society of Teachers of Family Medicine Group on Oral Health. 2011. *Smiles for life: A national oral health curriculum.* http://www.smilesforlife2.org (accessed January 6, 2011).

Solomon, E. S. 2007. Demographic characteristics of general dental practice sites. *General Dentistry* 55(6):552-558.

Sowter, J. R., and D. K. Raynor. 1997. The management of oral health problems in community pharmacies. *Pharmaceutical Journal* 259(6957):308-310.

Spielman, A. I., T. Fulmer, E. S. Eisenberg, and M. C. Alfano. 2005. Dentistry, nursing, and medicine: A comparison of core competencies. *Journal of Dental Education.* 69(11): 1257-1271.

Stanton, M. W., and M. K. Rutherford. 2003. *Dental care: Improving access and quality.* Rockville, MD: Agency for Healthcare Research and Quality.

Sullivan Commission. 2004. *Missing persons: Minorities in the health professions, a report of the Sullivan Commission on diversity in the healthcare workforce.* http://www.aacn.nche.edu/Media/pdf/SullivanReport.pdf (accessed January 24, 2011).

Sun, N., G. Burnside, and R. Harris. 2010. Patient satisfaction with care by dental therapists. *British Dental Journal* 208(5):E9.

Thind, A., K. A. Atchison, R. M. Andersen, T. T. Nakazono, and J. J. Gutierrez. 2008. Reforming dental education: Faculty members' perceptions on the continuation of pipeline program changes. *Journal of Dental Education* 72(12):1472-1480.

Thind, A., K. A. Atchison, T. T. Nakazono, J. J. Gutierrez, D. C. Carreon, and J. Bai. 2009. Sustainability of dental school recruitment, curriculum, and community-based pipeline initiatives. *Journal of Dental Education* 73(Supp. 2):S297-S307.

Thistlethwaite, J., and M. Moran. 2010. Learning outcomes for interprofessional education (IPE): Literature review and synthesis. *Journal of interprofessional care* 24(5):503-513.

Thomson, W. A., P. Ferry, J. King, C. M. Wedig, and G. B. Villarreal. 2010. A baccalaureate-MD program for students from medically underserved communities: 15-year outcomes. *Academic Medicine* 85(4):668-674.

Todd, B. A., A. Resnick, R. Stuhlemmer, J. B. Morris, and J. Mullen. 2004. Challenges of the 80-hour resident work rules: Collaboration between surgeons and nonphysician practitioners. *Surgical Clinics of North America* 84(6):1573-1586.

Tomar, S. L. 2005. *Dental public health training: Time for new models?* Presentation at the National Oral Health Conference, Pittsburgh, PA. May 3, 2005.

Tomar, S. L. 2006. An assessment of the dental public health infrastructure in the United States. *Journal of Public Health Dentistry* 66(1):5-16.

University of Bridgeport. 1998. *History of Fones School.* http://www1bpt.bridgeport.edu/dental/history.html (accessed November 3, 2010).

University of Maryland. 2010. *About the Baltimore College of Dental Surgery.* http://www.dental.umaryland.edu/z_dental_archives/aboutBCDS_old/ (accessed December 27, 2010).

U.S. Census Bureau. 2000. *Census 2000 EEO data tool.* http://www.census.gov/eeo2000/index.html (accessed January 7, 2011).

U.S. Census Bureau. 2002. *United States census 2000: U.S. Summary.* http://www.census.gov/prod/2002pubs/c2kprof00-us.pdf (accessed January 7, 2011).

USMLE (U.S. Medical Licensing Exam). 2010a. *2011 step 2 clinical knowledge: Content description and general information.* Philadelphia, PA: Federation of State Medical Boards of the United States and National Board of Medical Examiners.

USMLE. 2010b. *2011 step 3: Content description and general information.* Philadelphia, PA: Federation of State Medical Boards of the United States and National Board of Medical Examiners.

Veal, K., M. Perry, J. Stavisky, and K. D. Herbert. 2004. The pathway to dentistry for minority students: From their perspective. *Journal of Dental Education* 68(9):938-946.

Venezie, R., W. Vann, Jr., S. Cashion, and R. Rozier. 1997. Pediatric and general dentists' participation in the North Carolina Medicaid program: Trends from 1986 to 1992. *Pediatric Dentistry* 19(2):114-117.

Walker, M. P., S. I. Duley, M. M. Beach, L. Deem, R. Pileggi, N. Samet, A. Segura, and J. N. Williams. 2008. Dental education economics: Challenges and innovative strategies. *Journal of Dental Education.* 72(12):1440-1449.

Wall, T. P., and L. J. Brown. 2007. The urban and rural distribution of dentists, 2000. *Journal of the American Dental Association* 138(7):1003-1011.

Weinberg, M. A., and W. J. Maloney. 2007. Treatment of common oral lesions. *U.S. Pharmacist* 32(3):82-88.

Wendling, W. R. 2010. Private sector approaches to workforce enhancement. *Journal of Public Health Dentistry* 70(Supp. 1):S24-S31.

Wetterhall, S., J. D. Bader, B. B. Burrus, J. Y. Lee, and D. A. Shugars. 2010. *Evaluation of the dental health aide therapist workforce model in Alaska.* Research Triangle Park, NC: W.K. Kellogg Foundation, Rasmuson Foundation, Bethel Community Services Foundation.

WICHE (Western Interstate Commission for Higher Education). 2011. *Professional student exchange program (PSEP).* http://wiche.edu/psep (accessed January 11, 2011).

Wilder, R. S., J. A. O'Donnell, J. M. Barry, D. M. Galli, F. F. Hakim, L. J. Holyfield, and M. R. Robbins. 2008. Is dentistry at risk? A case for interprofessional education. *Journal of Dental Education* 72(11):1231-1237.

Williams, B. C., T. L. Remington, M. A. Foulk, and A. L. Whall. 2006. Teaching interdisciplinary geriatrics ambulatory care: A case study. *Gerontology and Geriatrics Education* 26(3):29-45.

Wing, P., M. H. Langelier, E. S. Salsberg, and R. S. Hooker. 2004. The changing professional practice of physician assistants: 1992 to 2000. *Journal of the American Academy of Physician Assistants* 17(1):37-40, 42, 45.

Wysen, K. H., P. M. Hennessy, M. I. Lieberman, T. E. Garland, and S. M. Johnson. 2004. Kids get care: Integrating preventive dental and medical care using a public health case management model. *Journal of Dental Education* 68(5):522-530.

4

HHS and Oral Health: Past and Present

Poor oral health remains a serious national health problem.

—Garth Graham, Deputy Assistant Secretary for Minority Health,
Office of Minority Health

Launch of the 2010 HHS Oral Health Initiative, April 26, 2010
(HHS, 2010f)

This chapter describes previous and current oral health reform efforts and oral health activities initiated at the federal level, focusing in particular on cross-agency initiatives within the U.S. Department of Health and Human Services (HHS). It also describes the current HHS Oral Health Initiative and provides recommendations for the future focus of this effort. Appendix B includes organizational charts of the key HHS agencies and divisions involved in oral health.

THE HISTORY OF HHS AND ORAL HEALTH

The earliest recognition of the impact of poor oral health in America dates back to concerns for the oral health of the nation's military, but the government's involvement in oral health care was limited. In the 18th and 19th centuries, the military considered oral health care to be the responsibility of the individual soldier, and this care was primarily provided by civilian dentists, or, on an emergency basis, by ill-trained army physicians (King and Hynson, 2007). By the mid-1800s, predecessors of the American Dental Association (ADA) began to press government leaders about the lack of access to oral health care for the nations' soldiers and sailors. Finally, in 1911, after numerous hearings and many failed bills, President Taft signed legislation creating the U.S. Army Dental Corps (King and Hynson, 2007).

Perhaps the U.S. government's first notable role in establishing the importance of oral health within federal-level health agencies was in 1931 when the U.S. Public Health Service (USPHS) created a Dental Hygiene Unit at the National Institutes of Health (NIH) and designated Dr. H.

Trendley Dean as the first dental research scientist (NIH, 2010). Dr. Dean examined the epidemiology of communities that presented with "mottled enamel" (i.e., fluorosis), but further research also suggested a benefit from fluoride in community drinking water on the prevalence of tooth decay. In 1944, a Dental Health Section was established for the first time within the Department of Health, Education, and Welfare (DHEW), predecessor to the modern-day HHS, under the Bureau of State Services, predecessor to the today's Health Resources and Services Administration (HRSA) (National Archives, 2010). In 1945, Grand Rapids, Michigan, with the support of Dr. Dean and the NIH, became the first city in the world to add a controlled level of fluoride to its community water supply (NIDCR, 2010f). On June 24, 1948, President Harry Truman signed Public Law 80-755, the National Dental Research Act, and thereby created the National Institute for Dental Research, predecessor to the current National Institute for Dental and Craniofacial Research (NIDCR), as well as the National Advisory Dental Research Council (NIH, 2010). By 1950, the results of the first 5 years of the Grand Rapids study confirmed that optimal water fluoridation was a safe, effective, and economical method for helping to prevent dental caries, and the Public Health Service adopted a policy of encouraging community water fluoridation (Lennon, 2006).

The 1960s

Strengthened by the success of the water fluoridation studies, by the mid-1960s, oral health care's position in the federal bureaucracy expanded when a Division of Dental Health (later called Division of Dentistry) was established within DHEW. Its director served as dental advisor to President Johnson's Office of Economic Opportunity, the agency responsible for administering programs such as Head Start (Diefenbach, 1969). The division administered a variety of programs centered on dental education, the dental workforce, dental caries prevention, and the use of fluorides. The work of the Division of Dental Health might be considered the first major oral health "initiative" conducted by the federal government.

At this time, programs such as Head Start discovered that oral health care was one of the services most requested by impoverished families (Diefenbach, 1969). Social Security Amendments of 1965 and 1967 required the inclusion of dental care in its program and also allowed for the development of special projects aimed at the oral health of children (Coker, 1969). At the same time, the advancing scientific understanding that tooth decay and periodontal disease are bacterial infections that can be controlled through preventive measures brought a growing sense of optimism that the prevalence of these conditions could be radically reduced over time. Through funding incentives, the Division of Dental Health sought to encourage dental schools to teach prevention and to establish departments of preventive dentistry. However, when the division's funding was later eliminated, virtually all of the participating dental schools either eliminated these departments or collapsed them into others.[1]

In the 1960s, the federal government also sought to improve access to oral health care through expansions and innovations in the oral health workforce. For example, the Health Professions Educational Assistance Act of 1963 provided the first federal support for dental education (Diefenbach, 1969).[2] The act (and later amendments) improved the financial base of existing dental schools, initiated new school construction, and sought to produce nearly 1,000 additional dental graduates within only a few years. In addition, the Health Manpower Act of 1968 provided even more funding to improve and expand training programs under Title VII of the Public Health Service Act.[3]

At this time, DHEW began to estimate the status of the dental workforce as part of its estimation of the health workforce (NCHS, 1968). DHEW was also actively involved in promoting workforce innovations (e.g., the use of nondentist personnel) such as dental auxiliary utilization, otherwise known as four-handed dentistry, and dental school-based training in expanded auxiliary management (TEAM) programs (Gladstone and Garcia, 2007; Johnson, 1969). These educational initiatives were designed to spur the adoption of team care in dentistry, with each member of the dental team working up to the capacity of his or her training, in order to provide more care at less cost. The Indian Health Service embraced the team care concept and demonstrated the effectiveness and efficiency of dental assistants in expanded functions in several sites, then expanded their utilization wherever it was practical (Abramowitz and Berg, 1973). In addition, an early innovation to integrate dental and nondental health care professionals is noted in the creation of craniofacial teams—in 1962, the National Institute for Dental Research funded the first multidisciplinary study of cleft palate at the University of Pittsburgh Health Center (NIH, 2010).

In an article appearing in the June 1969 issue of the *American Journal of Public Health and the Nation's Health*, Dr. Viron Diefenbach, then director of the Division of Dental Health of the Public Health Service, asserted that the 1960s would be remembered as a time of astounding scientific advances, and also one in which public policy began to address the striking inequalities in access to health care (Diefenbach, 1969). Specifically, he

---

[1] Personal Communication, A. Horowitz, University of Maryland, September 14, 2010.

[2] *Health Professions Educational Assistance Act of 1963*, Public Law 129, 88th Cong., 1st sess. (September 24, 1963).

[3] *Health Manpower Act of 1968*, Public Law 490, 90th Cong., 2d sess. (August 16, 1968).

expressed optimism for "revers[ing] the spiral of dental illness in the United States" (Diefenbach, 1969).

The 1970s

In the early 1970s, the federal government made substantial investments in the entire health care workforce. By the early 1970s, rural states had approached Congress about the worsening crisis due to the lack of health care professionals available to care for rural communities. In response, in 1970, the Emergency Health Personnel Act[4] created the National Health Service Corps (NHSC). Since 1972, the NHSC has assigned USPHS Commissioned Corps officers or civil servants to provide care in underserved areas (HRSA, 2010d). Amendments to this law in the 1970s and 1980s allowed for both scholarships and loan repayment in order to attract more health care professionals to serve in the NHSC (HRSA, 2010d). In addition, President Nixon signed the Comprehensive Health Manpower Training Act of 1971, which continued the federal government's involvement in the financing of health professions education, including dental education.[5] This law strove not just to increase numbers but also "to improve the distribution of such personnel—both geographically and by medical specialty—and to promote the more effective use of health manpower" (Woolley and Peters, 2011b). Later, President Ford signed the Health Professions Educational Assistance Act of 1976.[6] This law did not focus on increasing numbers, but rather on better distribution, both by specialty area as well as geographic location. The law included special provisions for education and training of general dentists and expanded function dental auxiliaries and revised and expanded the NHSC (Woolley and Peters, 2011a).

In addition to workforce investments, one major activity that did launch in the early 1970s was the National Caries Program (NCP). The program was housed within the NIH, and its goal was to substantially reduce the prevalence of dental caries in the United States (Harris, 1992). The NCP expenditures for the first year of operation exceeded $6 million, with $2 million in grants, $3 million in contracts, and $900,000 in laboratory and clinical research (Harris, 1992). The NCP continued until 1984.

While investments in the workforce overall were substantial and DHEW oral health activities had been successful, attention to oral health in particular was waning. A later review of HHS oral health programs found that

---

[4] *Emergency Health Personnel Act of 1970*, Public Law 623, 91st Cong., 2d sess. (December 31, 1970).

[5] *Comprehensive Health Manpower Training Act of 1971*, Public Law 157, 92d Cong., 1st sess. (November 18, 1971).

[6] *Health Professions Educational Assistance Act of 1976*, Public Law 484, 94th Cong., 2d sess. (October 12, 1976).

"the oral health activities of the department, and the resources devoted to those activities, have been disaggregated, dispersed, reduced drastically, or altogether eliminated since 1972" (Interim Study Group on Dental Activities, 1989). Since then, multiple agencies within HHS have been responsible for various programs related to oral health, and the need for integration of these activities across the department has become a recurring theme.

Healthy People (1979–Present)

In 1979, Surgeon General Julius B. Richmond issued *Healthy People: The Surgeon General's Report on Health Promotion and Disease Prevention*, which highlighted the dramatic impact of public health efforts in fighting communicable diseases and laid out a national agenda for the future role of public health efforts in noninfectious diseases—that is, health promotion and disease prevention (DHEW, 1979). This report highlighted dental health as a "prominent threat to the good health of children" and identified "fluoridation and oral heath" as one of 15 priority areas. It also illustrated goals along the age continuum, namely, to reduce deaths among infants, children, young adults and adults, and to reduce the number of sick days among older adults.

That same year, the Office of Disease Prevention and Health Promotion was established under the purview of Assistant Surgeon General Michael McGinnis, who also had borne responsibility for the development of the surgeon general's report.[7] In 1980, this office, working closely with the Centers for Disease Control and Prevention (CDC) and the other agencies of the USPHS, oversaw the production of *Promoting Health/Preventing Disease: Objectives for the Nation* (known as *Healthy People 1990*), which outlined 226 objectives to achieve significant improvements in the health of the nation by 1990 (USPHS, 1980). Objectives tended to be chosen, in part, based on whether they were measurable, whether improvement was considered possible or likely, whether there were science-based interventions, and whether they were easily understood both by health care professionals and the general public (Andersen and Mullner, 1990; McGinnis, 2010). While important, the presence of ongoing data sources was not a precondition for these objectives, with the expectation being that the objective would drive data collection[8] (McGinnis, 2010).

While *Healthy People 1990* had a mortality-based framework, *Healthy People 2000* focused on the broader goals of increasing the span of healthy life, reducing disparities, increasing access to preventive services, and age-

---

[7] Personal Communication, M. McGinnis, Institute of Medicine, July 30, 2011.

[8] As this did not fully come to fruition, *Healthy People 2020* required the existence of or the commitment to develop a tracking source.

specific targets (McGinnis, 2010). As the number of individual objectives was growing, *Healthy People 2000* identified about 20 priority areas, one of which was oral health (HHS, 1991). *Healthy People 2010* changed its focus yet again, to concentrate on increasing the quality and years of healthy life and eliminating health disparities. Oral health was identified as one of 28 "focus areas" (HHS, 2005).

Overall, the *Healthy People* goals are intended to be used as a guide for the nation, not just for the use of the federal government. Partners in the development of *Healthy People* goals and objectives include federal agencies, the Healthy People Consortium (an alliance of non-federal stakeholders committed to supporting *Healthy People* goals), and public-private partnerships developed through memorandums of understanding (MOUs). For *Healthy People 2010*, HHS had MOUs with the American Association for Dental Research and the Academy of General Dentistry (HHS, 2003b). (*Healthy People 2010* and *2020* are also discussed in general in Chapter 2 as well as later in this chapter.)

The 1980s

In 1980, the Division of Dentistry consolidated with Division of Associated Health Professions to form the Division of Associated and Dental Health Professions under the Bureau of Health Professions (National Archives, 2010). During the 1980s, federal activity was proceeding along many different tracks, largely in an uncoordinated manner. Preparations for the second national health objectives report (*Healthy People 2000*) were under way, which engaged the participation of agencies across the department. Also, in 1987, Congress directed the National Institute for Dental Research to develop a multiagency national plan for improving the oral health of adults (especially older adults) that would engage both the public and private sectors to address education, research, and delivery of oral health services (Gershen, 1991; Interim Study Group on Dental Activities, 1989; NIH, 2010). The Maternal and Child Health Bureau (MCHB) took the lead in conducting a workshop examining children's access to oral health care (HRSA, 1990).

Through the Omnibus Budget Reconciliation Act of 1989 (OBRA 1989),[9] Congress initiated significant changes in the MCHB block grant program. In addition, Congress codified previous regulatory requirements applicable to the Medicaid Early and Periodic Screening, Diagnosis and Treatment (EPSDT) benefits for individuals under age 21. Prior to 1989, dental coverage had been a regulatory requirement; the 1989 amendments

---

[9] *Omnibus Budget Reconciliation Act of 1989*, Public Law 239, 101st Cong., 1st sess. (December 19, 1989).

mandated dental services provided at intervals meeting reasonable standards of dental practice as well as at medically necessary intervals, and consisting of relief of pain and infections, restoration of teeth, and maintenance of dental health[10] (OIG, 1996). Finally OBRA 1989 also mandated that all state Medicaid programs increase their eligibility levels to 133 percent of the federal poverty level (FPL) and give states the option to increase it to 185 percent of the FPL.

The Meskin Report (1989)

As part of the appropriations process for fiscal year 1988, the congressional appropriations committees in both the House and the Senate mandated a study of the oral health activities of HHS (Interim Study Group on Dental Activities, 1989; USPHS, 1989). The objectives of that study, now known as the Meskin report (after chairman Lawrence H. Meskin), resemble the charge that has been put forward to this Institute of Medicine (IOM) committee—namely, "to address the identification of appropriate goals and priorities in oral health" and "to consider appropriate organizational and administrative arrangements for achieving maximum coordination" (Interim Study Group on Dental Activities, 1989). As a result of this mandate, HHS formed the Interim Study Group on Dental Activities to identify goals and priorities in the areas of oral health research, education, prevention, and service provision. The appointed study group consisted of 12 members representing both the public and private sectors, along with four HHS agency representatives who served as consultants. All 12 of the study group members were dentists, with the exception of then executive director of the ADA.

To inform this study, an inventory of oral health activities within HHS was conducted by a contractor and presented to HHS in January 1989 (USPHS, 1989). The group also solicited input from 30 individuals and organizations including the ADA, the American Association of Public Health Dentistry (AAPHD), the American Association of Dental Schools, state departments of health, and the World Health Organization. This process identified a number of needs within HHS, including:

- A strengthened central focus;
- An increased federal government leadership role;
- Better coordination among agencies;
- Identification of agencies' oral health goals;
- Dental presence in all agencies;
- Strengthened regional offices;

---

[10] 42 U.S.C. §1396d(r)(3).

- Greater input from states;
- Greater interaction with national dental organizations;
- More input from private dentistry;
- Increased access for underserved and special populations; and
- Greater prevention orientation (USPHS, 1989).

The Interim Study Group on Dental Activities submitted its report, *Improving the Oral Health of the American People: Opportunity for Action,* to the USPHS in March 1989, and this was subsequently submitted to the House of Representatives Appropriations Committee in May 1989 (Interim Study Group on Dental Activities, 1989; USPHS, 1989). The report began by noting the dramatic improvements in the scientific understanding of oral disease in the post–World War II era. It said that these developments had "caused a fundamental shift in the focus of dentistry from the repair and replacement of teeth to the prevention of disease and the preservation of the natural dentition for a lifetime" (USPHS, 1989). "Indeed," the report continued, "leaders in the dental community now talk of the prospect of essentially eliminating caries and periodontal disease in the early decades of the 21st century" (USPHS, 1989).

The question was how to realize this potential—specifically, how HHS could be structured to promote this objective. The study group found that

decentralization in recent years has resulted in severe fragmentation of the remaining oral health programs, decreased interagency communication, and limited opportunities for collaboration among the various [d]epartmental programs, despite the fact that they share the goal of improving the oral health of the [n]ation. Decreased collaboration leads to duplication of efforts in some areas and absence of efforts in other areas, and results in uncoordinated oral health programs which lack direction or purpose. The attainment of a unified program is hindered primarily by the lack of a clear focus for the [d]epartment's oral health activities. No single entity has been empowered and enabled to coordinate oral health activities. . . . The [s]tudy [g]roup was unable to identify within the [d]epartment . . . a discernible oral health policy. (USPHS, 1989)

The study group's recommendations (see Box 4-1) included that HHS name an individual to serve as the focal point of oral health activities throughout the department. This would be a full-time position within the USPHS at the level of the Office of the Assistant Secretary for Health. They stated that the individual needed to have clearly visible administrative and policy responsibility, serving as the principal oral health advisor to the secretary of HHS. The group recommended that the individual should be advised by a formally chartered committee with representatives primarily from the private sector, along with ex officio representatives from the U.S.

BOX 4-1
Meskin Report Recommendations

- Establish a focus for oral health activities in the Department of Health and Human Services with clearly visible administrative and policy responsibility.
- The individual serving as the focus for oral health activities in the DHHS should be advised by a formally chartered committee.
- Establish a strong, clearly identified, oral health presence in any DHHS agency that regularly conducts oral health activities.

SOURCE: USPHS, 1989.

Departments of Defense (DOD) and Veterans Affairs (VA). The group also emphasized that all HHS agencies with oral health activities should have a strong, clearly identified oral health presence.

The Oral Health Coordinating Committee (1990)

Due, in part, to the findings of the Meskin Report, on February 26, 1990, then Assistant Secretary for Health James Mason established the Oral Health Coordinating Committee (OHCC) to help coordinate federal activities in improving oral health (USPHS, 2002). The chief dental officer of the USPHS was delegated the leadership of the OHCC on behalf of the assistant secretary of health; however, this person had (and still has) full-time responsibilities elsewhere within HHS. The Meskin committee's recommendation that one person serve in a dedicated full-time role as a focal point for oral health policy within HHS was not adopted. The OHCC continues to draw its leadership and its staffing from the operating divisions within HHS, but it has neither line authority nor its own budget (Bailey, 2010). The Meskin committee had also recommended that the advisory committee have significant private-sector representation; however, the OHCC was not structured to include this point of view.

In 1996, the Office of the Inspector General (OIG) released a report indicating many children were not receiving EPSDT services that were supposed to be available through Medicaid (OIG, 1996). Approximately 80 percent of the states attributed the problem to a shortage of dentists willing to accept Medicaid patients. The OIG offered a single recommendation on how this should be addressed at the federal level: "The department should convene a work group that, at a minimum, would include the HCFA

[Health Care Financing Administration], HRSA, [the Administration for Children and Families], [the Office of Public Health and Science], and [the HHS Assistant Secretary for Planning and Evaluation] to develop an integrated approach to improve dental access and utilization for EPSDT eligible children (OIG, 1996)." The assistant secretary of health and the NIH responded that the existing OHCC could adequately serve this purpose without creating a new workgroup. The OIG agreed, and revised its recommendation to state that "with expanded membership, the existing PHS Oral Health Coordinating Committee Working Group could fulfill this need" (OIG, 1996). The recommendation indicated that the workgroup should consider ways to encourage professional volunteerism, support demonstrations aimed at increasing provider participation in Medicaid, and improve outreach to eligible families. Over the course of the remainder of the 1990s and then through most of the 2000s, however, the members of the OHCC served more as senior advisors rather than having a role in developing a plan as suggested by the OIG.

The HRSA-HCFA Initiative (1998–2001)

The HRSA-HCFA Oral Health Initiative aimed to improve collaboration at the national level in order to improve access to oral health care at the local level. Goals of the initiative were to

- Eliminate disparities and barriers to care,
- Respond to unmet needs for clinical services,
- Increase the number of dental professionals,
- Expand the dental public health infrastructure,
- Restructure and increase coordination among federal oral health programs, and
- Coordinate federal initiatives with key partners in the dental community (HHS, 2000c).

The initiative included three main types of activities: integrating activities within and between federal agencies, partnering with stakeholders, and sharing scientific data (HHS, 2000c). For example, HRSA and HCFA sought interagency collaborations to provide information to communities based on information gathered from efforts such as the National Health and Nutrition Examination Survey (NHANES) and *Healthy People* (HHS, 2000c). Other state and regional activities included oral health summits and workshops, regular conference calls with state dental directors, on-site reviews of state programs, recruitment of dental consultants, and solicitation of federal funds for dental programs (HHS, 2000c).

The HRSA-HCFA initiative continued for 3 years and was arguably one of the HHS's most successful and far-reaching oral health initiatives. In testimony to this IOM committee, the incoming president of the ADA, Raymond Gist, praised the HRSA-HCFA effort, saying that it was a "sweeping oral health initiative" (Gist, 2010). He said that the effort not only highlighted and boosted HRSA's oral health programs, it also recognized that HRSA needed to forge a closer relationship with (what is now) the Centers for Medicare and Medicaid Services (CMS) and programs such as Head Start. Longer-term objectives for the HRSA-HCFA initiative had been to "expand funding for dental programs in community health centers, increase the number of grants for sealant programs, expand the number of loans and scholarships for dental students willing to practice in underserved areas, support development of state infrastructures, provide GIS mapping for all states" to enable them to assess oral health care infrastructure at county and subcounty levels, "simplify the designations for Health Professional Shortage Areas, and change federal policies that restrict provider enrollment and access to care" (HHS, 2000c). However, the HRSA-HCFA initiative ended after the transition in administrations following the 2000 presidential election.

The Surgeon General's Report (2000)

On May 25, 2000, the USPHS issued its landmark report *Oral Health in America: A Report of the Surgeon General* (HHS, 2000b). The report alerted the nation of a "silent epidemic" of oral disease in America and brought attention to the deep disparities in oral health status as well as who receives adequate oral health care services nationwide. The report also helped to reframe the term *oral health*, so that it not only includes dental care and teeth but also overall oral health, including periodontal disease, oral cancer, and craniofacial issues such as cleft palate. In reviewing the existing body of knowledge on oral health issues at that time, the surgeon general noted that safe and effective measures existed to prevent the most common oral diseases—dental caries and periodontal disease. For example, the report noted that good oral hygiene practices such as simple brushing and flossing can prevent gingivitis and that the effectiveness of water fluoridation for the prevention of dental caries had been proven for decades. But the report also found that lifestyle choices such as tobacco use, excessive alcohol use, and poor dietary choices can be detrimental to oral health. Overall, the report's major message was that oral health is essential to general health and well-being and can be achieved by all Americans. However, not everyone is achieving the same degree of oral health (HHS, 2000b). In conjunction with the release of this report, the surgeon general held two meetings focusing on children's oral health. The "Surgeon General's Workshop," held March 19–21, 2000, involved 80 invited experts who were charged with developing an action plan (NIDCR, 2001). This was followed by a national, multidisciplinary meeting of more than 700 people on June 12–13, 2000, entitled "The Face of a Child: Surgeon General's Conference on Children and Oral Health," wherein the participants considered the recommendations of the workshop group (NIDCR, 2000, 2001).

The report called for the development of a national oral health plan and provided components of that plan that contributed to the development of the *National Call to Action to Promote Oral Health* (discussed below). The framework for the plan centered on efforts to change perceptions about oral health among providers, policy makers, and the public; strengthening the evidence base for oral health services; building an effective health infrastructure to meet oral health needs; removing barriers to care; and employing public–private partnerships. The surgeon general's report was highly discussed 10 years ago and continues to be heavily cited in the literature. In an examination of oral health policy development subsequent to the release of the surgeon general's report, Crall stated, "Evidence suggests that accomplishments in the area of oral health policy development have been modest but positive, but a significant amount of work remains to be done to address oral health disparities" (Crall, 2009). In a presentation to this committee, Dushanka Kleinman attributed the successful impact of *Oral Health in America* to the personal experience and interest of HHS leaders, a focus on oral health (not just dentistry), the ability to build on existing HHS activities, and the inclusion of and appeal to nontraditional partners (Kleinman, 2010). However, she also noted limitations due to the lack of an implementation plan with specific goals and measures, the lack of capacity within the federal health care workforce to work on and lead these issues, and the lack of an accountable central body at HHS.

The National Call to Action (2003)

Three years following the release of the surgeon general's report, HHS developed a *National Call to Action to Promote Oral Health* (HHS, 2003c). Partnering with voluntary and professional organizations, private and government agencies, foundations, and universities, HHS defined a vision to "advance the general health and well-being of all Americans by creating critical partnerships at all levels of society to engage in programs to promote oral health and prevent disease." The effort to advance this "National Call to Action" was again led by the NIDCR as the lead federal agency but also engaged senior oral health experts at several HHS agencies to assist in its development. In addition, the report defined goals to reflect those of *Healthy People 2010*, namely: promote oral health, improve quality of life, and eliminate oral health disparities. Finally, the report specified five necessary actions to improve oral health (see Box 4-2) under the as-

---

BOX 4-2
Five Actions of the *National Call to*
Action to Promote Oral Health

- Change perceptions of oral health.
- Overcome barriers by replicating effective programs and proven efforts.
- Build the science base and accelerate science transfer.
- Increase oral health workforce diversity, capacity, and flexibility.
- Increase collaborations.

SOURCE: HHS, 2003c.

---

sumption that all actions should be science based, culturally sensitive, integrated into overall health and well-being activities, and routinely evaluated. Nearly a decade later, while improvements have been made, these actions are still needed.

CURRENT ROLES OF INDIVIDUAL HHS DIVISIONS

In the sections below, the roles of individual HHS operating divisions and staff divisions are discussed. Examples are taken from public sources of information and given to highlight some of the major work of these entities but are not necessarily exhaustive of every role the entities have in improving oral health and oral health care. Appendix B includes a chart of the key HHS agencies currently involved in oral health.

Administration for Children and Families

Oral health activities in the Administration for Children and Families center on its Head Start program, which is operated through the Office of Head Start. The Administration for Children and Families requires Head Start programs to determine whether a child has received age-appropriate preventive dental care within 90 days of the child entering the Head Start program.[11]

If a child has not received appropriate care, the Head Start program must help the parents make arrangements for the child to receive it.[12] Ap-

---

[11] *Code of Federal Regulations*, Office of Human Development Services, Department of Health and Human Services, title 45, sec. 1304.20 (2009).

[12] Ibid.

propriate care is determined by the state's EPSDT program and periodicity schedule. Head Start programs must also obtain or arrange for testing, examination, and treatment for children with known or suspected dental problems, and develop and implement a follow-up plan for any problems identified. To foster access to oral health for children enrolled in Head Start, in 2006, the Office of Head Start invested $2 million in grants to 52 Head Start, Early Head Start, and Migrant/Seasonal Head Start programs for the Head Start Oral Health Initiative; grantees received supplemental funding for 4 additional years (Del Grosso et al., 2008). While grantees reported successfully developing partnerships with community organizations and providers who would serve Head Start children, educating staff about the importance of oral health, and incorporating oral health education into the curriculum, they reported that they likely could not sustain much of the oral health programming when the grant funding ended (Del Grosso et al., 2008). The Office of Head Start partners with other HHS agencies and outside organizations to improve access to oral health care services for children who participate in Head Start.

Agency for Healthcare Research and Quality

The Agency for Healthcare Research and Quality (AHRQ) contributes to oral health research by collecting data, funding both intramural and external research, and disseminating innovations in health care delivery. AHRQ collects information on oral health care needs, access, and expenditures through the Medical Expenditure Panel Survey (MEPS). MEPS contains two major parts: the household component and the insurance component (AHRQ, 2010). In the household component, MEPS asks individuals about demographic characteristics, oral health conditions, oral health status, access to dental care, charges and source of payments for dental care, satisfaction with care, and dental insurance coverage. Information from the household component is sometimes supplemented with information from the individuals' health care providers. In the insurance component, MEPS collects information from employers about the types of insurance plans they offer to their employees. AHRQ researchers use MEPS data for intramural research and also make the data available to researchers outside the federal government. AHRQ also funds extramural research on oral health care expenditures, insurance coverage, and access to care. AHRQ disseminates innovative practices in quality improvement through its Innovations Exchange website (www.innovations.ahrq.gov). Activities must meet certain criteria to be included on the site, including aiming to improve one of the domains of quality as defined by the IOM (effectiveness, efficiency, equity, patient-centeredness, safety, and timeliness). The website also includes a compilation of tools for assessing, measuring, promoting, and improving the quality of health care. AHRQ's role in convening the U.S. Preventive Services Task Force is discussed later in this chapter.

Centers for Disease Control and Prevention

At the CDC, most oral health activities occur in the National Center for Chronic Disease Prevention and Health Promotion (NCCDPHP), Division of Oral Health. Additionally, the National Center for Health Statistics (NCHS) collects important data on the oral health of the United States population through NHANES (see Chapter 2) and the National Health Interview Survey (NHIS), which collects information on dental visits and unmet dental needs; periodically it fields a module in oral health (CDC, 2010i; NCHS, 2010). The CDC analyzes these data and publishes reports on these analyses. The CDC's role in convening the Task Force on Community Preventive Services is discussed later in this chapter.

National Center for Chronic Disease Prevention and Health Promotion, Division of Oral Health

The NCCDPHP's activities fall into four categories: state support, monitoring oral health, research and education, and guidelines and recommendations (CDC, 2010b). Between 2009 and 2013, the NCCDPHP will provide support and funding to 19 state oral health programs to help them develop state oral health plans, monitor oral diseases and risk factors, and develop and evaluate disease prevention programs (CDC, 2010c). The NCCDPHP also provides training, resource development, and technical assistance to all states through partnerships with national organizations such as the Association of State and Territorial Dental Directors (ASTDD), the Children's Dental Health Project, and Oral Health America (CDC, 2010e). To supplement these activities, the NCCDPHP maintains an Oral Health Resources website that includes resources for enhancing state oral health infrastructure, links to state oral health plans, and surveillance data (CDC, 2010f).

The NCCDPHP monitors oral health indicators, such as oral diseases, use of preventive measures, and dental visits. Through the National Oral Health Surveillance System, the NCCDPHP collaborates with ASTDD to track nine indicators of oral health, including dental visits, untreated tooth decay, and dental sealants (CDC, 2010j). The NCCDPHP also works with states to track water fluoridation (CDC, 2010k). Building on this effort, and as part of HHS' new Oral Health Initiative (described later in this chapter), the NCCDPHP, the NCHS, and the NIDCR will develop a comprehensive National Oral Health Surveillance Plan (HHS, 2010g). The plan will allow HHS to create a "report card" for oral health in the United States

(HHS, 2010g). The role of the CDC in prevention is discussed further later in this chapter.

Centers for Medicare and Medicaid Services

As the largest insurer of children in the United States, Medicaid and the Children's Health Insurance Plan (CHIP) play a critical role in ensuring children's access to oral health services. Medicaid includes mandatory dental insurance for children through the EPSDT dental benefit.[13] States must provide dental care to children insured by Medicaid "at intervals which meet reasonable standards of . . . dental practice, as determined by the state after consultation with recognized . . . dental organizations involved in child health care."[14] States are also required to provide dental care to children insured by CHIP.[15] In contrast, while states may elect to provide dental coverage to adults insured by Medicaid, they are not required to do so.

As the federal administrator of state Medicaid and CHIP plans, CMS monitors state Medicaid programs through the CMS-416 form, which requires states to report specific measures, including the total number of children eligible for EPSDT who received any dental service, preventive dental services, and dental treatment services (CMS, 1999). In response to criticism from the Government Accountability Office that data collected through CMS-416 were incomplete, inconsistent, and often based on un-reliable information, CMS recently updated the form to include questions such as the number of children who receive an oral health service from a nondentist, the total number of children receiving any dental or oral health service, and the number of children (ages 6–9 years and 10–14 years) who have received a protective sealant on at least one permanent molar tooth (CMS, 2011; Mann, 2009).

CMS has two goals related to oral health. The first is to increase the rate of children who are enrolled in Medicaid or CHIP who receive any preventive dental service by 10 percent over a 5-year period (CMS, 2010c). This goal will be applied with respect to each state's measured access rate as well as to the overall national rate. CMS's second goal is to increase the national rate of children ages 6–9 and 10–14 who receive a dental sealant on a permanent molar tooth by 10 percent over a 5-year period (CMS, 2010c). The baseline and progress for these goals will be based on data from the CMS-416 form and from the annual CHIP report.

CMS is working to improve guidance to states on oral health issues.

---

[13] 42 U.S.C. §1396d(r)(3).

[14] Ibid.

[15] *Children's Health Insurance Program Reauthorization Act of 2009*, Public Law 3, 111th Cong., 1st sess. (February 4, 2009).

The agency has established two advisory groups—the CMS Oral Health Technical Advisory Group and the EPSDT work group—to guide their dental policies (Mann, 2009). The technical advisory group is examining the effects of recent legislation on oral health programs, considering improvements to the CMS-416 annual reports, providing guidance to states about the EPSDT dental benefit, and improving materials used to inform beneficiaries of their Medicaid dental benefits (GAO, 2009). The EPSDT work group will help the agency prioritize and design projects to improve EPSDT services, including dental services (Mann, 2009). CMS anticipates that the work group may assist the agency in updating the state Medicaid manual, and provide training and support to state Medicaid and CHIP programs. The work group will comprise representatives from other federal agencies, states, a variety of health care professions, consumer groups, advocacy organizations, and researchers (Mann, 2009). In addition, CMS will be reviewing state Medicaid dental programs for innovative practices that have increased access to dental care and will be sharing the information about those practices with other states (HHS, 2010g).

CMS is also working directly with families whose children are insured by Medicaid and CHIP to educate them about oral health and connect them with oral health professionals. The Children's Health Insurance Program Reauthorization Act (CHIPRA)[16] requires HHS to develop a program to educate parents of newborns whose birth was funded by Medicaid or CHIP about the risks and prevention of early childhood caries. To connect more children with Medicaid providers, CMS developed the Insure Kids Now! website, which includes a current list of dentists and health care providers in each state (CMS, 2010b).

In testimony to the IOM committee, CMS identified the following initiatives it plans to undertake:

- Identifying state Medicaid dental programs that have demonstrated higher dental utilization rates and unique initiatives, and sharing those via the CMS Medicaid Promising Practices website as well as through national meetings with state partners;
- Identifying and promoting use of quality measures for access and health outcomes related to oral health services through collaboration with the Dental Quality Alliance and AHRQ;
- Providing state peer-to-peer learning opportunities to share successful strategies and lessons learned from state activities implemented to improve utilization rates through national policy academies, all-state conference calls, and other mechanisms;

---

[16] *Children's Health Insurance Program Reauthorization Act of 2009*, Public Law 3, 111th Cong., 1st sess. (February 4, 2009).

- Identifying ways that federal and state governments can encourage the expansion of the availability and supply of qualified oral health care professionals, including new mid-level practitioners, through collaboration with other HHS agency partners, the IOM, and others involved in current research in this area;
- A "Call-to-Action" request to states to develop action plans for breaking down barriers to children receiving oral health services and providing extensive technical assistance to states;
- Encouraging State Medicaid and CHIP participation in partnerships with state and local oral health organizations, including provider groups, advocacy groups, dental health professional organizations, and dental schools through incentives such as possible funding for meetings and travel costs to promote cooperation and coordination of service delivery;
- Enhancing outreach to beneficiaries through several strategies, including: federal-state education materials that provide a consistent message and information on the importance of oral health care, public service announcements, encouraging cross-agency collaborations at the state level for broad distribution of educational materials, and encouraging public-private partnerships for implementing beneficiary incentives to obtain services through the potential provision of educational materials and related expenses for distribution of materials;
- Assessing opportunities for advancing oral health initiatives as part of the prevention initiatives created under the new Patient Protection and Affordable Care Act (ACA);[17]
- Assessing opportunities for advancing oral health initiatives as part of the health information technology provisions of CHIPRA and the American Recovery and Reinvestment Act of 2009 (ARRA);[18]
- Leveraging new CHIPRA quality grants to states to foster the development of additional state-level approaches to ensuring access and quality of oral health care;
- Enhancing federal guidance to states on ensuring children's access to preventive and follow-up care through EPSDT, including oral health;
- Developing a strategy for oversight and compliance reviews if needed to ensure that particularly those states that have the lowest dental utilization rates are taking steps to come into compliance with EPSDT program requirements, including oral health; and

---

[17] *Patient Protection and Affordable Care Act*, Public Law 148, 111th Cong., 2nd sess. (March 23, 2010).

[18] *American Recovery and Reinvestment Act*, Public Law 5, 111th Cong., 1st sess. (February 17, 2009).

- Ongoing CMS collaboration with other federal agencies, including the CDC and HRSA, to provide comprehensive support and incentives to state efforts (CMS, 2010c).

While CMS is greatly involved in the oral health care of children, it is significant to note that the Medicare program, the primary source of health care coverage for adults over age 65, largely excludes oral health care. Medicare coverage and exclusions are discussed in Chapter 3.

Food and Drug Administration

The U.S. Food and Drug Administration (FDA) has responsibility to protect and advance public health. Their role includes assurance of "the safety, efficacy, and security" of drugs, biological products, and medical devices; advancement of innovations that make medicines "more effective, safer, and more affordable"; and provide the public with the "accurate, science-based information" needed to improve health (FDA, 2011a). The scope of drugs, devices, and other products regulated by the FDA is quite broad: for example, e.g., drugs, medical devices, biological products, food supply, cosmetics, tobacco products, and products that emit radiation (FDA, 2011a). The FDA approval process is challenging due to a balance needed between getting newer products to the market quickly and identifying concerns for patient safety. In recent years, the FDA approval process has been criticized as being slow and ineffective, but there has also been recognition of the broadening charges to the FDA without commensurate funding (IOM, 2007a,b, 2010a,c, 2011).

As with health care in general, the FDA regulates oral health devices, drugs, and products. For example, by law, the FDA regulates dental devices, including diagnostic devices (e.g., X-ray systems), prosthetic devices (e.g., dental amalgam, implants), surgical devices (e.g., dental drills), therapeutic devices (e.g., orthodontic appliances), and many other products (e.g., toothbrushes, dental floss).[19] Other forms of regulation include approval and labeling of prescription drugs (e.g., injectible forms of anesthesia) and over-the-counter products (e.g., toothpastes) (FDA, 2011b). The FDA also issues alerts regarding recall of products with concerns for patient safety.

Health Resources and Services Administration

Many of HRSA's bureaus and offices provide funding for oral health care activities; Appendix B includes a chart of the key HRSA agencies in-

---

[19] *Code of Federal Regulations*, Food and Drug Administration, Department of Health and Human Services, title 21, sec. 872.1–872.6890 (2010).

volved in oral health. In her presentation to this IOM committee, HRSA Administrator Mary Wakefield noted that HRSA programs collectively provide some oral health services to more than 3 million people (Wakefield, 2010). She also noted the recent creation within her office of an Office of Special Health Affairs, and within that, the Office of Strategic Priorities. This office acts as the HRSA administrator's primary advisor on oral health (as well as other major health issues), sets HRSA goals, and coordinates oral health activities within HRSA as well as among HHS agencies and other federal agencies (Anderson, 2010).

HRSA also maintains and operates 10 regional offices through its Office of Regional Operations (HRSA, 2011e). In addition to supporting HRSA's basic mission of improving the health care safety net, increasing quality of care, reducing disparities, and advancing public health, the Office of Regional Operations has the following core functions: (1) provide leadership to regions, states, and territories regarding HRSA's mission, goals, priorities and initiatives; (2) assess environmental trends in health care and recommend ways to improve HRSA policies and programs; (3) foster collaborations between HRSA and state health care leaders; (4) improve HRSA's alignment with public and private programs that are pursuing common goals; (5) provide technical assistance to HRSA grantees; and (6) support the recruitment and retention of primary health care providers in the health professional shortage areas (HRSA, 2011e).

Bureau of Primary Health Care

The Bureau of Primary Health Care (BPHC) allocates capital and operating funds to federally funded community health centers that receive grants under §330 of the Public Health Service Act (HRSA, 2010a). Federally Qualified Health Centers (FQHCs) encompass both federally funded health centers and "look-alike" health centers that meet all of the §330 federal requirements but do not receive federal grants. Preventive dental services are a requirement of all federally funded health centers.[20] Health centers provide oral health care services to low-income individuals both directly and through referrals to private professionals.[21] BPHC also manages the Service Expansion in Oral Health grants that provided additional funding to FQHCs to expand oral health care services. FQHCs serve more than 3 million dental patients and employ approximately 2,300 dentists, 900 dental hygienists, and 4,300 other dental personnel (Anderson, 2010).

---

[20] 42 U.S.C. §254b(b)(A)(i)(III)(hh).
[21] 42 U.S.C. §254b.

Bureau of Clinician Recruitment and Service

The Bureau of Clinician Recruitment and Service manages the previously discussed NHSC, which provides scholarships and loan repayment to clinicians, including dentists and dental hygienists, who agree to serve for 2–4 years in health professional shortage areas (HRSA, 2010e). In FY 2009, 464 dentists and 66 dental hygienists served in the NHSC (Anderson, 2010).

Bureau of Health Professions

The Bureau of Health Professions (BHP) plays an important role in developing the oral health workforce. BHP sponsors grants to support the health workforce, through training and diversity grants for health professional schools and students, and grants to states to support oral health workforce activities (HRSA, 2011a). In addition, BHP designates the Health Professional Shortage Areas. BHP sponsors the Advisory Committee on Training in Primary Care and Dentistry, which makes recommendations about workforce policy and program development in BHP (see Chapter 3 for more information on recent recommendations from this committee).

The HIV/AIDS Bureau

The HIV/AIDS Bureau sponsors several activities to improve the oral health care of persons with HIV/AIDS through both education of students and residents as well as grant funding to increase opportunities for provision of oral health care to this population (HRSA, 2011d). For example, the Ryan White Special Projects of National Significance Oral Health Initiative funds 15 demonstration sites for up to 5 years to support organizations using innovative models of care to provide oral health care to HIV-positive, underserved populations in both urban and nonurban settings (Anderson, 2010).

Maternal and Child Health Bureau

The Maternal and Child Health Bureau (MCHB) sponsors two centers focused on oral health: the National Maternal and Child Oral Health Resource Center (OHRC) and the National Oral Health Policy Center (OHPC). The OHRC collaborates with federal, state, and local agencies, national and state organizations and associations, and foundations to gather, develop, and share information and materials on oral health (OHRC, 2010a). The OHRC also collects, reviews, and disseminates Head Start oral health technical and programmatic information and materials

(OHRC, 2010b). The OHPC at the Children's Dental Health Project provides information and support to federal, state, and local programs and policy makers to promote policies that address disparities in children's oral health (OHPC, 2010). The ACA authorized MCHB grants for early childhood home visitation programs designed to improve maternal and child health, among other goals.[22] This program, if adequately funded and managed, would be an opportunity to educate parents about the transmissibility and prevention of dental caries.

Indian Health Service

The Division of Oral Health of the Indian Health Service (IHS) provides oral health care and promotes oral health improvements for American Indians and Alaska Natives (AI/AN). The IHS directly employs dentists and dental hygienists through the USPHS and the Federal Civil Service, but it has struggled to recruit and retain this workforce (Halliday, 2010). Many AI/AN communities are small, which makes it difficult for them to support a full-time dentist, and they are geographically isolated, which makes them difficult for traveling dentists to reach. A majority of AN, for example, live in villages that are not connected to the rest of the state by roads (Nash and Nagel, 2005). A major challenge to the IHS system is the high staff vacancy rate (Blahut, 2009). In October 2010, there were 52 vacancies for dental professionals (including 3 dental hygiene positions) in IHS facilities (USPHS, 2010b).

In early 2010, the IHS began an Early Childhood Caries (ECC) Initiative (IHS, 2010b). Through the initiative, the IHS is working with community partners such as Head Start, the Women's, Infants, and Children's Program, and nurses, doctors, and community health representatives to reduce the prevalence of ECC in AI/AN children by 25 percent by fiscal year 2015. Other goals of the initiative are to increase access to dental care for 0- to 5-year old AI/AN children by 10 percent in FY 2010 and 50 percent by FY 2015; to increase the number of children 0–5 years old who receive a fluoride varnish treatment by 10 percent in FY 2010 and 25 percent by FY 2015; and to increase the number of sealants among children 0–5 years old by 10 percent in FY 2010 and 25 percent by 2015.

The IHS is piloting several other projects designed to improve the oral health of AI/AN populations, including using chemotherapeutics to treat ECC, nonsurgical intervention for the treatment of periodontal disease in diabetic and prediabetic patients, and implementing electronic dental re-

---

[22] *Patient Protection and Affordable Care Act*, Public Law 148, 111th Cong., 2nd sess. (March 23, 2010).

cords (IHS, 2010a).[23] Finally, the IHS has been involved in the use of dental therapists to care for AN communities (see Chapter 3).

National Institutes of Health

Most of the oral health activities at the NIH occur in the NIDCR. The NIDCR's work is guided by four goals articulated in its strategic plan: using the best science to solve problems in oral, dental, and craniofacial health; strengthening the pipeline of researchers dedicated to solving problems in oral, dental, and craniofacial health; identifying innovative clinical research avenues to improve oral, dental, and craniofacial health; applying rigorous, multidisciplinary research approaches to eliminate disparities in oral, dental, and craniofacial health (NIDCR, 2010d). Extramural and intramural research supported by the NIDCR provides much of the scientific basis for the practice of dentistry.

In excess of 75 percent of the NIDCR's budget funds extramural research grants (NIDCR, 2010b). The NIDCR supports extramural research in oral and craniofacial biology, clinical research, and translational genetics and genomics. Recently, the NIDCR has funded several notable projects in oral health disparities. In fiscal year 2009, oral health disparities activities made up 14 percent of NIDCR's extramural research budget.[24] These activities include five Centers for Research to Reduce Disparities in Oral Health, where researchers from diverse disciplines partner with communities to research disparities in early childhood caries and oral cancers (NIDCR, 2010a). Using funds from ARRA, the NIDCR funded several developmental projects on oral health disparities, including a study examining gaps in access to dental care for pregnant women, a study that examines how a low dental literacy population interprets dental health prevention information, a study that examines the acceptability and feasibility of a community-based Latino lay health worker, or *promotora*, and a study that examines the predictors and outcomes of the age of a child at the first preventive dental visit for children enrolled in Medicaid.[23] The remainder of NIDCR's budget is used for intramural research and research management and support among its eights branches (NIDCR, 2010e).

The NIDCR and the CDC Division of Oral Health cosponsor the Dental, Oral, and Craniofacial Data Resource Center, which provides several resources for the research and policy-making communities, including a catalog of surveys related to oral health, descriptions of national and state oral

---

[23] Personal communication, C. Halliday, Indian Health Service, June 7, 2010.

[24] Written testimony of NIDCR to the Committee on an Oral Health Initiative is in the committee's public access file.

health surveys, and a tool for generating tables and statistical analysis based on the national and state oral health surveys (NIDCR and CDC, 2010).

The NIH offers several loan repayment programs for health professionals (including dentists) in which, in exchange for repayment of student loans, the professionals agree to perform relevant research over a given period of time. This research may be performed outside of the NIH at qualified locations or within the NIH (for NIH employees) (NIH, 2009b).

Office of the Assistant Secretary for Health

The Office of the Assistant Secretary for Health, formerly known as the Office of Public Health and Science, has a major role in oral health care in that it oversees the Commissioned Corps of the USPHS. The Surgeon General directly oversees the operation of the USPHS. The USPHS has 6,500-plus professionals (including dentists) who lead the nation's public health programs and advance public health science (USPHS, 2010a). As of 2008, there were 376 dentists serving in the USPHS (USPHS, 2008). The primary areas dental officers work in within the USPHS are clinical dentistry (including direct patient care), dental forensics (in disasters), and oral health education (USPHS, 2010e). USPHS dental officers may work within HHS agencies (e.g., IHS, HRSA) or within agencies (e.g., U.S. Coast Guard, Bureau of Prisons). As part of the USPHS compensation package, dental officers may be eligible for repayment of dental school loans (USPHS, 2010d).

The surgeon general appoints a chief professional officer for each of the individual professional categories of the USPHS Commissioned Corps. The role of the chief dental officer is to provide leadership and coordination for dental officers and to advise the Office of the Surgeon General and HHS on the recruitment, assignment, deployment, retention, and career development of USPHS dentists (USPHS, 2008). Chief dental officers have 4-year terms, and they typically retain substantial responsibilities in the agency from which they were selected. For example, Dr. William Bailey, the current chief dental officer, serves in a dual role as a dental officer within CDC's Division of Oral Health (ADA, 2010).

Within the USPHS, the Dental Professional Advisory Committee (DePAC) "provides advice and consultation . . . on issues related to professional practices and personnel activities of Civil Service and Commissioned Corps dentists" (USPHS, 2010c). The DePAC provides this assistance to the surgeon general, the chief dental officer of the USPHS, and dental program directors. Membership of the DePAC reflects many of the USPHS agencies and operating divisions. Their goals include assistance in recruitment, training, and use of USPHS dentists; development of reports and position papers; promotion of utilization of oral health professionals; promotion of cooperation and communication among oral health professionals; and promotion of oral health in all USPHS agencies and programs.

The assistant secretary of health has another major role in oral health as the colead for a new HHS oral health initiative that is discussed later in this chapter.

ROLE OF HHS IN PREVENTION

Chapter 2 documented the evidence base establishing the key role of prevention in many oral diseases. HHS plays a key role in promoting the adoption of evidence-based preventive oral health services, including those provided at the national, state, community, and personal levels. The previous sections have already touched upon some ways in which HHS promotes prevention in oral health care, such as FDA's role in regulating oral health products and therapies. Two other significant roles include AHRQ's convening of the USPSTF and CDC's convening of the TFCPS. The USPSFT reviews clinical research to assess the merits of preventive interventions. The USPSTF makes recommendations about which services should be incorporated into routine medical care, based on the strength of the evidence (USPSTF, 2010). Table 4-1 highlights a number of recent recommendations, conclusions, and statements made by the USPSTF that relate to craniofacial and oral health for both children and adults. The committee notes that significant time has passed since the USPSTF determined that there was insufficient evidence to make recommendations for routine risk assessment of children and oral cancer screening for adults. It urges the task force to consider whether sufficient evidence has been published since 2004 to make conclusive recommendations.

The CDC convenes the TFCPS, which is similar to the USPSTF but focuses on community preventive services (Task Force on Community Preventive Services, 2010). Table 4-2 describes oral health–related community-level interventions recommended by the TFCPS.

Other CDC Activities

The NCCDPHP supports research that investigates and improves prevention of oral diseases. Recently, the NCCDPHP supported research on the effectiveness of dental sealants (Griffin et al., 2008, 2009; Oong et al., 2008). The NCCDPHP also publishes guidelines and recommendations for best practices in oral health (CDC, 2010d). It promotes water fluoridation, has established infection control guidelines for practitioners, and has made recommendations for a variety of prevention programs, including school-based dental sealant programs, population-based interventions to prevent and control dental caries and oral and pharyngeal cancers,

TABLE 4-1
USPSTF Oral Health-Related Recommendations, Conclusions, and Statements

Date	Recommendation/Conclusion/Statement	USPSTF Grade
May 2009	Recommend all women planning or capable of pregnancy take a daily supplement containing 0.4 to 0.8 mg (400 to 800 ug) of folic acid.	A
April 2009	Recommend clinicians ask all adults about tobacco use and provide tobacco cessation interventions for those who use tobacco products.	A
April 2009	Recommend clinicians ask all pregnant women about tobacco use and provide augmented, pregnancy-tailored counseling for those who smoke.	A
April 2004	Recommend primary care clinicians prescribe oral fluoride supplementation at currently recommended doses to preschool children older than 6 months of age whose primary water source is deficient in fluoride.	B
April 2004	Conclude that the evidence is insufficient to recommend for or against routine risk assessment of preschool children by primary care clinicians for the prevention of dental disease.	1 Statement
February 2004	Conclude that the evidence is insufficient to recommend for or against routinely screening adults for oral cancer.	1 Statement
1996	The USPSTF recognizes the importance of preventing dental and periodontal disease. However, it has determined that there is no new evidence regarding the role of the primary care clinician in counseling for dental services. The USPSTF will not update its 1996 recommendation.	

SOURCE: USPSTF, 2010.

and sports-related craniofacial injuries (CDC Fluoride Recommendations Work Group, 2001; Gooch et al., 2009; Kohn et al., 2003; Task Force on Community Preventive Services, 2001). The CDC also provides grants and technical assistance to states for developing oral health infrastructure, including water fluoridation (CDC, 2010h). The ACA included several provisions that will improve the CDC's ability to assist the states in preventing

TABLE 4-2
TFCPS Oral Health–Related Recommendations

Preventing Dental Caries	
Community water fluoridation	Recommended
State- or community-wide sealant promotion	Insufficient evidence
School-based or -linked sealant delivery programs	Recommended

Preventing Oral and Pharyngeal Cancers	
Population-based interventions for early detection	Insufficient evidence

Preventing Oral and Pharyngeal Cancers	
Population-based interventions to encourage use of helmets, facemasks, and mouth guards in contact sports	Insufficient evidence

SOURCE: CDC, 2010g.

oral disease, if funded.[25] The bill requires the CDC to establish a 5-year oral health campaign related to prevention and award grants to all states, territories, Indians, Indian tribes, tribal organizations, and urban Indian organizations to develop school-based sealant programs. In addition, the ACA will improve the surveillance capabilities of the CDC and states by authorizing oral health infrastructure grants to all states and improvements to the oral health components of several national health surveys.

ROLE OF HHS IN HEALTH LITERACY

Chapter 2 documented the basics of health literacy and the status of the oral health literacy of both health care professionals and the general public. The federal government has a role to play in improving oral health literacy and has several specific actions that target the general health literacy of both the public and health care professionals.

AHRQ Health Literacy Universal Precautions Toolkit

AHRQ developed the Health Literacy Universal Precautions Toolkit to help primary care providers improve communication with people of all literacy levels (DeWalt et. al., 2010). The toolkit provides methods to improve spoken communication, written communication, self-management,

---

[25] *Patient Protection and Affordable Care Act*, Public Law 148, 111th Cong., 2nd sess. (March 23, 2010).

and supportive systems, and is aimed at all employees in a primary care office, from the receptionist to the physician. Examples of tools include using the teach-back method, in which health care professionals ask the patient to repeat back information to assure that the patient understands; assessing the phone system and procedures to ensure that telephone communications are friendly and understandable for all patients; designing easy-to-read materials; creating patient-centered action plans; and connecting patients to community resources. Because it is often unclear to professionals which patients have low health literacy, the toolkit encourages them to take "universal precautions," in other words, to use the tools with all patients regardless of their perceived literacy level.

Healthy People 2010/2020 Health Communications Objectives

Recognizing the importance of health communication to improving public health and health care, HHS has included health communications objectives in the last two versions of *Healthy People*. *Healthy People 2010* included six health communications objectives, which *Healthy People 2020* has expanded to 13 (see Box 4-3) (HHS, 2000a, 2010c). Encouragingly, two of the *Healthy People 2010* goals were archived because the objectives have been met. The new goals reflect the increased use of health information technology and the advent of personalized medicine.

HHS National Action Plan to Improve Health Literacy

In May 2010, HHS released the National Action Plan to Improve Health Literacy, which aims to situate health literacy improvement in the context of public health. Over a 3-year period, more than 700 individuals and organizations representing health care, public health, education, consumers, social services, communication, and the media participated in the effort. The plan starts out with a vision for a society that

- Provides everyone access to accurate and actionable health information,
- Delivers person-centered health information and services, and
- Supports lifelong learning and skills to promote good health (HHS, 2010i).

In addition, the plan defines seven goals to improve health literacy (see Box 4-4).

While not specific to oral health, this plan is certainly important to the attention needed to effect an improvement of oral health literacy for both

---

BOX 4-3
Healthy People 2020: **Health Communication and Health Information Technology Proposed Objectives**

1. Improve the health literacy of the population.
2. Increase the proportion of persons who report that their health care providers have satisfactory communication skills.
3. Increase the proportion of persons who report that their health care providers always involved them in decisions about their health care as much as they wanted.
4. Increase the proportion of patients whose doctor recommends personalized health information resources to help them manage their health.
5. Increase the proportion of persons who use electronic personal health management tools.
6. Increase individuals' access to the Internet.
7. Increase the proportion of adults who report having friends or family members whom they talk with about their health.
8. Increase the proportion of quality, health-related websites.
9. Increase the proportion of online health information seekers who report easily accessing health information.
10. Increase the proportion medical practices that use electronic health records.
11. Increase the proportion of meaningful users of health information technology.
12. Increase the proportion of crisis and emergency risk messages intended to protect the public's health that demonstrate the use of best practices.
13. Increase social marketing in health promotion and disease prevention.

SOURCE: HHS, 2010c.

---

patients and professionals, especially considering that oral health is a part of general health.

National Standards on Culturally and Linguistically Appropriate Services

Recognizing the increasing diversity of the U.S. population and the increasing disparities in health status and access to health care for diverse populations, the HHS Office of Minority Health published National Standards on Culturally and Linguistically Appropriate Services (CLAS standards) in 2001 (see Box 4-5). Organizations both inside and outside HHS have adopted the CLAS standards as a tool to evaluate the cultural

BOX 4-4
Goals of the National Action Plan
to Improve Health Literacy

1. Develop and disseminate health and safety information that is accurate, accessible, and actionable.
2. Promote changes in the health care system that improve health information, communication, informed decision making, and access to health services.
3. Incorporate accurate, standards-based, and developmentally appropriate health and science information and curricula in child care and education through the university level.
4. Support and expand local efforts to provide adult education, English language instruction, and culturally and linguistically appropriate health information services in the community.
5. Build partnerships, develop guidance, and change policies.
6. Increase basic research and the development, implementation, and evaluation of practices and interventions to improve health literacy.
7. Increase the dissemination and use of evidence-based health literacy practices and interventions

SOURCE: HHS, 2010i.

competence of health care. For example, while the use of CLAS standards is not mandatory in Medicare, in 2008, Congress asked the OIG to examine Medicare provider and plan compliance with these standards (OIG, 2010). The Joint Commission, which accredits a variety of health care organizations and programs, also incorporated the CLAS standards into its accreditation requirements (The Joint Commission, 2008).

Web-Based Information and Training

HRSA already has made the effort to share and disseminate information on cultural competence. On its own website, HRSA maintains a portal on "Cultural Competency and Health Literacy Resources for Health Care Providers" (http://www.hrsa.gov/culturalcompetence/). This website is a repository for assessment tools, culture- and language-specific information, technical assistance, and training curricula. The website also includes web-based training tools. The Office of Minority Health also maintains content on its website related to cultural competency that includes training tools "for physicians and others" (OMH, 2010).

Public Education

In part, improving the knowledge of individuals needs to start with the education of children in the importance of oral health. In 2002, the House of Delegates of the Academy of General Dentistry adopted a policy in this regard:

> Resolved, that the Academy of General Dentistry advocates incorporation of oral health education into primary and secondary curricula with measurable outcomes, as a proven and cost-effective disease prevention and universal health promotion program. (Halpern, 2010)

The 2004 IOM report *Health Literacy: A Prescription to End Confusion* noted that "the U.S. educational systems offer a primary point of intervention to improve the quality of literacy and health literacy" (IOM, 2004). The report also noted that "public educational systems in the United States are influenced by national policy and funding, but remain under the jurisdiction of and are funded by states and localities." While most elementary, middle, and high schools require health education classes, these programs lack consistency (IOM, 2004). In addition, given the breadth of topics that need to be covered in these classes, many teachers are unprepared to teach specific topics (Peterson et al., 2001). The percentage of states that require school districts to teach health education increased from 61 percent to 75 percent between 2000 and 2006 (Kann et al., 2007). In 2006, 74.5 percent of elementary schools, 54.6 percent of middle schools, and 55.1 percent of high schools included oral and dental health as a required part of the health education curriculum (Kann et al., 2007).

The National Center for Education Statistics, part of the Department of Education, collects data and produces reports on the status of American education (http://nces.ed.gov/). The Department of Education may be able to play a role in providing guidance to states on best practices for improving health literacy through the public school system. (See later in this chapter for more on the role of the Department of Education in oral health.)

Grants for Oral Health Literacy Research

NIH and AHRQ have partnered to fund grants for health literacy research (NIH, 2011). These grants were first announced in 2004 and have been renewed through 2013 (NIH, 2006, 2011). In the past, these grants have been used to fund research on a wide variety of health literacy topics, including developing instruments for oral health literacy assessment, assessing the oral health knowledge, opinions, and practices among Latinos, and assessing the health promotion activities in a dental clinic (NIH, 2009c).

BOX 4-5
National Standards for Culturally and Linguistically
Appropriate Services in Health Care

Standard 1: Health care organizations should ensure that patients/consumers receive from all staff members effective, understandable, and respectful care that is provided in a manner compatible with their cultural health beliefs and practices and preferred language.

Standard 2: Health care organizations should implement strategies to recruit, retain, and promote at all levels of the organization a diverse staff and leadership that are representative of the demographic characteristics of the service area.

Standard 3: Health care organizations should ensure that staff at all levels and across all disciplines receive ongoing education and training in culturally and linguistically appropriate service delivery.

Standard 4: Health care organizations must offer and provide language assistance services, including bilingual staff and interpreter services, at no cost to each patient/consumer with limited English proficiency at all points of contact, in a timely manner during all hours of operation.

Standard 5: Health care organizations must provide to patients/consumers in their preferred language both verbal offers and written notices informing them of their right to receive language assistance services.

Standard 6: Health care organizations must assure the competence of language assistance provided to limited English proficient patients/consumers by interpreters and bilingual staff. Family and friends should not be used to provide interpretation services (except on request by the patient/consumer).

Standard 7: Health care organizations must make available easily understood patient-related materials and post signage in the languages of the commonly encountered groups and/or groups represented in the service area.

ROLE OF HHS IN EDUCATION AND TRAINING

HHS is involved in training the oral health workforce and the health workforce more broadly. Several agencies within HHS continue to support training and educating the oral health workforce, particularly the workforce that cares for underserved populations, including children, older adults, and

Standard 8: Health care organizations should develop, implement, and promote a written strategic plan that outlines clear goals, policies, operational plans, and management accountability/oversight mechanisms to provide culturally and linguistically appropriate services.

Standard 9: Health care organizations should conduct initial and ongoing organizational self-assessments of CLAS-related activities and are encouraged to integrate cultural and linguistic competence-related measures into their internal audits, performance improvement programs, patient satisfaction assessments, and outcomes-based evaluations.

Standard 10: Health care organizations should ensure that data on the individual patient's/consumer's race, ethnicity, and spoken and written language are collected in health records, integrated into the organization's management information systems, and periodically updated.

Standard 11: Health care organizations should maintain a current demographic, cultural, and epidemiological profile of the community as well as a needs assessment to accurately plan for and implement services that respond to the cultural and linguistic characteristics of the service area.

Standard 12: Health care organizations should develop participatory, collaborative partnerships with communities and use a variety of formal and informal mechanisms to facilitate community and patient/consumer involvement in designing and implementing CLAS-related activities.

Standard 13: Health care organizations should ensure that conflict and grievance resolution processes are culturally and linguistically sensitive and capable of identifying, preventing, and resolving cross-cultural conflicts or complaints by patients/consumers.

Standard 14: Health care organizations are encouraged to regularly make available to the public information about their progress and successful innovations in implementing the CLAS standards and to provide public notice in their communities about the availability of this information.

SOURCE: OMH, 2001.

people with special needs (Ng et al., 2008). HRSA provides grants to dental and hygiene schools and residency programs through Title VII and workforce grants to states. CMS provides graduate medical education (GME) funding to hospitals and dental schools for training dental residents through Medicare. NIH supports dental researchers through grants and fellowships.

HHS also supports some interdisciplinary training and care through Title VII grants as well as funding from recent health reform legislation.

Public investment in dental education is driven by the belief that education has a broad impact on the number and quality of dentists that are available to serve the oral health needs of the population. Federal support for dental education allowed dental schools to expand dramatically between 1960 and 1980; 13 new dental schools were built, and graduating classes grew from 3,775 in 1970–1971 to 5,756 in 1982–1983 (HRSA, 2005). Government support, however, has lagged recently. In 2005, HRSA released a report stating that "federal and state involvement in matters concerning the adequacy of the dental workforce has been intermittent, uncoordinated, and inconsistent" (HRSA, 2005).

Title VII Support for Training

Title VII training grants for dentistry currently take two forms: grants to increase the workforce that is prepared to care for vulnerable populations, and grants to diversify the workforce, though the public policy goals of the Title VII grants have varied over time. When the grants were established in the Health Professions Educational Assistance Act of 1963,[26] Congress intended them to expand the supply and diversity of dentists and physicians due to concern over access to and maldistribution of practitioners (HRSA, 2005; Reynolds, 2008). This commitment to expanding and diversifying the health workforce continued through the mid-1970s with passage of the Health Professions Educational Assistance Amendments of 1965,[27] the Health Manpower Act of 1968,[28] and the Comprehensive Health Manpower Training Act of 1971[29] (Reynolds, 2008). Funding during this era was often tied to increasing class size: schools were given funds for construction, enhancing curriculum, and faculty support in exchange for a promise to enroll more students. Beginning in the mid-1970s, the focus of Title VII shifted to addressing the shortage of primary care providers, including dentists, especially in underserved areas (HRSA, 2005; Reynolds, 2008). The Health Professions Educational Assistance Act of 1976[30] required Title VII grant recipients to either require dental students

---

[26] *Health Professions Educational Assistance Act of 1963*, Public Law 129, 88th Congress, 1st sess. (September 24, 1963).

[27] *Health Professions Educational Assistance Amendments of 1965*, Public Law 290, 89th Cong., 1st sess. (October 22, 1965).

[28] *Health Manpower Act of 1968*, Public Law 490, 90th Cong., 2d sess. (August 16, 1968).

[29] *Comprehensive Health Manpower Training Act of 1971*, Public Law 157, 92d Cong., 1st sess. (November 18, 1971).

[30] *Health Professions Educational Assistance Act of 1976*, Public Law 484, 94th Cong., 2d sess. (October 12, 1976).

to rotate in underserved and urban communities or dedicate a percentage of residency slots to general dentistry training, dramatically expanded the National Health Service Corps, and provided significant funding to train dental auxiliaries (Reynolds, 2008). This commitment to primary care continued throughout the 1980s, although it had limited success in encouraging practitioners to work in underserved areas (HRSA, 2005; Reynolds, 2008). Most recently, Title VII funding has focused on developing a workforce that is prepared to care for vulnerable populations and promoting diversity in the health professions (Reynolds, 2008). For example, all Title VII grants are now subject to grant scoring mechanisms that give preference to departments that train primary care practitioners or who provide most of their care to patients in medically underserved communities. Additionally, since 1998, all grant applications have had to propose curricula targeting vulnerable populations (Reynolds, 2008).

Title VII has been successful at expanding residencies in general and pediatric dentistry, which were, until recently, the only dental disciplines for which the grants were available. Between 72 and 75 percent of the growth in general dentistry residencies between 1977 and 1995 can be attributed to Title VII support (Duffy et al., 1997). Title VII–funded dental residencies have been successful at recruiting and training underrepresented minorities, and graduates of Title VII–funded medical residencies are more likely to provide care to underserved communities and populations and more prepared to provide culturally competent care (Edelstein et al., 2003; Green et al., 2008; HHS, 2003a).

The ACA significantly expanded the number of grants available for dental training. Title VII funds are now available for

- Dental public health residencies in addition to general and pediatric dentistry;
- Dental hygiene programs in general, pediatric, and public health dentistry;
- Predoctoral training programs in general, pediatric, and public health dentistry;
- Faculty development programs in general, pediatric, and public health dentistry;
- Technical assistance to pediatric dentistry training programs;
- Financial assistance to dentists who plan to teach or are teaching in general, pediatric, or public health dentistry; and
- Faculty loan repayment programs for general, pediatric, and public health dentists who agree to serve as full-time faculty.

Previously, training grants for dentistry were grouped together with grants for medicine in Title VII, section 747, of the Public Health Service

Act. The ACA removes dentistry from section 747 and creates a new section 748: Training in General, Pediatric, and Public Health Dentistry. As a result of the significant expansion of dental training grants, HRSA's Advisory Committee on Training in Primary Care Medicine and Dentistry advised the Secretary of Health and Human Services to create a separate Advisory Committee in General, Pediatric, and Public Health Dentistry (HHS, 2010h).

Several Title VII grants are specifically targeted to increase the diversity of the health care workforce. Dental schools with significant enrollment of underrepresented minority students are eligible for Centers of Excellence grants to improve recruitment and training of minority students. Each center must agree to develop a competitive applicant pool; enhance academic performance; support faculty development to train, recruit, and retain underrepresented minority faculty; address minority health issues through clinical education and curriculum; facilitate research in minority health; and train students in community-based settings that provide a significant amount of care to underrepresented minorities.[31] Health Careers Opportunity Program grants are available to dental and dental hygiene schools to establish or extend programs to identify, recruit, and support students from disadvantaged backgrounds.[32] Scholarships for Disadvantaged Students grants provide funding to dental and dental hygiene schools for financial aid to disadvantaged students.[33] Individuals from disadvantaged backgrounds who agree to serve as faculty for at least 2 years at dental and dental hygiene schools are eligible for the Faculty Loan Repayment Program.[34]

Grants to States for Training

HRSA also supports the training of the oral health workforce through grants to states for innovative programs to address the dental workforce needs of designated dental health professional shortage areas.[35] States can use these grants a number of ways, including to recruit oral health professionals, to expand dental residencies, to support service expansion, and to establish faculty recruitment programs. In the past, states have increased the availability of school, community, and mobile-based oral health care; developed cultural competence curriculum for allied health professionals; and implemented school-based sealant programs, among many others (HRSA, 2011a).

---

[31] 42 U.S.C. §293.
[32] 42 U.S.C. §293c.
[33] 42 U.S.C. §293a.
[34] 42 U.S.C. §293b
[35] 42 U.S.C. §256g.

GME Support for Training

GME payments are also available to train dental residents who train inside the hospital.[36] Hospitals used to be able to receive GME for dental residents who trained at affiliated institutions outside the hospital, including dental school–based residency programs (HCFA, 1989).[37] However, in 2003, CMS issued a regulation clarifying it would no longer make any GME payments for residents whose training had historically been paid for by dental schools (CMS, 2003). Dental schools could not substitute GME payments for alternative sources of funding.[38] As a result of this rule, 26 dental schools lost funding for most or all of their residency programs, while the 6 additional schools that had GME agreements were not affected (Bresch, 2010).

A special type of GME funding is available for independent children's teaching hospitals, which are generally not eligible for standard GME funding. In 2000, Congress established the Children's Hospitals Graduate Medical Education Payment Program, which provides children's teaching hospitals with funding to train health professionals who focus on children's unique health care needs (HRSA, 2011c). This funding is available to train both dental and medical residents.[39]

Support from HHS Divisions

Both the NIH and the NIDCR support dental researchers through loan repayment, fellowships, and scholarships. NIH loan repayment programs include support for clinical researchers, pediatric researchers, health disparities researchers, and clinical researchers from disadvantaged backgrounds. The NIDCR also sponsors scholarships for students who are pursuing dual D.D.S./D.M.D.-Ph.D. programs. HRSA's Bureau of Health Professions funds dental public health residency training grants to support approved residencies in dental public health (HRSA, 2010c). The CDC's NCCDPHP sponsors a dental public health residency with the goal of producing dental public health specialists that can work in a variety of settings, such as in health agencies, research settings, or financing systems, to improve the oral health of populations (CDC, 2010a). In addition, the CDC trains health professionals, including dentists, in applied epidemiology through fellow-

---

[36] *Code of Federal Regulations*, Centers for Medicare and Medicaid Services, Department of Health and Human Services, title 42, sec. 413.75 (2009).

[37] *Balanced Budget Act of 1997*, Public Law 33, 105th Cong., 1st sess. (August 5, 1997):34621.

[38] *Code of Federal Regulations*, Centers for Medicare and Medicaid Services, Department of Health and Human Services, title 42, sec. 413.81 (2009).

[39] 42 U.S.C. §256e.

ships and the Epidemic Intelligence Service (CDC, 2011). The IHS is also involved in training dentists and dental students. The IHS runs a comprehensive continuing dental education program for its staff, and it trains dental students through an externship program for second- and third-year students (Halliday, 2010).

The USPHS offers Commissioned Officer Student Training and Extern Programs (COSTEP) to a variety of students (including dental students) (USPHS, 2011). The *junior* version of the program is offered to students at the baccalaureate level and above to gain experience working in public health settings (usually during summer vacations). Students are compensated for their time. In the *senior* version of the program, students near graduation are given financial assistance toward their education in return for an obliged period of service to the USPHS after graduation.

Interdisciplinary Training

The value of interdisciplinary care was discussed in Chapter 3, and HHS plays a role in promoting interdisciplinary team care through training grants. Some recent and ongoing examples of HHS' efforts to promote interdisciplinary training include: $29.5 million from the ACA and the ARRA to fund interdisciplinary geriatric training (HHS, 2010e), and the Title VII interdisciplinary, community-based grant programs, which are designed to promote interdisciplinary care and increase access to care for underserved populations and in underserved areas.[40] In its most recent report to the secretary and Congress, the Advisory Committee on Training in Primary Care and Dentistry recommended additional funding for training programs that promote interprofessional practice (HHS, 2010b).

HHS COLLABORATIONS WITH THE PRIVATE SECTOR

While this report focuses on the role HHS alone has in improving the oral health of the nation, the committee notes that there are many opportunities for HHS to partner with multiple other stakeholders, such as those in the private sector (including consumers). The need for effective public-private partnerships has been a central theme across time as HHS has sought to improve oral health care. For example, the Meskin Commission in 1989 had predominately private-sector representation, along with collaborators from various federal agencies. In addition, the Meskin report called for greater interaction with national dental organizations within the department and more input from private dentistry (Interim Study Group on Dental Activities, 1989).

---

[40] 42 U.S.C. §§294 et seq.

Healthy People (discussed previously throughout this report) represents a successful collaboration between the public and private sectors to develop national goals and objectives. Another example of a public-private partnership is the Friends of the NIDCR, created in 1998 (upon the 50th anniversary of the NIDCR) to "educate the public and key decision makers about the importance of investing in the NIDCR" (FNIDCR, 2010a). As a non-for-profit 501(c)(3), the foundation brings together a coalition of key stakeholders, including advocacy groups, dental schools and societies, corporations, and individuals to educate Congress and the administration about the importance of oral health research. Another example is the partnership between the CDC and the Association of State and Territorial Dental Directors to establish the previously discussed National Oral Health Surveillance System. This system can track state-level data that can be used to monitor progress toward *Healthy People* goals, justify budget allocations, and guide state policy development (Crall, 2009; Malvitz et al., 2009).

As the professional organization representing about 70 percent of practicing dentists in the United States (Gist, 2010), the ADA is a key partner for HHS. The ADA is actively involved in lobbying the government regarding oral health issues. In 2010, the ADA spent $2.6 million on lobbying related to funding for community-based prevention, the recruitment of dentists, and improving the Medicaid dental program, especially for low-income adults, making it the fourth largest lobbying group among all health professional groups (Center for Responsive Politics, 2009, 2010a,b).

The ADA has convened several summits that included stakeholders from both the public and private sectors. For example, in 2007 they convened the American Indian/Alaskan Native Oral Health Access Summit (ADA, 2007). In 2009, they convened the Access to Dental Care Summit, which included representatives from state dental societies, the dental industry, dental specialty interest groups, federal programs, health care policy makers, other health care professions, dental education and research institutions, consumer advocacy groups, finance organizations, ADA leadership, volunteer dental leaders, and safety net dental providers (ADA, 2009). Overall, participants sought to identify common ground for the future in areas such as workforce development, financing, prevention, literacy, quality assessment, and better collaboration between professions. From 2001 to 2008, the Office of Head Start partnered with MCHB and the Association of State and Territorial Dental Directors to foster collaboration between Head Start programs and state oral health programs. During the course of the collaboration, state oral health programs reported becoming more actively involved in Head Start programs and all 50 states developed Head Start oral health action plans (Geurink and Isman, 2009). In 2007, the Office of Head Start began a collaborative effort with the American Academy of Pediatric Dentistry on a Dental Home Initiative. The goal of the initiative was to establish dental homes for all Head Start children, to develop oral health leadership and infrastructure at the regional and state levels, and to expand oral education for Head Start children, families, and staff. However, in 2010, the Office of Head Start announced it would not exercise the two remaining option years for the American Academy of Pediatric Dentistry's partnership on the project (AAPD, 2010).

Recently, two efforts have arisen to promote the sharing of health data and encourage innovation in the use of the data. First, HHS' Community Health Data Initiative is an effort to provide the public with free access to "easily accessible, standardized, structured, downloadable data on health care, health, and determinants of health performance at the national, state, and county levels, as well as by age, gender, race/ethnicity, and income (where available)" (HHS, 2011a). This will include data from CMS and *Healthy People*, including data that have not been available to the public in the past. HHS hopes to use this effort to encourage all interested parties to use the data in innovative ways that will benefit the public as a whole. HHS compares this effort to that of the National Oceanic and Atmospheric Administration, which openly shares weather data that users can turn into websites, applications, and other useful tools for the public domain (HHS, 2011a). Similarly, the Blue Button Initiative, a partnership between CMS and the VA, will aim to promote public innovation related to improving the use of personal health information (CMS, 2010a).

Finally, there is a history of consumer involvement within HHS agencies as the department has sought to advance oral health for patients. For example, the National Institute for Dental Research and later the NIDCR sought (and continues to seek) the input of patient advocacy organizations in conducting its research work (NIDCR, 2008). Patient advocacy organizations also voluntarily partner with and participate through foundations such as the Friends of NIDCR (FNIDCR, 2010b). This reflects the recent movement toward patient-centeredness and shared decision making (IOM, 2001).

ROLES OF OTHER FEDERAL AGENCIES

The committee also notes that other parts of the federal government are responsible for the delivery of oral health care as well as collection of oral health data for their relevant populations. The following sections highlight just some areas in which other federal departments are involved in oral health.

Department of Agriculture

The U.S. Department of Agriculture (USDA) is most notably involved in oral health through its Special Supplemental Nutrition Program for Women, Infants, and Children (WIC) that "provides federal grants to states for supplemental foods, health care referrals, and nutrition education for low-income pregnant, breastfeeding, and non-breastfeeding postpartum women, and to infants and children up to age five who are found to be at nutritional risk" (USDA, 2010b). WIC is often the first contact with the health care system for low-income children and their mothers (Mitchell, 2010). WIC has been a tremendous source of education for young mothers about nutrition and immunization and could be a great setting to educate on oral health as well. WIC is administered by the Food and Nutrition Service of the USDA, providing grants to 90 state agencies who administer the program at more than 10,000 WIC clinics (Mitchell, 2010). In addition to the educational services they provide, WIC agencies work to improve the linkage between their clients and outside health care professionals— including dentists—through referrals to the provider networks they have developed. At a 2010 IOM workshop on planning a WIC research agenda, speakers addressed the research needed to ensure WIC's continued effectiveness, including "how to include oral health screening, fluoride treatment, dental sealant application, and other basic oral-health examination and referrals as part of WIC services, considering that poor oral health is a silent epidemic, especially in the pediatric population" (IOM, 2010b).

The USDA's Food and Nutrition Information Center also provides educational services to its clients. For example, one recent document provided information on toddler nutrition, including links to numerous resources (NAL, 2009). Among the educational materials included were links to a CDC website that detailed the steps to follow in caring for the teeth of a child. The USDA document included resources from the American Academy of Pediatrics (AAP) that described good oral health practices and strategies for keeping teeth healthy throughout childhood. The document also provided links to materials from the Kansas Head Start Association regarding appropriate containers (e.g., to avoid baby bottle tooth decay) and included advice on making better food and drink choices.

Every 5 years, the USDA and HHS work collaboratively to produce national Dietary Guidelines for Americans. In 2005, a key recommendation for carbohydrates was "[r]educe the incidence of dental caries by practicing good oral hygiene and consuming sugar- and starch-containing foods and beverages less frequently" (HHS and USDA, 2005). The USDA runs the National School Lunch Program; these meals must meet the relevant recommendations of the Dietary Guidelines for Americans (USDA, 2010a). However, the federal regulations for the program concentrate on fat content, caloric intake, and recommended daily allowances of certain nutrients, and not on the presence or frequency of cariogenic foods.

Department of Commerce

The National Institute of Standards and Technology (NIST), an agency of the U.S. Department of Commerce, and the ADA have a dental research collaboration that dates back many decades. This collaboration has led to the development of many instruments and materials that have been used daily in dental practice. Inventions resulting from the partnership include the panoramic X-ray machine, resin composite filling materials, and dental bonding systems (NIST, 2010b).

NIST currently operates the Dental Materials Project, funded by NIDCR, which seeks to facilitate a better approach to dental materials design (NIST, 2010a). While the materials used in dental restorations have been improving, many still must be replaced because the restoration materials degrade or secondary dental caries develop under the restoration. The goal of the Dental Materials Project is to develop methods to assess the performance of and improve the longevity of restorations *in vitro*, where bacteria and other environmental factors may affect the restoration materials in different ways (NIST, 2010a).

Department of Defense

Throughout the years, the prevalence of oral disease and dental emergencies emerged as a major concern in military recruitment, retention, and readiness for deployment. During the Civil War, many recruits had to be turned away because they didn't have adequate dentition to bite off the end of the paper cartridges of gun powder (as was needed in order to load their weapons) (King and Hynson, 2007). During the Vietnam War, field commanders complained of loss of soldiers due to dental emergencies; this led to the development of programs to improve care on both a routine and an ad hoc basis (King and Hynson, 2007).

By the early 1990s, the army had developed a classification system for "dental readiness," which defined an oral health standard (associated with a decreased risk of dental emergency) that was required for deployment of troops (King and Hynson, 2007). In 2005, about 33 percent of all military personnel needed dental work before they could be deployed (up from 16 percent in 1998), ranging from 22 percent of those serving in the Air Force to 46 percent of those serving in the Marine Corps (Bray et al., 2006).

In 2005, approximately 81 percent of all military personnel reported having a dental check within the previous year (down from 90 percent in 2002) (Bray et al., 2003, 2006). Among those who had not had a visit, the most common reasons given were the inability to get time off at work, the inability to get an appointment with a military dentist, and personal aversion to visiting a dentist (Bray et al., 2006).

The Military Health System

The Military Health System (MHS) is a global network that provides health care services to the military, both in military and in civilian settings. Aside from health care services, the MHS fosters innovative research, education, and training programs (DOD, 2010). The MHS is also responsible for assuring the oral health of all uniformed DOD personnel, including determination of readiness for deployment based on oral health status (DOD, 2002). TRICARE, a major component of the MHS, is the health care program primarily for members of the uniformed services,[41] retirees, their families, and some members of the National Guard and Reserve. The program includes dental care as part of the medical benefit for active duty service members (TRICARE, 2010).

TRICARE also offers two voluntary dental benefit programs. The TRICARE Dental Program offers benefits for family members of the active duty military, as well as National Guard and Reserve members and their eligible families (TRICARE, 2010). The TRICARE Retiree Dental Program offers benefits for military retirees and their eligible family members, National Guard and Reserve members and their eligible family members, and several other categories of personnel (e.g., Medal of Honor recipients) (Humana Military, 2010; TRICARE, 2010). Both are administered by private companies (United Concordia Companies Inc. and Delta Dental of California, respectively) and provide access to a nationwide network of dentists. Program benefits cover a range of diagnostic and preventive services, oral surgery, as well as endodontic, prosthodontic, and periodontic services. Approximately 1.9 million people are currently enrolled in the TRICARE Dental Program (United Concordia, 2010).

Department of Education

The U.S. Department of Education (DOE) is ultimately responsible for the quality of education of oral health care professionals. Institutional accreditation is used as one method to protect the public from poorly trained health professionals. IOM's *Dental Education at the Crossroads* (1995) said "the accreditation of U.S. dental education programs is a private func-

---

[41] The seven uniformed services of the U.S. government include the U.S. Army, U.S. Marine Corps, U.S. Navy, U.S. Air Force, U.S. Coast Guard, U.S. Public Health Service Commissioned Corps, and the National Oceanic and Atmospheric Administration Commissioned Corps.

tion with a public purpose" (IOM, 1995). The DOE currently delegates responsibility for accrediting dental schools and dental programs to the Commission on Dental Accreditation (CODA), which is housed in the ADA (DOE, 2010). (The role of the DOE in general public education was discussed earlier in this chapter; oral health education and training of the health care professions was reviewed in Chapter 3.)

Department of Homeland Security

The U.S. Department of Homeland Security is notably involved in the delivery of oral health care in that the U.S. Coast Guard (USCG) is located within the department. The USCG employs 58 dentists (USPHS dental officers detailed to the Department of Homeland Security) in their 30 clinics (USCG, 2009). USCG dentists provide a range of dental services primarily to active members of the USCG or other military services; therefore, very few clinics offer care for pediatric or geriatric patients. Commissioned dental officers are eligible for residency training as well as both sign-on bonuses and special pay bonuses.

In addition, the Department of Homeland Security provides and oversees the health care of detainees in custody of the U.S. Immigration and Customs Enforcement (ICE) or the U.S. Customs and Borders Protection through the ICE Health Service Corps (DHS, 2010). The ICE Health Service Corps (formerly the Division of Immigration Health Services) uses USPHS commissioned officers, federal civil servants, and contractors directly provide or oversee the health care (including dental care) for about 32,000 detainees (DHS, 2011b). In FY2010, the ICE Health Service Corps provided nearly 33,000 dental visits (DHS, 2011a).

Department of Justice

The Federal Bureau of Prisons (BOP) within the U.S. Department of Justice (DOJ) hires dentists and dental hygienists (or uses USPHS commissioned officers) to provide a range of dental services for the inmates of the nation's federal prisons.[42] As of August 2010, there were almost 210,000 individuals incarcerated in a variety of settings (BOP, 2010b). The BOP identifies a "constant need" for dental officers (BOP, 2010a). As of August 2010, there were eight vacancies listed for dental hygienists and 39 vacancies for dentists (USPHS, 2010b). BOP has made strides in advancing technology for the oral health care of its population. For example, in FY 2008, the BOP transitioned to the use of digital dental radiography and successfully developed an electronic medical record that integrated the am-

---

[42] This section speaks only to the federal prison system.

bulatory medical record and the dental record (BOP, 2008). Overall, there is little recent peer-reviewed literature on the oral health and oral health care of prisoners across the United States, but it indicates poor oral health status among inmates, including racial and ethnic disparities (Treadwell and Formicola, 2005).

Department of Labor

The Bureau of Labor Statistics (BLS) within the U.S. Department of Labor provides detailed statistical measures of the nation's employment and economic status. It is the principal fact-finding agency for the federal government in the broad field of labor economics (BLS, 2011a). BLS' *Occupational Outlook Handbook* (BLS, 2011b) provides detailed information on specific types of employment, including working conditions, necessary training, advancement potential, job outlook and earnings for over 250 different occupations (approximately 9 out of 10 jobs in the economy). BLS also publishes a measure of the fastest-growing occupations in the United States.

BLS information was used in this report to document labor trends among dentists, dental hygienists, dental assistants, and laboratory technicians as well as other providers such as physician assistants and pharmacists. It also provided an assessment of the growth projections for various oral health job classifications. In addition, BLS provided information on the oral health care benefits provided by employers and consumer out-of-pocket expenditures.

Department of Veterans Affairs

The U.S. Department of Veterans Affairs arguably runs one of the nation's largest health care systems. More than 8 million veterans are enrolled in the VA health care system, and in FY 2010, more than 5.6 million individuals received care in this system (National Center for Veterans Analysis and Statistics, 2011). The VA provides health care in over 1,400 sites, including 152 medical centers (VA, 2011a,b). Criteria of eligibility for outpatient dental care in the VA differ from the guidelines used for determining other health care benefits and have several different classifications through which the extent of benefits are determined. For inpatient care (veterans in hospital, nursing home, and domiciliary settings), veterans may receive dental services that are "professionally determined by a VA dentist, in consultation with the referring physician, to be essential to the management of the patient's medical condition under active treatment" (VA, 2010). The VA has an integrated medical and dental electronic record system and requires the use of diagnostic codes for oral health care.

Environmental Protection Agency

The Environmental Protection Agency (EPA) regulates levels of fluoride in community drinking water. The EPA's involvement in monitoring water quality dates back to 1974 with the enactment of the Safe Drinking Water Act (EPA, 2011a). The agency is required to determine safe levels of potential drinking water contaminants, or its maximum contaminant level goals. Fluoridation is not required by the EPA; in fact, it is prohibited by the Act from requiring the addition of any substance to drinking water for preventive health care purposes (EPA, 2011b). The decision to fluoridate a water supply is made by the state or local municipality. The CDC does provide recommendations about the optimal levels of fluoride in drinking water in order to prevent tooth decay.

In early 2011, the EPA released new fluoride risk and exposure assessments and announced its intent to review the national drinking water regulations for fluoride. The assessments addressed recommendations made by the National Research Council (NRC) of the National Academies of Science in a 2006 report titled, *Fluoride in Drinking Water: A Scientific Review of EPA's Standards* (NRC, 2006). The NRC's report recommended that EPA update its risk assessment to include new data on the health risks of fluoride and better estimates of total fluoride exposure.

CURRENT REFORM EFFORTS

A Revitalized Oral Health Coordinating Committee (2009)

In 2009, newly appointed Assistant Secretary for Health Dr. Howard Koh asked the OHCC, located in the USPHS, to "regroup" (Bailey, 2010). Membership to the OHCC occurs through nomination by HHS operating divisions, staff divisions, or agencies with oral health functions. Other entities will also be included in the OHCC, such as national dental organizations and other federal agencies (e.g., DOD, VA, BOP, DOE) (Bailey, 2010).

Overall, the purpose of the OHCC is to "assist the USPHS in meeting its responsibility to promote the oral health of the American public: through coordination of a broad spectrum of oral health policy, research, and programs; within the USPHS; across federal agencies; and between public and private sectors" (Bailey, 2010). The specific functions of the OHCC are quite broad, especially given that the OHCC itself has not been allocated any funding and its membership all serve in full-time positions elsewhere in the department. The new charter enumerates 16 functions for the OHCC (Bailey, 2010):

1. Provide policy direction for the USPHS through preparation, review, and evaluation of relevant USPHS and agency documents,

with particular attention to the *Healthy People 2010/2020* National Oral Health Objectives; the 2000 surgeon general's report and the National Call to Action; and recommendations from other relevant oral health workshops and reports.

2. Propose goals, objectives, and approaches for promoting oral health and preventing oral, dental, and craniofacial diseases throughout the life span.
3. Propose goals, objectives, and approaches for reducing and/or eliminating oral health disparities.
4. Promote oral health workforce development.
5. Coordinate planning, implementation, and evaluation of departmental oral health research, policy, surveillance, services, education, and health promotion activities.
6. Promote oral health initiatives and serve as liaison to relevant federal and nonfederal agencies.
7. Encourage relevant nonfederal organizations to participate with the OHCC in planning, implementing, and evaluating joint public- and private-sector initiatives to improve the oral health of the nation.
8. Provide consultation to the assistant secretary for health and the surgeon general on oral health matters.
9. Promote the integration of oral health care into primary care and encourage collaboration between primary care and oral health services providers.
10. Promote the translation of oral health research into practice.
11. Provide leadership in supporting a National Oral Health Agenda that focuses on continually improving oral health outcomes, workforce development, and enhancing access to oral health services.
12. Promote the application of science-based new technologies into oral health care and practice, including harnessing the full potential of health information technology.
13. Examine and make recommendations regarding the financing of oral health care, including federal payment policies for Medicaid, CHIPRA, and locations designated as being health professional shortage sites.
14. Collaborate with the nation's leading quality experts on the development of performance and quality measures for use by federal programs.
15. Provide a written annual report to the assistant secretary for health as to OHCC activities and progress of oral health initiatives relative to national oral health.
16. Provide the HHS secretary with periodic updates on the state of oral health in the nation.

Part of the OHCC's role is to coordinate agency activity, but with no dedicated staff, it will be very difficult for the OHCC to achieve all of the functions listed above.

The HHS Oral Health Initiative (2010)

In April 2010, HHS Assistant Secretary Koh announced the initiation of a department-wide effort within HHS to improve the nation's oral health (HHS, 2010f). The HHS Oral Health Initiative 2010 (OHI 2010) is co-led by Koh and HRSA Administrator Dr. Mary Wakefield, and is supported both by the OHCC (which would help coordinate programs) and the HHS Office of Minority Health. The OHI 2010 once again calls on the department to "improve coordination and integration among programs to maximize outputs" (HHS, 2010g). In addition to realigning existing resources, it established nine new oral health activities (two of which are IOM reports—see Box 4-6). It is notable that AHRQ plays a large role in the collection of oral health data, and might have a role in advancing ef-

---

BOX 4-6
HHS Oral Health Initiative 2010

Administration for Children and Families (ACF)
　　Head Start Dental Home Initiative
Centers for Disease Control and Prevention (CDC) and National Institutes of Health (NIH)
　　National Oral Health Surveillance Plan
Centers for Medicare and Medicaid Services (CMS)
　　Review of Innovative State Medicaid Dental Programs
Health Resources and Services Administration (HRSA)
　　National Study on an Oral Health Initiative (IOM)
　　National Study on Oral Health Access to Services (IOM)
Indian Health Service (IHS)
　　The Early Childhood Caries Initiative
National Institutes of Health (NIH)
　　Clinical and Translational Science Program
Office of Minority Health
　　A Cultural Competency E-Learning Continuing Education Program
　　　for Oral Health Professionals
The Office on Women's Health
　　Oral Health as Part of Women's Health Across the Life Span

SOURCE: HHS, 2010g.

forts toward quality assessment efforts in oral health, yet it is not explicitly involved in the OHI 2010.

Drawing upon the surgeon general's report, the department has indicated that the key message of the OHI 2010 will be "Oral health is integral to overall health." Once again, HHS voices a desire to work with national and state partners and continues building upon previous efforts. However, the department's literature on OHI 2010 does not specify how the existing HHS programs will be coordinated or how the new activities will be integrated with the older ones. The specific goals (e.g., outcomes) and strategies are also not clear, aside from indicating that "the initiative utilizes a systems approach to create and finance programs to

- Emphasize oral health promotion/disease prevention,
- Increase access to care,
- Enhance the oral health workforce, and
- Eliminate oral health disparities" (HHS, 2010g).

American Recovery and Reinvestment Act (2009)

The American Recovery and Reinvestment Act of 2009 (ARRA) included provisions that affect delivery and access to oral health services, as well as investment in oral health research. ARRA investments that affect oral health fall into four major categories: training grants, health information technology, health centers, and research funding from the NIDCR. ARRA invested $500 million in training the health workforce, including dentistry (HRSA, 2009). The training grants included in excess of $800,000 for dental public health residencies and $50 million for equipment to enhance training for health professionals (HRSA, 2009, 2010b). ARRA also included $20 billion to develop health information technology infrastructure and incentive payments to practices that adopt information technology, including dental offices.

ARRA authorized $2 billion for investments in community health centers, including $1.5 billion for construction, renovation, and equipment, and $500 million for services (HHS, 2011b). Some of this money was used to build dental facilities and hire oral health personnel (Patrick, 2010). HRSA's Bureau of Primary Health Care reported that ARRA funds supported 565 dental professionals between July and September 2010 (NACHC, 2011).

The NIDCR distributed $101 million of ARRA funds for dental and craniofacial research. The funds supported 141 new or competing 2-year research grants, 128 administrative supplements to existing NIDCR grants, and research projects in 33 states (NIDCR, 2010c). Nearly a quarter of the funds were used to support NIH Challenge Grants in Health and Science

Research. These grants were created in ARRA and were designed to support research in very specific areas where NIH identified knowledge gaps, scientific opportunities, new technologies, data generation, or research methods that would benefit from an influx of funds to quickly advance the area in significant ways. A number of oral health topics were identified, including validating dental caries risk assessment guidelines, treatment and outcomes for cleft palate/cleft lip, infrastructure for comparative effectiveness studies in oral health and craniofacial conditions, and novel self-healing smart dental and biorestorative materials (NIH, 2009a). ARRA funds also allowed the NIDCR to provide faculty recruitment grants to seven dental schools, allowing each to hire two new faculty members (NIDCR, 2010c).

Patient Protection and Affordable Care Act (2010)

On March 23, 2010, President Obama signed the ACA. The law contains many significant provisions for the oral health of the nation. However, most of these provisions are not yet funded. The provisions explicitly related to oral health are contained in Table 4-3. While the committee notes the significance of these provisions, they recognize the reality of the current economic situation and that not all of these provisions may ultimately receive the needed funding.

Strategic Plan (FY 2010–2015)

Every 3 years, HHS updates its strategic plan to address the department's mission, which is "to enhance the health and well-being of Americans by providing for effective health and human services and by fostering sound, sustained advances in the sciences underlying medicine, public health, and social services" (HHS, 2010j). In the most recent iteration of this plan, the secretary identified five overarching goals (see Box 4-7).

Each of these goals has several objectives as well as strategies for achieving those objectives, including examples for oral health. For example, for Goal 1, the plan identifies one objective as ensuring access to quality, culturally competent care for vulnerable populations. A listed strategy is "Increase access to primary oral healthcare services and to oral disease preventive services by expanding access to health centers, school-based health centers, and Indian Health Service-funded health programs that have comprehensive primary oral health care services, and state and community-based programs that improve oral health, especially for children and pregnant women" (HHS, 2010j). For Goal 2, one strategy includes "Strengthen oral health research and use evidence-based oral health promotion and disease prevention to clarify the interrelationships between oral disease and other medical diseases" (HHS, 2010j). Finally, under Goal 5, the plan

TABLE 4-3
Key Oral Health Provisions in the ACA

	Section	Summary	Appropriated?
Coverage and access	Oral health services for children— Sec. 1201, 1302	Requires health plans offered through state exchanges, and the individual or small group market to cover pediatric oral health care	n/a
	Stand alone dental plans— Sec. 1311	Allows insurers to offer stand-alone dental plans through state exchanges, as long as the plans cover pediatric oral health care	Yes
	Expanded Medicaid eligibility— Sec. 2001	Requires states to expand Medicaid eligibility to residents at or below 133% of the federal poverty level	No
	Medicare Advantage—Sec. 3202	Requires Medicare Advantage plans to use rebates to pay for dental services, among other items	n/a
	School based health centers— Sec. 4101	Establishes a grant program for school based health centers, and requires grantees to provide referrals to, and follow-up for, oral health services	Yes
	Indian health care improvement— Sec. 10221	Allows Indian tribes or tribal organizations to use the dental health aide therapist program, if the state in which the tribe is located has authorized new and emerging oral health practitioners	n/a
Workforce	Health Care Workforce Commission— Sec. 5101	Establishes a National Health Care Workforce Commission to assess the adequacy of the health care workforce; the oral health workforce is identified as a high priority area.	No; the President's FY 2012 budget requests $3 million
	Training in general, pediatric, and public health dentistry— Sec. 5303	Expands Title VII training grant programs for dentistry, including newly authorized funding for dental schools, financial assistance to dental and dental hygiene students, and pediatric dentistry residencies, among others	No; the President's FY 2012 budget requests an additional $19 million for oral health training

continued

TABLE 4-3 *Continued*

	Section	Summary	Appropriated?
Workforce, *continued*	Alternative dental health care providers demonstration project— Sec. 5304	Authorizes the secretary to award grants for demonstration programs to train or employ alternative dental health care providers in order to increase access for rural and underserved populations	No
	Primary care residency programs— Sec. 5508	Establishes grant program for newly established or expanded "teaching health centers," which are community-based care centers that operate primary care residency programs, including general and pediatric dental residencies. Also describes payment mechanisms for residents working in teaching health centers	No; the President's FY 2012 budget requests $10 million
Prevention	Oral health care prevention campaign— Sec. 4102	Requires the CDC to establish a 5-year oral health campaign for prevention of oral diseases	No
	Dental caries disease management— Sec. 4102	Requires the CDC to award demonstration grants to research the effectiveness of research-based dental caries disease management	No
	School based sealant programs— Sec. 4102	Requires the CDC and HRSA to award grants to all states, territories, Indians, Indian tribes, tribal organizations, and urban Indian organizations to develop school-based sealant programs	No
Infrastructure and surveillance	Oral health infrastructure— Sec. 4102	Requires the CDC to enter into cooperative agreements with states, territories, and Indian tribes or tribal organizations to improve oral health infrastructure	No
	Oral healthcare surveillance (PRAMS)— Sec. 4102	Requires the secretary to improve the Pregnancy Risk Assessment Monitoring System (PRAMS) for oral health and requires states to report oral health measures in PRAMS	No

TABLE 4-3 Continued

	Section	Summary	Appropriated?
Infrastructure and surveillance, *continued*	Oral healthcare surveillance (NHANES)— Sec. 4102	Requires the National Health and Nutritional Examination Survey (NHANES) to include tooth-level surveillance	No
	Oral health care surveillance (MEPS)— Sec. 4102	Requires the Medical Expenditure Panel Survey (MEPS) to report on dental utilization, expenditure, and coverage	No; the President's FY 2012 budget requests $10 million
	Oral healthcare surveillance (NOHSS)— Sec. 4102	Authorizes funding to increase the participation in the National Oral Health Surveillance System (NOHSS) from 16 states to all 50 states, territories, and the District of Columbia	No; the President's FY 2012 budget requests $10 million

SOURCE: Patient Protection and Affordable Care Act, Public Law 148, 11th Cong., 2nd sess. (March 23, 2010).

identifies this strategy: "Expand the primary oral healthcare team and promote models that incorporate new providers, expanded scope of existing providers, and utilization of medical providers to provide evidence-based oral health preventive services" (HHS, 2010j). Many of the other goals, objectives, and strategies do not explicitly call out to oral health but are implicit to quality oral health care.

Healthy People 2020

Recently, HHS released the objectives for *Healthy People 2020* (see Box 4-8). There will be four overarching goals for *Healthy People 2020*: eliminating health disparities; increasing life expectancy and the quality of life for people of all ages; eliminating preventable disease, disability, injury, and premature death; and creating social and physical environments that promote good health for all (Koh, 2010). The first two were retained from *Healthy People 2010*; the last two are new for 2020. In addition to the overarching goals, 17 objectives specific to oral health have been proposed. Many of these objectives were retained from *Healthy People 2010*, but two new objectives have also been added.

BOX 4-7
Goals of HHS Strategic Plan FY 2010–2015

Goal 1: Transform health care.
Goal 2: Advance scientific knowledge and innovation.
Goal 3: Advance the health, safety, and well-being of the American people.
Goal 4: Increase efficiency, transparency, and accountability of HHS programs.
Goal 5: Strengthen the nation's health and human services infrastructure and workforce.

SOURCE: HHS, 2010j.

BOX 4-8
Healthy People 2020: **Oral Health Proposed Objectives**

Oral Health of Children and Adolescents
- Reduce the proportion of children and adolescents who have dental caries experience in their primary or permanent teeth.
- Reduce the proportion of children and adolescents with untreated dental decay.

Oral Health of Adults
- Reduce the proportion of adults with untreated dental decay.
- Reduce the proportion of adults who have ever had a permanent tooth extracted because of dental caries or periodontal disease.
- Reduce the proportion of adults aged 45–74 with moderate or severe periodontitis.
- Increase the proportion of oral and pharyngeal cancers detected at the earliest stage.

Access to Preventive Services
- Increase the proportion of children, adolescents, and adults who used the oral health care system in the past year.
- Increase the proportion of low-income children and adolescents who received any preventive dental service during the past year.
- Increase the proportion of school-based health centers with an oral health component.

- Increase the proportion of local health departments and Federally Qualified Health Centers that have an oral health component.
- Increase the proportion of patients that receive oral health services at Federally Qualified Health Centers each year.

Oral Health Interventions
- Increase the proportion of children and adolescents who have received dental sealants on their molar teeth.
- Increase the proportion of the U.S. population served by community water systems with optimally fluoridated water.
- Increase the proportion of adults who receive preventive interventions in dental offices.

Monitoring and Surveillance Systems
- Increase the number of states and the District of Columbia that have a system for recording and referring infants and children with cleft lips and cleft palates to craniofacial anomaly rehabilitative teams.
- Increase the number of states and the District of Columbia that have an oral and craniofacial health surveillance system.

Public Health Infrastructure
- Increase the number of health agencies that have a public dental health program directed by a dental professional with public health training.

SOURCE: HHS, 2010d.

KEY FINDINGS AND CONCLUSIONS

The committee noted the following key findings and conclusions:

- Oral diseases can affect all Americans, and vulnerable and under-served populations are especially at risk. Therefore, the prioritization of oral health as a key issue for HHS falls in line with its basic mission.
- HHS has had some notable successes in improving oral health in the past, yet that prior work has not had the necessary transformative impact on oral health.
- HHS needs to capitalize on its prior efforts and then build on that work to elevate the priority and visibility of oral health in all relevant divisions of HHS.
- The oral health activities of HHS are spread throughout the agency with little communication and coordination between divisions.
- The failure of previous HHS initiatives to produce significant results resulted from a lack of coordination, a lack of clear goals, a lack of resources, and a lack of high-level accountability.
- HHS has many unique opportunities to influence the oral health system, particularly through education grants, fostering payment innovation, promoting research, coordinating with other agencies that collect oral health data, and developing quality measures.
- The ACA has many authorized provisions related to oral health, but most remain unfunded.
- HHS has many opportunities to partner with the private sector (e.g., professional societies) as well as other parts of the public sector (e.g., states, other federal agencies).

REFERENCES

AAPD (American Academy of Pediatric Dentistry). 2010. *Head start dental home initiative.* http://www.aapd.org/headstart/ (accessed June 15, 2010).

Abramowitz, J., and L. E. Berg. 1973. A four-year study of the utilization of dental assistants with expanded functions. *Journal of the American Dental Association* 87(3):623-635.

ADA (American Dental Association). 2007. *American Indian and Alaska Native oral health access summit: Summary report.* Santa Ana Pueblo, NM: American Dental Association.

ADA. 2009. *Proceedings of the March 23-25, 2009, access to dental care summit.* Chicago, IL: American Dental Association.

ADA. 2010. *Dr. Bailey named PHS dental chief.* http://www.ada.org/news/4309.aspx (accessed February 25, 2011).

AHRQ (Agency for Healthcare Research and Quality). 2010. *Medical expenditure panel survey: Survey background.* http://www.meps.ahrq.gov/mepsweb/about_meps/survey_back.jsp (accessed November 24, 2010).

Andersen, R., and R. Mullner. 1990. Assessing the health objectives of the nation. *Health Affairs* 9(2):152-162.

Anderson, J. R. 2010. *HRSA oral health programs*. Presentation at 2010 Dental Management Coalition, Annapolis, MD. June 27, 2010.

Bailey, W. 2010. *The United States Public Health Service Oral Health Coordinating Committee*. Presentation at meeting of the Committee on an Oral Health Initiative, Washington, DC. June 28, 2010.

Blahut, P. 2009. *Access to dental care, IHS dental program*. Presentation at IOM workshop on the U.S. Oral Health Workforce in the Coming Decade, Washington, DC. February 9, 2009.

BLS (Bureau of Labor Statistics). 2011a. *About us*. http://www.bls.gov/bls/infohome.htm (accessed February 23, 2011).

BLS. 2011b. *Occupational outlook handbook, 2010-2011 edition*. http://www.bls.gov/oco/ (accessed February 23, 2011).

BOP (Bureau of Prisons). 2008. *State of the bureau 2008*. U.S. Department of Justice. Washington, DC.

BOP. 2010a. *Medical and mental health care career opportunities*. http://www.bop.gov/jobs/hsd/index.jsp (accessed October 26, 2010).

BOP. 2010b. *Quick facts about the Bureau of Prisons*. http://www.bop.gov/about/facts.jsp#1 (accessed October 26, 2010).

Bray, R. M., L. L. Hourani, K. L. Rae, J. A. Dever, J. M. Brown, A. A. Vincus, M. R. Pemberton, M. E. Marsden, D. L. Faulkner, and R. Vandermaas-Peeler. 2003. *2002 Department of Defense survey of health-related behaviors among military personnel*. Research Triangle Park, NC: RTI International.

Bray, R. M., L. L. Hourani, K. L. R. Olmsted, M. Witt, J. M. Brown, M. R. Pemberton, M. E. Marsden, B. Marriott, S. Scheffler, R. Vandermaas-Peeler, B. Weimer, S. Calvin, M. Bradshaw, K. Close, and D. Hayden. 2006. *2005 Department of Defense survey of health-related behaviors among active duty military personnel*. Research Triangle Park, NC: RTI International.

Bresch, J. 2010. *Critical importance of HHS to dental education and training*. Presentation at meeting of the Committee on an Oral Health Initiative, Washington, DC. June 28, 2010.

CDC (Centers for Disease Control and Prevention). 2010a. *CDC dental public health residency program*. http://www.cdc.gov/oralhealth/residency_program.htm (accessed October 25, 2010).

CDC. 2010b. *Division of oral health: About us*. http://www.cdc.gov/oralhealth/about.htm (accessed November 24, 2010).

CDC. 2010c. *Division of oral health: CDC funded states*. http://www.cdc.gov/oralhealth/state_programs/cooperative_agreements/index.htm (accessed November 24, 2010).

CDC. 2010d. *Division of oral health: Guidelines and recommendations*. http://www.cdc.gov/oralhealth/guidelines.htm (accessed November 24, 2010).

CDC. 2010e. *Division of oral health: Infrastructure development tools*. http://www.cdc.gov/oralhealth/state_programs/infrastructure/index.htm (accessed November 24, 2010).

CDC. 2010f. *Division of oral health: State-based programs*. http://www.cdc.gov/oralhealth/state_programs/index.htm (accessed November 24, 2010).

CDC. 2010g. *Guide to community preventive services: Oral health*. http://www.thecommunityguide.org/oral/index.html (accessed January 2, 2011).

CDC. 2010h. *Infrastructure development tools*. http://www.cdc.gov/oralhealth/state_programs/infrastructure/index.htm (accessed January 6, 2011).

CDC. 2010i. *National health interview survey: Questionnaires, datasets, and related documentation 1997 to the present*. http://www.cdc.gov/nchs/nhis/quest_data_related_1997_forward.htm (accessed December 22, 2010).

CDC. 2010j. *National oral health surveillance system*. http://www.cdc.gov/nohss/ (accessed November 24, 2010).

CDC. 2010k. *National oral health surveillance system: Fluoridation status.* http://apps.nccd. cdc.gov/nohss/FluoridationV.asp (accessed November 24, 2010).

CDC. 2011. *Epidemic intelligence service.* http://www.cdc.gov/eis/index.html (accessed January 7, 2011).

CDC Fluoride Recommendations Work Group. 2001. Recommendations for using fluoride to prevent and control dental caries in the United States. *MMWR Recommendations and Reports* 50(RR14).

Center for Responsive Politics. 2009. *Dentists: Background.* http://www.opensecrets.org/lobby/background.php?lname=H1400&year=2010 (accessed February 25, 2011).

Center for Responsive Politics. 2010a. *American Dental Association: Client profile, summary 2010.* http://www.opensecrets.org/lobby/clientsum.php?lname=American+Dental+Assn &year=2010 (accessed February 25, 2011).

Center for Responsive Politics. 2010b. *Health professionals: Industry profile, 2010.* http://www.opensecrets.org/lobby/indusclient.php?lname=H01&year=2010 (accessed February 25, 2011).

CMS (Centers for Medicare and Medicaid Services). 1999. *Form CMS-416: Annual EPSDT participation report.* https://www.cms.gov/cmsforms/downloads/cms416.pdf (accessed October 25, 2010).

CMS. 2003. Medicare program; proposed changes to the hospital inpatient prospective payment systems and fiscal year 2004 rates. *Federal Register* 68(96):27212-27214.

CMS. 2010a. *Blue Button Initiative.* https://www.cms.gov/NonIdentifiableDataFiles/12_Blue ButtonInitiative.asp (accessed January 10, 2011).

CMS. 2010b. *Insure kids now!* http://www.insurekidsnow.gov/ (accessed December 22, 2010).

CMS. 2010c. *Written testimony of CMS to the Committee on an Oral Health Initiative.*

CMS. 2011. *Form CMS-416: Annual EPSDT participation report.* http://www.cms.gov/MedicaidEarlyPeriodicScrn/downloads/416_12_10.pdf (accessed September 19, 2011).

Coker, C. F. 1969. Current trends in dental care delivery systems: Comprehensive health services for children and youth. *American Journal of Public Health and the Nation's Health* 59(6):909-914.

Crall, J. J. 2009. Oral health policy development since the surgeon general's report on oral health. *Academic Pediatrics* 9(6):476-482.

Del Grosso, P., A. Brown, S. Silva, J. Henderson, N. Tein, and D. Paulsell. 2008. *Strategies for promoting prevention and improving oral health care delivery in Head Start: Findings from the oral health initiative evaluation.* Princeton, NJ: Mathematica Policy Research, Inc.

DeWalt, D. A., L.F. Callahan, V.H. Hawk, K. A. Broucksou, A. Hink, R. Rudd, and C. Brach. 2010. Health literacy Universal Precautions toolkit. Rockville, MD, Agency for Healthcare Research and Quality.

DHEW (Department of Health, Education, and Welfare). 1979. *Healthy People: The surgeon general's report on health promotion and disease prevention.* Washington, DC: U.S. Department of Health, Education, and Welfare.

DHS (Department of Homeland Security). 2010. *Enforcement and removal operations: ICE Health Service Corps—detainee covered services.* http://inshealth.org/ManagedCare/IHSC%202010%20Detainee%20Covered%20Service%20Package_12-28-10.pdf (accessed February 16, 2011).

DHS. 2011a. *Fact sheet: ERO—detainee health care—FY2010.* http://www.ice.gov/doclib/news/library/factsheets/pdf/ihs-fy10.pdf (accessed February 16, 2011).

DHS. 2011b. *ICE Health Service Corps.* http://www.ice.gov/about/offices/enforcement-removal-operations/ihs/ (accessed February 16, 2011).

Diefenbach, V. L. 1969. The dental health future: Prognosis positive. *American Journal of Public Health and the Nation's Health* 59(6):919-922.

DOD (Department of Defense). 2002. *Policy on standardization of oral health and readiness classifications.* https://secure.ucci.com/non-ldap/forms/addp/forms/readiness-policy.pdf (accessed January 3, 2011).

DOD. 2010. *What is the MHS?* http://www.health.mil/About_MHS/index.aspx (accessed November 5, 2010).

DOE (Department of Education). 2010. *College accreditation in the United States: Specialized accrediting agencies.* http://www2.ed.gov/admins/finaid/accred/accreditation_pg7.html#health (accessed December 22, 2010).

Duffy, R., R. Weaver, and K. Hayes. 1997. General dentistry grant program: 1976-1996. *Journal of Dental Education* 61(10):804.

Edelstein, B., D. Krol, P. Ingargiola, and A. De Biasi. 2003. *Assessing pediatric dentistry Title VII training program success.* Washington, DC: American Academy of Pediatric Dentistry Foundation.

EPA (Environmental Protection Agency). 2011a. *Basic information about fluoride in drinking water.* http://water.epa.gov/drink/contaminants/basicinformation/fluoride.cfm#four (accessed February 23, 2011).

EPA. 2011b. *Questions and answers on fluoride.* http://water.epa.gov/lawsregs/rulesregs/regulatingcontaminants/sixyearreview/upload/2011_Fluoride_QuestionsAnswers.pdf (accessed February 23, 2011).

FDA (Food and Drug Administration). 2011a. *About FDA: What we do.* http://www.fda.gov/AboutFDA/WhatWeDo/default.htm (accessed February 22, 2011).

FDA. 2011b. *Drugs@FDA.* http://www.accessdata.fda.gov/scripts/cder/drugsatfda/index.cfm (accessed February 22, 2011).

FNIDCR (Friends of the NIDCR). 2010a. *Friends of the National Institute of Dental and Craniofacial Research* http://fnidcr.org/about/index.html (accessed November 16, 2010).

FNIDCR. 2010b. *Friends of the National Institute of Dental and Craniofacial Research.* http://www.fnidcr.org/index.html (accessed December 22, 2010).

GAO (Government Accountability Office). 2009. *State and federal actions have been taken to improve children's access to dental services, but gaps remain.* Washington, DC: U.S. Government Accountability Office.

Gershen, J. A. 1991. Geriatric dentistry and prevention: Research and public policy. *Advances in Dental Research* 5:69-73.

Geurink, K., and B. Isman. 2009. *Association of State and Territorial Dental Directors Head Start oral health project evaluation report: 2001-2008.* Sparks, NV: Association of State and Territorial Dental Directors.

Gist, R. 2010. *Oral testimony of Dr. Raymond Gist, president-elect of the American Dental Association.* Presentation at meeting of the Committee on an Oral Health Initiative, Washington, DC. March 31, 2010.

Gladstone, R., and W. M. Garcia. 2007. Dental hygiene: Reflecting on our past, preparing for our future. *Access.* November 2007.

Gooch, B. F., S. O. Griffin, S. K. Gray, W. G. Kohn, R. G. Rozier, M. Siegal, M. Fontana, D. Brunson, N. Carter, D. K. Curtis, K. J. Donly, H. Haering, L. F. Hill, H. P. Hinson, J. Kumar, L. Lampiris, M. Mallatt, D. M. Meyer, W. R. Miller, S. M. Sanzi-Schaedel, R. Simonsen, B. I. Truman, and D. T. Zero. 2009. Preventing dental caries through school-based sealant programs: Updated recommendations and reviews of evidence. *Journal of the American Dental Association* 140(11):1356-1365.

Green, A. R., J. R. Betancourt, E. R. Park, J. A. Greer, E. J. Donahue, and J. S. Weissman. 2008. Providing culturally competent care: Residents in HRSA Title VII funded residency programs feel better prepared. *Academic Medicine* 83(11):1071-1079.

Griffin, S. O., E. Oong, W. Kohn, B. Vidakovic, B. F. Gooch, J. Bader, J. Clarkson, M. R. Fontana, D. M. Meyer, R. G. Rozier, J. A. Weintraub, and D. T. Zero. 2008. The effectiveness of sealants in managing caries lesions. *Journal of Dental Research* 87(2):169-174.

Griffin, S. O., S. K. Gray, D. M. Malvitz, and B. F. Gooch. 2009. Caries risk in formerly sealed teeth. *Journal of the American Dental Association* 140(4):415-423.

Halliday, C. 2010. *Oral testimony of Dr. Chris Halliday, director of the Indian Health Service Division of Oral Health.* Presentation at meeting of the Committee on an Oral Health Initiative, Washington, DC. June 28, 2010.

Halpern, D. 2010. *Testimony before the IOM oral health initiative committee.* Presentation at meeting of the Committee on an Oral Health Initiative, Washington, DC. March 31, 2010.

Harris, R. R. 1992. *Dental science in a new age: A history of the National Institute of Dental Research.* Ames, IA: Iowa State University Press.

HCFA (Health Care Financing Administration). 1989. Medicare program; changes in payment policy for direct graduate medical education costs. *Federal Register* 54(188):40286.

HHS (Department of Health and Human Services). 1991. *Healthy People 2000: National health promotion and disease prevention objectives.* Washington, DC: Government Printing Office.

HHS. 2000a. *Healthy People 2010: Understanding and improving health.* 2nd ed. Washington, DC: U.S. Government Printing Office.

HHS. 2000b. *Oral health in America: A report of the surgeon general.* Rockville, MD: U.S. Department of Health and Human Services.

HHS. 2000c. *Summary minutes.* Paper read at 162nd Meeting of the National Advisory Dental and Craniofacial Research Council, Bethesda, MD.

HHS. 2003a. *Advisory committee on training in primary care medicine and dentistry: Training culturally competent primary care professionals to provide high quality healthcare for all Americans: The essential role of Title VII, section 747, in the elimination of healthcare disparities.* Washington, DC: U.S. Department of Health and Human Services.

HHS. 2003b. *Memorandum of understanding (MOU) goals.* http://www.healthypeople.gov/ Implementation/mous/ (accessed November 16, 2010).

HHS. 2003c. *National call to action to promote oral health.* Rockville, MD: U.S. Department of Health and Human Services.

HHS. 2005. *Healthy People 2010 fact sheet.* http://www.healthypeople.gov/About/hpfactsheet. pdf (accessed November 16, 2010).

HHS. 2010b. *Advisory committee on training in primary care medicine and dentistry: The redesign of primary care with implications for training.* Rockville, MD: U.S. Department of Health and Human Services.

HHS. 2010c. *Healthy People 2020: Health communication and health information technology.* http://www.healthypeople.gov/2020/topicsobjectives2020/objectiveslist.aspx?topicid=18 (accessed December 27, 2010).

HHS. 2010d. *Healthy People 2020: Oral health objectives.* http://www.healthypeople. gov/2020/topicsobjectives2020/objectiveslist.aspx?topicid=32 (accessed December 27, 2010).

HHS. 2010e. *HHS awards $159.1 million to support health care workforce training.* http:// www.hhs.gov/news/press/2010pres/08/20100805a.html (accessed January 7, 2011).

HHS. 2010f. *HHS launches oral health initiative.* http://www.hhs.gov/ash/news/20100426. html (accessed November 17, 2010).

HHS. 2010g. *HHS oral health initiative 2010.* http://www.hrsa.gov/publichealth/clinical/ oralhealth/hhsinitiative.pdf (accessed August 19, 2010).

HHS. 2010h. *Letter from advisory committee training in primary care medicine and dentistry to Secretary Sebelius.* May 19, 2010.

HHS. 2010i. *National action plan to improve health literacy.* Washington, DC: U.S. Department of Health and Human Services.

HHS. 2010j. *Strategic plan and priorities.* http://www.hhs.gov/secretary/about/priorities/priorities.html (accessed December 29, 2010).

HHS. 2011a. *Community health data initiative.* http://www.hhs.gov/open/plan/open governmentplan/initiatives/initiative.html (accessed January 10, 2011).

HHS. 2011b. *Recovery act funding for community health centers.* http://www.hhs.gov/recovery/programs/hrsa/index.html (accessed September 19, 2011).

HHS and USDA (Department of Health and Human Services and U.S. Department of Agriculture). 2005. *Dietary guidelines for Americans.* Washington, DC: U.S. Department of Health and Human Services and U.S. Department of Agriculture.

HRSA (Health Resources and Services Administration). 1990. *Equity and access for mothers and children: Strategies from the public health service workshop on oral health of mothers and children.* Rockville, MD: U.S. Department of Health and Human Services.

HRSA. 2005. *Financing dental education: Public policy interests, issues and strategic considerations.* Washington, DC: U.S. Department of Health and Human Services.

HRSA. 2009. *American Recovery and Reinvestment Act: Residency training in dental public health program questions and answers.* Rockville, MD: U.S. Department of Health and Human Services.

HRSA. 2010a. *Bureau of primary health care.* http://www.hrsa.gov/about/organization/bureaus/bphc/ (accessed December 22, 2010).

HRSA. 2010b. *Equipment to enhance training for health professionals.* http://bhpr.hrsa.gov/grants/equipment/index.html (accessed January 5, 2011).

HRSA. 2010c. *Health professions: Public health.* http://bhpr.hrsa.gov/grants/public.htm (accessed December 22, 2010).

HRSA. 2010d. *National health service corps: History.* http://nhsc.hrsa.gov/about/history.htm (accessed November 15, 2010).

HRSA. 2010e. *NHSC loan repayment.* http://nhsc.hrsa.gov/loanrepayment/ (accessed December 22, 2010).

HRSA. 2011a. *BHPR grants: Oral health workforce activities FY 2010 grantee abstracts.* http://bhpr.hrsa.gov/grants/10oralhealthabstracts.htm (accessed January 10, 2011).

HRSA. 2011b. *Bureau of health professions.* http://www.hrsa.gov/about/organization/bureaus/bhpr/index.html (accessed September 15, 2011).

HRSA. 2011c. *Children's hospitals graduate medical education payment program.* http://www.hrsa.gov/bhpr/childrenshospitalgme/ (accessed January 10, 2011).

HRSA. 2011d. *HIV/AIDS bureau.* http://www.hrsa.gov/about/organization/bureaus/hab/index.html (accessed September 15, 2011).

HRSA. 2011e. *Office of regional operations.* http://www.hrsa.gov/about/organization/bureaus/oro/index.html (accessed February 23, 2011).

Humana Military. 2010. *Tricare dental benefits.* http://www.humana-military.com/south/bene/tools-resources/bulletins-newsletters/standard-2009/dental.asp (accessed November 5, 2010).

IHS (Indian Health Service). 2010a. *IHS electronic dental record.* http://www.doh.ihs.gov/EDR/index.cfm?fuseaction=help.faqs (accessed December 22, 2010).

IHS. 2010b. Introducing the Indian health service early childhood caries initiative. *IHS Dental Explorer.* February 2010.

Interim Study Group on Dental Activities. 1989. *Improving the oral health of the American people: Opportunity for action.* Rockville, MD: Department of Health and Human Services.

IOM (Institute of Medicine). 1995. *Dental education at the crossroads: Challenges and change.* Washington, DC: National Academy Press.

IOM. 2001. *Crossing the quality chasm: A new health system for the 21st century.* Washington, DC: National Academy Press.

IOM. 2004. *Health literacy: A prescription to end confusion.* Washington, DC: The National Academies Press.

IOM. 2007a. *Challenges for the FDA: The future of drug safety, workshop summary.* Washington, DC: The National Academies Press.

IOM. 2007b. *The future of drug safety: Promoting and protecting the health of the public.* Washington, DC: The National Academies Press.

IOM. 2010a. *Enhancing food safety: The role of the Food and Drug Administration.* Washington, DC: The National Academies Press.

IOM. 2010b. *Planning a WIC research agenda.* Washington, DC: The National Academies Press.

IOM. 2010c. *Public health effectiveness of the FDA 510(k) clearance process: Balancing patient safety and innovation, workshop report.* Washington, DC: The National Academies Press.

IOM. 2011. *Public health effectiveness of the FDA 510(k) clearance process: Measuring postmarket performance of other select topics, workshop report.* Washington, DC: The National Academies Press.

Johnson, D. W. 1969. Dental manpower resources in the United States. *American Journal of Public Health and the Nation's Health* 59(4):689-693.

The Joint Commission. 2008. *Crosswalk of the Office of Minority Health's national standards for culturally and linguistically appropriate services (CLAS) and The Joint Commission's 2009 standards for the hospital accreditation program.* Oakbrook Terrace, IL: The Joint Commission.

Kann, L., S. K. Telljohann, and S. F. Wooley. 2007. Health education: Results from the school health policies and programs study 2006. *Journal of School Health* 77(8):408-434.

King, J. E., and R. G. Hynson. 2007. *Highlights in the history of U.S. Army dentistry.* Falls Church, VA: U.S. Army.

Kleinman, D. V. 2010. *Implementing oral health in America: Lessons learned.* Presentation at meeting of the Committee on an Oral Health Initiative, Washington, DC. March 31, 2010.

Koh, H. 2010. A 2020 vision for Healthy People. *New England Journal of Medicine* 362(18): 1653-1656.

Kohn, W. G., A. S. Collins, J. L. Cleveland, J. A. Harte, K. J. Eklund, and D. M. Malvitz. 2003. Guidelines for infection control in dental health-care settings—2003. *MMWR Recommendations and Reports* 52(RR17):1-61.

Lennon, M. A. 2006. One in a million: The first community trial of water fluoridation. *Bulletin of the World Health Organization* 84(9):759-760.

Malvitz, D. M., L. K. Barker, and K. R. Phipps. 2009. Development and status of the national oral health surveillance system. *Preventing Chronic Disease* 6(2).

Mann, C. R. 2009. *Access to dental services for Medicaid Recipients.* Testimony before the House Committee on Oversight & Government Reform, Subcommittee on Domestic Policy, U.S. House of Representatives, Washington, DC. October 7, 2009.

McGinnis, J. M. 2010. *Healthy People: A three decade retrospective.* Paper presented at Society for Public Health Education, Denver, CO. November 5, 2010.

Mitchell, P. 2010. Paper read at National Oral Health Conference, April 27, St. Louis, MO.

NACHC (National Association of Community Health Centers). 2011. *More patients gain access to health center care thanks to stimulus funds.* http://www.nachc.com/client/documents/Stimulus%20Funds%20One%20Pager%20March%202011.pdf (accessed September 19, 2011).

NAL (National Agricultural Library). 2009. *Toddler nutrition and health resource list.* http://www.nal.usda.gov/fnic/pubs/bibs/gen/toddler.pdf (accessed November 16, 2010).

Nash, D. A., and R. J. Nagel. 2005. Confronting oral health disparities among American Indian/Alaska Native children: The pediatric oral health therapist. *American Journal of Public Health* 95(8):1325-1329.

National Archives. 2010. *Records of the health resources and services administration (HRSA): Record group 512 (1935-93).* http://www.archives.gov/research/guide-fed-records/groups/512.html (accessed October 21, 2010).

National Center for Veterans Analysis and Statistics. 2011. *Utilization.* http://www.va.gov/vetdata/Utilization.asp (accessed September 19, 2011).

NCHS (National Center for Health Statistics). 1968. Health manpower: United States—1965-1967. *Vital and Health Statistics* 14(1).

NCHS. 2010. *National Health and Nutrition Examination Survey: 1999-2010 survey content.* Hyattsville, MD: U.S. Department of Health and Human Services.

Ng, M., P. Glassman, and J. Crall. 2008. The impact of Title VII on general and pediatric dental education and training. *Academic Medicine* 83(11):1039.

NIDCR (National Institute for Dental and Craniofacial Research). 2000. *The face of a child: Surgeon general's workshop and conference on children and oral health.* http://www.nidcr.nih.gov/NR/rdonlyres/E7E614B5-5A03-48B6-9CD9-75B38111AFC3/0/registration.pdf (accessed February 18, 2011).

NIDCR. 2001. *The face of a child: Surgeon general's workshop and conference on children and oral health—proceedings.* http://www.nidcr.nih.gov/NR/rdonlyres/ED6FB3B5-CEF4-4175-938D-5049D8A74F66/0/SGR_Conf_Proc.pdf (accessed February 18, 2011).

NIDCR. 2008. *Director's report to council: January 2008.* http://www.nidcr.nih.gov/aboutus/councils/nadcrc/directorsreport/archiveofdirectorsreports/january2008.htm (accessed December 22, 2010).

NIDCR. 2010a. *Centers for research to reduce disparities in oral health.* http://www.nidcr.nih.gov/Research/NIDCR_Centers_and_Research_Networks/CentersforResearchtoReduceDisparities/ (accessed December 22, 2010).

NIDCR. 2010b. *FY 2011 congressional justification.* http://www.nidcr.nih.gov/AboutUs/BudgetCongressionalStatements/CongressionalJustifications/FY2011Congressional Justification/ (accessed September 27, 2010).

NIDCR. 2010c. *NIDCR completes its commitment of American Recovery and Reinvestment Act funds.* http://www.nidcr.nih.gov/Research/ResearchResults/NewsReleases/CurrentNewsReleases/ARRAFunding.htm (accessed January 5, 2011).

NIDCR. 2010d. *NIDCR strategic plan 2009-2013.* www.nidcr.nih.gov/Research/ResearchPriorities/StrategicPlan (accessed September 27, 2010).

NIDCR. 2010e. *Overview: Research conducted at NIDCR.* http://www.nidcr.nih.gov/Research/NIDCRLaboratories/OverviewDIR/ (accessed December 22, 2010).

NIDCR. 2010f. *The story of water fluoridation.* http://www.nidcr.nih.gov/oralhealth/topics/fluoride/thestoryoffluoridation.htm (accessed December 22, 2010).

NIDCR and CDC. 2010. *Dental, oral, and craniofacial data resource center.* http://drc.hhs.gov/ (accessed December 22, 2010).

NIH (National Institutes of Health). 2006. PAR-04-116. http://grants.nih.gov/grants/guide/pa-files/PAR-04-116.html (accessed February 28, 2011).

NIH. 2009a. *American Recovery and Reinvestment Act of 2009: Challenge grant applications: Omnibus of broad challenge areas and specific topics.* Bethesda, MD: U.S. Department of Health and Human Services.

NIH. 2009b. *Loan repayment programs.* http://lrp.info.nih.gov/index.aspx (accessed October 26, 2010).

NIH. 2009c. Research underway in health literacy supported by NIH. http://www.nih.gov/icd/od/ocpl/resources/healthlitfull.htm (accessed February 28, 2011).

NIH. 2010. *The NIH almanac: National Institute of Dental and Craniofacial Research.* http://www.nih.gov/about/almanac/organization/NIDCR.htm (accessed November 1, 2010).

NIH. 2011. PAR-10-133: Understanding and promoting health literacy. http://grants.nih.gov/grants/guide/pa-files/PAR-10-133.html (accessed February 28, 2011).

NIST (National Institute of Standards and Technology). 2010a. *Dental materials.* http://www.nist.gov/mml/polymers/biomaterials/dental.cfm (accessed February 23, 2011).

NIST. 2010b. *From Dental Materials to Panoramic X-Rays: The NIST-ADA Dental Research Collaboration.* http://www.nist.gov/public_affairs/colloquia/20081205.cfm (accessed February 23, 2011).

NRC (National Research Council). 2006. *Fluoride in drinking water: A scientific review of EPA's standards.* Washington, DC: The National Academies Press.

OHRC (National Maternal and Child Oral Health Resource Center). 2010a. *About us.* http://www.mchoralhealth.org/about/index.html (accessed December 22, 2010).

OHRC. 2010b. *Head Start.* http://www.mchoralhealth.org/HeadStart/index.html (accessed December 22, 2010).

OIG (Office of Inspector General). 1996. *Children's dental services under Medicaid: Access and utilization.* Washington, DC: Department of Health and Human Services.

OIG. 2010. *Guidance and standards on language access services: Medicare plans.* Washington, DC: U.S Department of Health and Human Services.

OMH (Office of Minority Health). 2001. *National standards for culturally and linguistically appropriate services in health care.* Washington, DC: U.S. Department of Health and Human Services.

OMH. 2010. *Office of Minority Health: Cultural competency.* http://minorityhealth.hhs.gov/templates/browse.aspx?lvl=1&lvlID=3 (accessed February 23, 2011).

Oong, E. M., S. O. Griffin, W. G. Kohn, B. F. Gooch, and P. W. Caufield. 2008. The effect of dental sealants on bacteria levels in caries lesions: A review of the evidence. *Journal of the American Dental Association* 139(3):271-278.

Patrick, D. L. 2010. *Governor Patrick celebrates groundbreaking of new Whittier Street health center.* http://www.mass.gov/?pageID=gov3pressrelease&L=1&L0=Home&sid=Agov3&b=pressrelease&f=100914_whittier_street_hc&csid=Agov3 (accessed January 5, 2011).

Peterson, F. L., R. J. Cooper, and J. M. Laird. 2001. Enhancing teacher health literacy in school health promotion: A vision for the new millennium. *Journal of School Health* 71(4):138-144.

Reynolds, P. P. 2008. A legislative history of federal assistance for health professions training in primary care medicine and dentistry in the United States, 1963-2008. *Academic Medicine* 83(11):1004-1014.

TFCPS (Task Force on Community Preventive Services). 2001. Promoting oral health: Interventions for preventing dental caries, oral and pharyngeal cancers, and sports-related craniofacial injuries. *MMWR Recommendations and Reports* 50(RR21):1-13.

TFCPS. 2010. *The community guide.* http://www.thecommunityguide.org/index.html (accessed October 29, 2010).

Treadwell, H. M., and A. J. Formicola. 2005. Improving the oral health of prisoners to improve overall health and well-being. *American Journal of Public Health* 95(10):1677-1678.

TRICARE. 2010. *Tricare prime handbook: August 2010.* http://www.tricare.mil/tricaresmartfiles/Prod_435/TRICARE_Prime_Handbook_Update_040811.pdf (accessed August 17, 2011).

United Concordia. 2010. *Tricare dental program.* http://www.tricaredentalprogram.com/tdptwo/enrollee/about_ucci.jsp (accessed November 5, 2010).

USCG (U.S. Coast Guard). 2009. *Human resources: Dental.* http://www.uscg.mil/HEALTH/cg1122/dental.asp (accessed October 26, 2010).

USDA (U.S. Department of Agriculture). 2010a. *National school lunch program.* http://www.fns.usda.gov/cnd/Lunch/AboutLunch/NSLPFactSheet.pdf (accessed December 30, 2010).

USDA. 2010b. *Women, infants, and children.* http://www.fns.usda.gov/wic/ (accessed October 26, 2010).

USPHS (U.S. Public Health Service). 1980. *Promoting health/preventing disease: Objectives for the nation.* Washington, DC: U.S. Department of Health and Human Services.

USPHS. 1989. *Final report to the house of representatives appropriation committee on oral health activities.* Washington, DC: Department of Health and Human Services.

USPHS. 2002. *Oral health coordinating committee annual report: October 2001-October 2002.* http://www.phs-dental.org/depac/minutes/10-01to10-02.doc (accessed November 17, 2010).

USPHS. 2008. *About the commissioned corps: Leadership.* http://www.usphs.gov/aboutus/leadership.aspx (accessed October 26, 2010).

USPHS. 2010a. *About the Commissioned Corps: Questions.* http://www.usphs.gov/aboutus/questions.aspx#whatis (accessed August 1, 2011).

USPHS. 2010b. *Dental category of the United States Public Health Service: Vacancies.* http://www.phs-dental.org/depac/vacancies.html (accessed October 26, 2010).

USPHS. 2010c. *Dentists in the United States Public Health Service: Depac.* http://www.phs-dental.org/depac/depac.html (accessed October 26, 2010).

USPHS. 2010d. *Profession: Dentist—pay/benefits.* http://www.usphs.gov/profession/dentist/activities.aspx/compensation.aspx (accessed September 15, 2011).

USPHS. 2010e. *Profession: Dentist—what we do.* http://www.usphs.gov/profession/dentist/activities.aspx (accessed October 26, 2010).

USPHS. 2011. *Student opportunities.* http://www.usphs.gov/student/ (accessed February 17, 2011).

USPSTF (U.S. Preventive Services Task Force). 2010. *USPSTF recommendations.* http://www.uspreventiveservicestaskforce.org/uspstopics.htm (accessed October 29, 2010).

VA (Veterans Affairs). 2010. *VA health care eligibility & enrollment.* http://www4.va.gov/healtheligibility/coveredservices/SpecialBenefits.asp (accessed October 25, 2010).

VA. 2011a. *About VHA.* http://www.va.gov/health/aboutVHA.asp (accessed September 19, 2011).

VA. 2011b. *Medical centers.* http://www.va.gov/health/MedicalCenters.asp (accessed September 19, 2011).

Wakefield, M. 2010. *Oral testimony of Mary Wakefield.* Presentation at meeting of the Committee on an Oral Health Initiative, Washington, DC. June 28, 2010.

Woolley, J. T., and G. Peters. 2011a. *The American Presidency Project: Gerald Ford—statement on signing the Health Professions Educational Assistance Act of 1976.* http://www.presidency.ucsb.edu/ws/?pid=3223 (accessed February 18, 2011).

Woolley, J. T., and G. Peters. 2011b. *The American Presidency Project: Richard Nixon—statement on signing the health manpower and nurse training bills.* http://www.presidency.ucsb.edu/ws/index.php?pid=6452#axzz1TVIk6Y5L (accessed July 29, 2011).

5

A New Oral Health Initiative

The U.S. Department of Health and Human Service's (HHS') commitment to improving the oral health of the nation has fluctuated; while there have been notable successes, these efforts have not led to oral health parity in health care overall. Substantial inequities remain across population subgroups, and many Americans continue to suffer from avoidable and treatable oral diseases. The expressed intent of the surgeon general's report *Oral Health in America* was "to alert Americans to the full meaning of oral health and its importance in relation to general health and well-being" (HHS, 2000). Now, more than a decade later, scientific investments demonstrate significant dividends in some areas and some progress in children's oral health has been made; yet many of the concerns raised in that report remain (Mertz and Mouradian, 2009; Mouradian et al., 2009; Slayton and Slavkin, 2009).

LEARNING FROM THE PAST

Through extensive research, testimony, and their own professional experiences, the members of the Institute of Medicine (IOM) Committee on an Oral Health Initiative considered why prioritization of oral health continues to be a challenge in HHS. In any initiative to improve oral health and oral health care, HHS' challenge will be to marshal its resources in a way that produces a significant impact in the lives of people all across the country. Given that HHS' resources are limited, the scope of the challenge is substantial, and many solutions will require the involvement of multiple stakeholders, one of the most important roles HHS can play is in providing leadership and direction for the rest of the country.

The 2000 surgeon general's report (HHS, 2000) presented the state of the science in oral health, called attention to the oral health care challenge facing the country, and outlined a framework for future action. While the report is still widely discussed today, it did not lead to a direct and immediate change in the government's approach to oral health. This disappointing outcome may have been due to broader environmental factors, including grave and immediate national crises (e.g., 9/11, Hurricane Katrina); changes in the economy that affect state and federal budgets (e.g., recessions); competing health policy priorities (e.g., obesity); a tendency to blame individual behaviors alone for poor oral health; a lack of political will; or simply the long-standing failure to recognize oral health as an integral part of overall health. But certainly part of the explanation lies in "gaps in leadership and the failure to unite a critical mass of key stakeholders with sufficient common interests, political will, and resources to effect fundamental policy change" (Crall, 2009). Within HHS, changes in administrations (with concomitant changes in priorities), workforce turnover (including agency administrators), lack of oral health "champions," insufficient funding and staffing, and the lack of oral health parity may all have contributed to the disappointing results.

THE NEW ORAL HEALTH INITIATIVE

As was discussed in Chapter 1, this committee was challenged by a statement of task that called for them to devise a "potential" oral health initiative, and then the subsequent announcement of the Oral Health Initiative 2010 (OHI 2010). The committee was mindful of the existence of the OHI 2010 but did not let its existence limit its considerations of what such an initiative should be. Therefore, in the rest of this chapter, the committee outlines seven recommendations that as a whole comprise what will be referred to as the *new* Oral Health Initiative (NOHI) (to distinguish it from and build upon the current initiative). In considering a potential HHS oral health initiative, the committee developed a set of organizing principles (see Box 5-1) based on areas in greatest need of attention as well as approaches that have the most potential for creating improvements. It will be HHS' responsibility to adapt the current structure of the OHI 2010 to these principles and the recommendations that follow.

The committee concluded that these principles will help move the nation toward achieving the goals and objectives set by *Healthy People 2020*, which represents the best long-term set of benchmarks for judging the success of the NOHI. *Healthy People 2020* is an existing and well-accepted set of benchmarks for the country developed by a strong collaboration of

---

BOX 5-1
Organizing Principles for a New Oral Health Initiative

1. Establish high-level accountability.
2. Emphasize disease prevention and oral health promotion.
3. Improve oral health literacy and cultural competence.
4. Reduce oral health disparities.
5. Explore new models for payment and delivery of care.
6. Enhance the role of nondental health care professionals.
7. Expand oral health research, and improve data collection.
8. Promote collaboration among private and public stakeholders.
9. Measure progress toward short-term and long-term goals and objectives.
10. Advance the goals and objectives of *Healthy People 2020*.

---

partners. The committee suggests that creating a new set of long-term goals would only contribute to the redundancy and fragmentation that is often criticized regarding government programming. In essence, attainment of *Healthy People 2020* goals and objectives is the continuing mission of the NOHI. The committee further notes that this approach should not be limited to the goals and objectives of the oral health section, but it also should embrace the goals and objectives of the health communication and health information technology section of *Healthy People 2020*.

Building upon *Healthy People* gives the NOHI a framework for sustainability as well as the ability to change goals and objectives depending upon achievements in improving oral health. More importantly, as better measures of quality in oral health are developed, more sophisticated goals can be set. The committee also notes that shorter-term and intermediate goals and objectives will also be needed along the way toward these larger goals.

Establishing High-Level Accountability

All Americans, especially those from vulnerable and underserved populations, are at risk of suffering compromised health. This is particularly important because HHS describes itself as "the United States government's principal agency for protecting the health of all Americans and providing essential human services, especially for those who are least able to help themselves" (HHS, 2010a).

The committee concluded that previous HHS efforts to improve oral health have largely suffered from lack of high-level accountability, a lack of coordination among HHS agencies, a lack of resources, and a lack of sustained interest. Considering the impact of oral diseases and disorders on the nation, its relevance to every American, and the importance of strong, accountable leadership, the committee recommends:

> **RECOMMENDATION 1:** The secretary of HHS should give the leader(s) of the new Oral Health Initiative (NOHI) the authority and resources needed to successfully integrate oral health into the planning, programming, policies, and research that occur across all HHS programs and agencies:
> - Each agency within HHS that has a role in oral health should provide an annual plan for how it will integrate oral health into existing programs within the first year.
> - Each agency should identify specific opportunities for public-private partnerships and collaborating with other agencies inside and outside HHS.
> - The leader(s) of the NOHI should coordinate, review, and implement these plans.
> - The leaders(s) of the NOHI should incorporate patient and consumer input into the design and implementation of the NOHI.

The identification of specific leadership for the NOHI would create a robust level of accountability. Because there was not enough evidence to determine exactly who the leader(s) of the NOHI should be, the committee concluded that the secretary should ultimately determine the leader of the NOHI; presumably this could be the current co-leads, the head of the Oral Health Coordinating Committee (OHCC), a new office or officer dedicated to oral health, or another person who is given distinct authority. In any case, as discussed earlier, lack of strong and consistent leadership, insufficient funding, and inadequate staffing all contributed to the ineffectiveness of previous efforts. Therefore, the committee recommends the named leader be given enough authority and resources to carry out his or her duties. If this effort is to be led by the OHCC, then clearly financial support will be needed where it currently has none.

Toward the goal of fully integrating oral health into overall health, instead of merely listing existing or planned oral health activities, the committee recommends that each relevant operating and staff division provide clear directions and goals for integrating oral health into all of its relevant programs within the first year of the NOHI. Aside from their individual abilities, each division should look for clear opportunities to partner with other entities, both within and outside of HHS. The committee urges that these individual plans focus on the issues laid out in the framework for the

NOHI and include measurable objectives. These objectives could focus on shorter-term or intermediate measures of departmental performance such as implementation of new programs and collaborations or demonstrated impact on oral health status and access. The leader(s) of the NOHI would be responsible for oversight of all of these plans, including looking for overarching areas for collaboration and learning both within HHS and with external partners.

Finally, in concert with the IOM definition of *quality*,[1] which includes patient-centeredness as a goal, the committee recommends the NOHI pursue a focus on patient-centered (and community-centered) care and therefore seek ways to ensure that the patient's and consumer's perspectives (including those of private-sector and other public-sector stakeholders) is recognized and appreciated in future oral health planning.

Focusing on Prevention

Among the most important contributions that HHS can make to improve oral health is to promote the use of regimens and services that have been shown to promote oral health, prevent oral diseases, and help manage these diseases. Too often, oral health care focuses more intently on treating disease once it has already become manifest. A focus on prevention may help to reduce the overall need for treatment, reduce costs, and improve the capacity of the system to care for those in need.

HHS plays a key role in promoting the adoption of evidence-based preventive oral health services, including those provided at the national, state, community, and individual levels. For example, as discussed in Chapter 4, the U.S. Preventive Services Task Force assesses the evidence about clinical preventive services while the Task Force on Community Preventive Services does the same for community-based preventive services. In addition to its role in assessing preventive services, HHS and the federal government as a whole directly provide (or oversee the provision of) a significant amount of oral health care.

The committee concluded that (1) preventive services and counseling have a strong evidence base for promoting oral health and preventing disease; and (2) HHS is a key provider of oral health care, especially for vulnerable and underserved populations through the safety net. Therefore, the committee recommends:

RECOMMENDATION 2: All relevant HHS agencies should promote and monitor the use of evidence-based preventive services in oral health

---

[1] In 2001, the IOM defined six dimensions of quality: safety, effectiveness, patient-centeredness, timeliness, efficiency, and equity (IOM, 2001).

(both clinical and community based) and counseling across the life span by

- Consulting with the U.S. Preventive Services Task Force and the Task Force on Community Preventive Services to give priority to evidentiary reviews of preventive services in oral health;
- Ensuring that HHS-administered health care systems (e.g., Federally Qualified Health Centers, Indian Health Service) provide recommended preventive services and counseling to improve oral health;
- Providing guidance and assistance to state and local health systems to implement these same approaches; and
- Communicating with other federally administered health care systems to share best practices.

This recommendation is in alignment with the HHS Strategic Plan for FY 2010–2015 that promotes "the incorporation of oral healthcare services and oral disease prevention into primary healthcare delivery sites" and "policies to integrate oral health into primary care, including prevention and improved health literacy" (HHS, 2010c). Overall, the plan states "Improved availability of oral health services, including disease prevention, treatment, and health promotion and education, should be promoted for poor and underserved populations as well as for the population at large."

A first step for the U.S. Preventive Services Task Force and the Task Force on Community Preventive Services would be to reexamine modalities that have been looked at previously but had insufficient evidence (see Chapter 4). The committee encourages the provision of preventive services in HHIS-administered health care systems by any and all health care professionals who are competent to do so; for example, physicians, nurses, and others could be involved either through direct provision of care (e.g., fluoride varnish) or through examination, risk assessment, and appropriate referrals as needed. Assistance to state and local health systems could include both financial assistance and technical assistance, through the sharing of best practices. Consideration will also be needed for the adequacy of and support needed for the public health infrastructure to support these activities—both at the federal and the state level. HRSA's regional offices might be one option to provide technical assistance at the state and local levels. The Centers for Disease Control and Prevention's (CDC's) grants to states for supporting public health infrastructure also could help encourage these activities.

Improving Oral Health Literacy

Overall, evidence suggests that the general oral health literacy of both individuals and all types of health care professionals is poor, especially in understanding the causes and prevention of oral diseases and how to communicate about these issues. For example, despite decades of evidence regarding the infectious nature of dental caries and the value of fluoride in preventing dental caries, both professional and patient knowledge regarding these issues remains lacking. In addition, poor oral health literacy contributes to poor access because individuals may not understand the importance of oral health care or their options for accessing such care.

The committee concluded that the oral health literacy of individuals, communities, and all types of health care providers remains low. This includes knowing how to prevent and manage oral diseases, the impact of poor oral health, how to navigate the oral health care system, and best techniques in patient–provider communication. Therefore, the committee recommends:

RECOMMENDATION 3: All relevant HHS agencies should undertake oral health literacy and education efforts aimed at individuals, communities, and health care professionals. These efforts should include, but not be limited to,

- Community-wide public education on the causes and implications of oral diseases and the effectiveness of preventive interventions;
  - o Focus areas should include
    - The infectious nature of dental caries,
    - The effectiveness of fluorides and sealants,
    - The role of diet and nutrition in oral health, and
    - How oral diseases affect other health conditions.
- Community-wide guidance on how to access oral health care; and
  - o Focus areas should include using and promoting websites such as the National Oral Health Clearinghouse and www.health care.gov.
- Professional education on best practices in patient–provider communication skills that result in improved oral health behaviors.
  - o Focus areas should include how to communicate to an increasingly diverse population about prevention of oral cancers, dental caries, and periodontal disease.

As described in relation to the previous recommendation, this current recommendation aligns with the HHS Strategic Plan for FY 2010–2015 that calls for improvements in oral health literacy and oral health promotion and education (HHS, 2010c). In her presentation to this committee, Dr. Marcia Brand, deputy administrator of the Health Resources and Services Administration (HRSA), noted that as part of the statement of task, HHS was interested in learning more about how to increase public awareness and communicate specific messages of the relationship between good oral health and good overall health (Brand, 2010). She also noted that HRSA was interested in the oral health literacy of all types of health care professionals, including what types of messages could be sent to them regarding prevention of oral diseases (and how to communicate these messages). The committee did not find enough evidence specifically in the oral health literacy and behavioral change literature to recommend exact strategies for delivering needed messages; therefore, it has given examples within the recommendation of the areas that have the most evidence supporting the need for outreach in these areas. (Research in oral health behavioral change will be discussed later in these recommendations.) The committee intends the highlighting of these areas to provide direction for HHS. In addition, the CDC might consider targeting these areas if the CDC oral health campaign related to prevention authorized in the Affordable Care Act (see Chapter 4) is eventually funded. The committee fully supports the funding of this national campaign to promote awareness of oral health promotion and disease prevention. In addition, this type of campaign represents another opportunity where input from other public and private stakeholders would be valuable, especially in learning about successes and failures of other individual campaigns. Finally, the committee recognizes that any literacy and education efforts should be carried out in accordance with standards for culturally and linguistically appropriate services.

Enhancing the Delivery of Oral Health Care

To meet the oral health care needs of the U.S. population, several workforce changes are needed. Dental professionals need more training in community-based settings in order to learn more about caring for underserved and vulnerable populations. Nondental health care professionals (e.g., nurses, pharmacists, physician assistants, physicians) are often not prepared to provide basic oral health care. This may include being able to recognize disease, teaching patients about self-care, or providing basic preventive services. In addition, both dental and nondental health care professionals need better training in collaborative efforts, including the appropriate use of referrals in both directions, and more research will be needed to understand best approaches. For example, examinations of team-based care may need to consider how health information technology might be used, such as through the integration of medical and dental electronic records. The emergence of new types of dental professionals and the use of existing professionals in expanded roles, as discussed in previous chapters, has been contentious for decades. Other health care professions have expanded roles for existing professionals in high-risk situations, and these efforts have also been accompanied by political tension between professions. While the evidence in this country on the quality of oral health care provided by health professionals who are not dentists is early and limited, without further research and evaluation, including a comparison of the quality of that care as compared to the care of dentists, better workforce models cannot be developed. Finally, particular attention is needed for underrepresented minority groups who often suffer from disparities in oral health. Health care professionals who are themselves from underrepresented minority groups often care for a larger proportion of patients from these populations. However, the racial and ethnic makeup of the dental professions has not changed markedly over time, and while programs such as bridge and pipeline programs have had some successes, newer models and methods of attracting a diverse student body need to be explored.

The committee concluded that (1) nondental health care professionals are well situated to play an increased role in oral health care, but they require improved education and training; (2) interprofessional, team-based care has the potential to improve care-coordination, patient outcomes, and produce cost-savings, yet dental and nondental health care professionals are largely not trained to work in this manner; (3) new dental professionals and existing professionals with expanded duties may have a role to play in expanding access to care; and (4) efforts to broaden the diversity of the oral health care workforce have not produced marked changes.

While the regulation of health care professions occurs at the state level, HHS has a role to play in both the education and training of the health care workforce (as noted in Chapter 4) as well as the demonstration and testing of new innovative workforce models for specific needs (as noted in Chapter 3 and through elements of the Affordable Care Act and the HHS Strategic plan, both described in Chapter 4). These issues all require innovative research and demonstration efforts in order to more fully develop the evidence base on their value and best use. Therefore, the committee recommends:

RECOMMENDATION 4: HHS should invest in workforce innovations to improve oral health that focus on
- Core competency development, education, and training, to allow for the use of all health care professionals in oral health care;
- Interprofessional, team-based approaches to the prevention and treatment of oral diseases;
- Best use of new and existing oral health care professionals; and
- Increasing the diversity and improving the cultural competence of the workforce providing oral health care.

This recommendation aligns with the HHS Strategic Plan for FY 2010–2015. One of the five identified goals of the plan is "Strengthen the nation's health and human service infrastructure and workforce" through objectives that address improving cultural competence and expanding care teams (including the use of new types of professionals). In fact, the plan has an explicit strategy for oral health: "Expand the primary oral health care team and promote models that incorporate new providers, expanded scope of existing providers, and utilization of medical providers to provide evidence-based oral health preventive services, where appropriate" (HHS, 2010c).

In addition to the training and composition of the oral health work-force, more needs to be done to consider alternatives to how oral health care can be delivered and financed to improve availability and scope of oral health coverage and care. Chapter 3 gives an overview to the financing of oral health care. Dental coverage is strongly associated with receiving oral health care, yet many Americans, especially older adults, do not have this coverage. The separation of dental coverage from overall health care coverage reinforces the separation of oral health from overall health. The committee concluded that oral health care is so integral to the overall health of individuals and the population that financing of these services would ideally be part of every health plan. However, the committee also recognizes the current political and economic infeasibility of seeking to have all oral health services covered under health care plans.

The committee found that not enough research has been done to determine if alternative payment mechanisms might be more efficient to finance oral health care and pay for delivery of the most effective services in the most efficient manner, or to determine if the delivery of preventive services would result in long-term cost savings (which would have implications for the scope of coverage). Some consideration might be needed for how the current compensation system drives the delivery of oral health care. For example, like in general health care, fee-for-service payment structures often reinforce the delivery of treatment services rather than preventive care. Like in general health care financing, exploration is likely needed for how alternative payment structures such as the bundling of payments and pay for performance might affect care delivery.

Also like in the general health care system, incentives may be needed to encourage oral health care providers to work in underserved areas or with underserved populations, such as increased payments for Medicaid providers or reimbursement for services performed by nondental health care professionals. Chapter 3 describes the delivery of oral health care services, yet also recognizes that distinct segments of the American public are not well served by the current system and that alternative solutions need to be explored (as discussed in the previous recommendation). As more members of the overall health care workforce become competent and licensed to deliver care, research will be needed for how they will work and be reimbursed.

In January 2010, the Advisory Committee on Training in Primary Care Medicine and Dentistry said, "CMS needs to work with primary care leadership organizations to develop strategies to redefine how to deliver and reimburse primary care (HHS, 2010b)." It added,

> CMS should pilot and evaluate reimbursement strategies that compensate for nontraditional approaches to care such as group visits, telephone and electronic communication, care management, and incorporation of nontraditional provider types (such as patient educators, patient navigators, and community health workers).

They suggested that such approaches could both improve outcomes and contain costs.

The committee concluded that (1) distinct segments of the U.S. population have challenges with accessing care in typical settings of care; (2) lack of dental coverage contributes to access problems; (3) newer financing mechanisms might help contain costs and improve health outcomes; and (4) new delivery models need to be explored to improve efficiency. Therefore, the committee recommends:

RECOMMENDATION 5: CMS should explore new delivery and payment models for Medicare, Medicaid, and CHIP to improve access, quality, and coverage of oral health care across the life span.

The committee notes that one option for how CMS could explore some of these models is through the Center for Medicare and Medicaid Innovation (the "Innovation Center"), which was established within HHS under a provision of the Affordable Care Act of 2010. The Innovation Center is focused on achieving improvements in three areas:

1. Better care for people (improving patient care across inpatient and outpatient settings, and developing ways to make care safer, more patient-centered, more efficient, more effective, more timely, and more equitable);
2. Care coordination (developing new models for transprofessional collaboration); and
3. Improved community care models (initiatives designed to improve the health of communities (e.g., obesity and heart disease) (Berwick, 2010).

The Innovation Center will help to identify, support, and evaluate models of care that improve the quality of care while also lowering costs. This includes demonstration projects on the effectiveness of team care and the impact of more coordinated payments (Carey, 2010; CMS, 2010b).

As with the previous recommendations, this recommendation aligns with the HHS Strategic Plan for 2010–2015 for its focus on improving how care is delivered. In addition, the plan identifies an overarching goal to "transform health care," including specific objectives to create new models for health delivery and payment that promote effective care and reduce costs (HHS, 2010c).

Expanding Research

Throughout the evidence-gathering process for this report, the committee noted a significant lack of robust evidence related to many different aspects of oral health care. While Chapter 2 highlighted significant oral health disparities between different populations, not enough is known about the best ways to decrease these disparities. Similarly, Chapter 2 describes the basics of health literacy practices and principles, including its relationship to disease management and behavioral change. The chapter highlights that although methods of preventing oral disease are well established, knowledge of these methods is still limited, both on the part of the public and even many professionals. In addition, not enough evidence yet exists to determine the best methods for changing behaviors in oral health specifically. Chapter 3 notes that very little evidence exists for the quality of oral health services. Very few measures of quality exist for oral health, leading to little evidence not only about the quality of the services themselves but also about their ultimate relationship to long-term improvements in oral health. Quality assessment efforts in oral health lag far behind analagous efforts in medicine. Finally, in Chapter 4 the committee describes the role of many other federal agencies in the oral health care of a significant number of Americans. The committee recognizes that these other agencies all have data collection systems and that consolidation of the data collected by these multiple sources would be useful in performing secondary research in oral health by many types of researchers. However, much effort would be needed to make all of these data usable.

Based on the findings in all of these chapters, the committee concluded that a more robust evidence base in oral health is needed overall. The committee concluded that efforts are needed most toward (1) generating new evidence on best practices; (2) improving the usefulness of existing data; and (3) evaluating the quality of oral health care (including outcomes).

Therefore, the committee recommends:

RECOMMENDATION 6: HHS should place a high priority on efforts to improve open, actionable, and timely information to advance science and improve oral health through research by

- Leveraging resources for research to promote a more robust evidence base specific to oral health care, including, but not limited to,
  o oral health disparities, and
  o best practices in oral health care and oral health behavior change;
- Working across HHS agencies— in collaboration with other federal departments (e.g., Department of Defense, Veterans Administration) involved in the collection of oral health data—to integrate, standardize, and promote public availability of relevant databases; and
- Promoting the creation and implementation of new, useful, and appropriate measures of quality oral health care practices, cost and efficiency, and oral health outcomes.

In terms of "leveraging resources," the committee supports the direction of new funding toward research, but in recognizing that this is a time of limited resources, it emphasizes that HHS should prioritize oral health research when deciding upon distribution of existing resources. While the committee fully supports fundamental research that underpins oral health, again, in a time of limited (or diminishing) resources, the committee asserts that research in disparities, best practices, and behavioral change are areas that are especially lacking in evidence and could have a great impact on long-term goals. Research on oral health disparities is especially needed to understand best approaches to reducing those disparities. The research into best practices in oral health should be interpreted broadly because many areas of research are still needed related to individual procedures, oral health literacy, interprofesssional approaches, and many other areas, all of which contribute to oral health overall. In addition, part of this research will require consideration of how to transfer oral health research results into use by appropriate user groups.

As previously noted, the committee sees that in addition to the need for new primary research, many databases already exist in multiple places, but they are not currently structured in a manner that allows for full integration of these data. Examples of data sets that include oral health information include the Medical Expenditure Panel Survey, the National Health and Nutrition Examination Survey, the Pregnancy Risk Assessment Monitoring System, and the National Health Interview Survey, among many others. Nearly all of the data sets are supported, at least in part, by different branches of the federal government. Some of these, however, do not have recent data.

The primary purpose here would be for secondary research on the vast amounts of existing data that are not being used efficiently. In addition to the publicly available data sets, there are many other data sets that exist and contain useful data. While the committee recognizes that some data may not be able to be shared (e.g., sensitive data such as in cases of military databases), these data, whenever possible, should be made available to all researchers. For example, HHS' Community Health Data Initiative and CMS's and the VA's Blue Button Initiative are current efforts to share standardized data with the public regarding health and health care in order to foster better public understanding of health care performance and personal health as well as to promote innovative use of the data for the public's benefit (CMS, 2010a; HHS, 2011a).

Finally, many challenges lie ahead for the development of more robust measures in oral health, including the lack of a universally used diagnostic coding system as well as challenges in collecting data from single practice settings. While HHS can require the use of diagnostic codes in their own systems, they cannot mandate their use in the private sector. Overall, the federal government has a great opportunity to assist in this process, both because of the wealth of existing data as well as because of its role in operating large systems of care.

Measuring Progress

Finally, the committee concluded that an effective NOHI needs an ongoing process for maintaining accountability, and for measuring progress toward achieving specific goals of improved oral health. Therefore, the committee recommends:

> RECOMMENDATION 7: To evaluate the NOHI the leader(s) of the NOHI should convene an annual public meeting of the agency heads to report on the progress of the NOHI, including
> * Progress of each agency in reaching goals;
> * New innovations and data;
> * Dissemination of best practices and data into the community; and
> * Improvement in health outcomes of populations served by HHS programs, especially as they relate to *Healthy People 2020* goals and specific objectives. HHS should provide a forum for public response and comment and make the final proceedings of each meeting available to the public.

The committee makes this recommendation with the intention that progress made on the NOHI is shared transparently with any and all interested parties. This is an opportunity not only to measure progress in implementing new programs and policies but also to share best practices in the prevention and treatment of oral diseases, to share new knowledge (based on new research and demonstration projects), develop consistent messages about oral health, and to monitor oral health outcomes related to the efforts of HHS. Overall, the committee envisions that this meeting be an opportunity to report on both short-term and intermediate goals (as set by the individual agencies, as discussed in Recommendation 1) and progress on *Healthy People 2020* goals and objectives (the overall mission of the NOHI). In addition, HHS needs to develop a mechanism to get public feedback on the programs they are responsible for, ensuring that consumers have a meaningful voice. The committee could not recommend the exact interval of this meeting, recognizing both the time needed for the start-up of new projects as well as the time needed to collect and evaluate new data. The committee also does not intend for this recommendation to preclude additional meetings that HHS might hold internally without a public presence.

LOOKING TO THE FUTURE

In her presentation to this committee, Dr. Mary Wakefield, Administrator of HRSA, responded to questions from this committee regarding the types of recommendations that might be most valuable for HHS. She recognized that a balance of specificity and generality would be needed but that the recommendations should be "actionable"—that is, recommendations that could be acted upon immediately but might have several methods of implementation and thereby give flexibility. This committee asserts that the framework and details of the previously outlined recommendations does just this. The committee recognizes that many of the recommendations made are not necessarily "new." However, as the title of this report suggests, the challenges and strategies illuminated by *Oral Health in America* represent and remain the areas that have the strongest evidence for effecting the needed changes.

As this committee looks to the future of HHS' involvement in oral health, questions arise regarding both the long-term viability of maintaining oral health as a priority issue and the likelihood of the recommendations of this report coming to fruition. In this vein, the committee has identified three key areas that are needed for future success: strong leadership, sustained interest, and the involvement of multiple stakeholders.

The Importance of Leadership

The foundation of the OHI 2010 provides many indications that leadership for oral health is currently strong. The OHI 2010 is broader than many previous efforts in that it involves many more HHS agencies and programs at multiple levels, which may result in more buy-in departmentally.

As the NOHI further calls for each agency to develop individual annual plans and short-term goals, it involves individuals at the staff level, who often drive programmatic activity, a structure that veterans of previous initiatives have said can be helpful. However, this also presents the challenge of organizing and directing a multitude of agencies within HHS that are highly independent and autonomous and may not always act in concert. In her presentation to this committee, Dr. Wakefield noted that they were working on signing a memorandum of agreement among CDC, CMS, and HRSA to facilitate cross-agency work (Wakefield, 2010). The new NOHI represents an additional challenge in that this committee calls for the increased involvement of and collaboration with leaders from the private sector and other segments of the public sector. These leaders are needed partners to help improve cross-sector communication and coordination in order to achieve significant improvements in oral health.

It appears that the current leadership at HHS is capable of meeting these challenges. The OHI 2010 is rooted in strong, high-level interest in that the Assistant Secretary for Health and the Administrator for CMS co-lead the effort. In another example, in her presentation to this committee, Dr. Brand noted that HRSA had recently created an Office of Special Health Affairs within its Office of Strategic Priorities that would focus on two cross-cutting areas: oral health and behavioral health (Brand, 2010).

However, while leadership to promote oral health within HHS itself appears strong, some have criticized the erosion of oral health expertise and leadership within HHS. During the public workshop of the committee's second meeting, a discussion ensued about whether a formal dental leadership position should be created in every agency. It was noted that creating a multitude of new positions might not necessarily be matched with enough individuals interested in entering government service, that positions for all types of health care professionals were being eliminated in public agencies to some degree, and that previous successes relied more on the interest from the workers on the ground level. However, the committee does support the need for individuals within HHS from all sectors of health care who are well versed in oral health issues (both dental and nondental professionals) and have an interest in promoting oral health.

Sustaining Interest

Regardless of how an initiative is structured, much of its long-term viability depends on the interests and efforts of the individuals leading the agencies and HHS, which can change in unpredictable ways over time. For example, a key factor may be whether it can survive a change in presidential administrations, particularly one involving a change in parties. In her presentation to this committee, Dr. Wakefield noted that while there hasn't been a formal focus on oral health across HHS, they saw the OHI 2010 as an opportunity to leverage assets and interests to improve the recognition of the importance of oral health to individuals and populations (Wakefield, 2010). Tragically, sustained interest is seen and promulgated in the case of Deamonte Driver. Driver's death in 2007 remains a high-profile example of the worst-case scenario for poor oral health. To date, Driver's story brings an awareness to these issues that facts or figures cannot achieve. Long-term viability depends on HHS itself making and keeping oral health a priority issue.

In spite of evidence for the likelihood of sustained interest, several warning signs have arisen recently that could contribute to a loss of momentum. First, in a February 2011 letter from the Secretary of HHS to state governors regarding state budget concerns, she highlighted areas where states could save money, including modifying benefits. The letter noted that "while some benefits, such as hospital and physician services, are required to be provided by State Medicaid programs, many services, such as prescription drugs, dental services, and speech therapy, are optional" (HHS, 2011b). The committee does recognize that in times of economic challenges, such as we have now, many important health and health care issues are competing for a limited pool of dollars. However, the burden of oral disease, including both the economic and the social impact, needs to be recognized as one of the grand challenges in the health of our nation. Additionally, in early 2011, the CDC released the report *CDC Health Disparities and Inequalities in the United States—2011* in which oral disease was not addressed at any level. The committee urges CDC to include oral health in subsequent reports.

More significantly, in early 2011, the committee learned of the proposed downgrading of the CDC's Division of Oral Health (within the National Center for Chronic Disease Prevention and Health Promotion) into a branch of the Division of Adult and Community Health (ADA, 2011). Such a change raises two serious concerns. First is that the Division of Adolescent and School Health does not list oral health among the "important topics that affect the health and well-being of children and adolescents" (CDC, 2011) despite the surgeon general's finding that dental caries was the "the single most common chronic childhood disease" (HHS, 2000). Therefore, placement of oral health into the Division of Adult and Community Health is likely to impede CDC's ability to give direct attention to the oral health needs of the U.S. population across the life span. The second concern is that such a decision implies that CDC is placing a low priority on oral health. This may be true of other HHS agencies as well. For example, the committee noted that the Administration on Aging does not have any specific initiatives related to the oral health of older adults. The success of the NOHI requires the active involvement of every agency within HHS. Similar to the need for consistent messages to patients about the importance of oral health, HHS needs consistent messaging within its own organization that oral health is a priority.

Engaging Stakeholders

Finally, an important ingredient for the success of the NOHI is public-private partnerships and grassroots involvement. As stated in Chapter 1, an HHS initiative cannot on its own change the entire oral health care system. While the committee agrees that HHS should look for ways to be a leader for the rest of the country, they also need to be mindful of opportunities to partner with and learn from other stakeholders. For example, the committee recognizes the efforts occurring in the private sector that should not be supplanted or ignored. Throughout the recommendations for the NOHI, there are examples and opportunities for HHS to work with other stakeholders to combine efforts, share best practices, and pool resources. Collective efforts in the different sectors are also key to the successful implementation of systems and services at the community level. There is also an explicit effort both in the administrative structure of the NOHI and in the reporting process to engage consumers and their communities so that efforts remain patient and community focused, and that HHS remains openly accountable to the people they serve.

The committee recognizes that bringing disparate sectors together to effect significant change is a daunting task, but it is one well suited to the mission and responsibilities of HHS. Every effort needs to be made by HHS to collaborate with and learn from the private sector; other public sector entities at the local, state, and national levels; and patients themselves toward achieving the goal of improving the oral health care and, ultimately, the oral health of the entire U.S. population. There are many reasons that HHS can and should be a leader in improving oral health and oral health care. However, most important is the burden that oral diseases are placing on the health and well-being of the American people.

REFERENCES

ADA (American Dental Assocation). 2011. *CDC decision to downgrade Division of Oral Health a bad move, ADA protests.* http://www.ada.org/advocacy.aspx#top (accessed February 24, 2011).

Berwick, D. 2010. *Introducing the CMS Center for Medicare & Medicaid Innovation—and innovations.cms.gov.* http://www.healthcare.gov/news/blog/InnovationCenter.html (accessed December 29, 2010).

Brand, M. 2010. *Oral testimony of Dr. Marcia Brand, Deputy Administrator of the Health Resources and Services Administration.* Presentation at meeting of the Committee on an Oral Health Initiative, Washington, DC. March 31, 2010.

Carey, M. A. 2010. *New Medicare/Medicaid projects aimed at cheaper, better care.* http://www.kaiserhealthnews.org/Stories/2010/November/17/cms-innovation-center-berwick.aspx (accessed January 9, 2011).

CDC (Centers for Disease Control and Prevention). 2011. *Healthy youth: Health topics.* http://www.cdc.gov/healthyyouth/healthtopics/index.htm (accessed February 28, 2011).

CMS (Centers for Medicare and Medicaid Services). 2010a. *Blue Button Initiative.* https://www.cms.gov/NonIdentifiableDataFiles/12_BlueButtonInitiative.asp (accessed January 10, 2011).

CMS. 2010b. *CMS introduces new Center for Medicare and Medicaid Innovation, initiatives to better coordinate health care.* http://innovations.cms.gov/innovations/pressreleases/pr110910.shtml (accessed December 29, 2010).

Crall, J. J. 2009. Oral health policy development since the surgeon general's report on oral health. *Academic Pediatrics* 9(6):476-482.

HHS (Department of Health and Human Services). 2000. *Oral health in America: A report of the surgeon general.* Rockville, MD: U.S. Department of Health and Human Services.

HHS. 2010a. *About HHS.* http://www.hhs.gov/about/ (accessed December 29, 2010).

HHS. 2010b. *Advisory committee on training in primary care medicine and dentistry: The redesign of primary care with implications for training.* Rockville, MD: U.S. Department of Health and Human Services.

HHS. 2010c. *Strategic plan and priorities.* http://www.hhs.gov/secretary/about/priorities/priorities.html (accessed December 29, 2010).

HHS. 2011a. *Community health data initiative.* http://www.hhs.gov/open/plan/opengovernmentplan/initiatives/initiative.html (accessed January 10, 2011).

HHS. 2011b. *Sebelius outlines state flexibility and federal support available for Medicaid.* http://www.hhs.gov/news/press/2011pres/01/20110203c.html (accessed February 24, 2011).

IOM (Institute of Medicine). 2001. *Crossing the quality chasm: A new health system for the 21st century.* Washington, DC: National Academy Press.

Mertz, E., and W. E. Mouradian. 2009. Addressing children's oral health in the new millennium: Trends in the dental workforce. *Academic Pediatrics* 9(6):433-439.

Mouradian, W. E., R. L. Slayton, W. R. Maas, D. V. Kleinman, H. C. Slavkin, D. DePaola, C. Evans, and J. Wilentz. (2009) Progress in children's oral health since the surgeon general's report on oral health. *Academic Pediatrics.* 9(6):374-379.

Slayton, R. L., and H. C. Slavkin. 2009. Commentary: Scientific investments continue to fuel improvements in oral health (May 2000–2009). *Academic Pediatrics* 9(6):383-385.

Wakefield, M. 2010. *Oral testimony of Dr. Mary Wakefield, Administrator of the Health Resources and Services Administration.* Presentation at meeting of the Committee on an Oral Health Initiative, Washington, DC. June 28, 2010.

Appendix A

Acronyms

AADR	American Association for Dental Research
AAP	American Academy of Pediatrics
AAPD	American Academy of Pediatric Dentistry
AAPHD	American Association of Public Health Dentistry
ACA	Patient Protection and Affordable Care Act
ADA	American Dental Association
ADHA	American Dental Hygienists' Association
AGD	Academy of General Dentistry
AHRQ	Agency for Healthcare Research and Quality
AI/AN	American Indians and Alaska Natives
ASH	Assistant Secretary for Health
ASTDD	Association of State and Territorial Dental Directors
BHP	Bureau of Health Professions
BLS	Bureau of Labor Statistics
BOP	Federal Bureau of Prisons
BPHC	Bureau of Primary Health Care
CDA	certified dental assistant
CDC	Centers for Disease Control and Prevention
CDHC	community dental health coordinator
CDT	certified dental technician
CHIP	Children's Health Insurance Program
CHIPRA	Children's Health Insurance Program Reauthorization Act

CLAS	National Standards on Culturally and Linguistically Appropriate Services
CMS	Centers for Medicare and Medicaid Services
CODA	Commission on Dental Accreditation
COSTEP	Commissioned Officer Student Training and Extern Programs
CRNA	certified registered nurse anesthetist
DDS	Doctor of Dental Surgery
DePAC	Dental Professional Advisory Committee
DHEW	Department of Health, Education, and Welfare
DMD	Doctor of Dental Medicine
DOD	U.S. Department of Defense
DOE	U.S. Department of Education
DOJ	U.S. Department of Justice
DQA	Dental Quality Alliance
ECC	early childhood caries
EFDAs	expanded function dental assistants
EPA	Environmental Protection Agency
EPSDT	Early and Periodic Screening, Diagnosis, and Treatment
FDA	U.S. Food and Drug Administration
FPL	federal poverty level
FQHCs	Federally Qualified Health Centers
FTC	Federal Trade Commission
GAO	U.S. Government Accountability Office
GME	Graduate Medical Education
HCFA	Health Care Financing Administration
HHS	U.S. Department of Health and Human Services
HRSA	Health Resources and Services Administration
ICD	International Statistical Classification of Diseases and Related Health Problems
ICE	U.S. Immigration and Customs Enforcement
IHS	Indian Health Service
IMB	Into the Mouths of Babes
IOM	Institute of Medicine
MCHB	Maternal and Child Health Bureau
MEPS	Medical Expenditure Panel Survey

MHS	Military Health System
MOU	memorandum of understanding
NCHS	National Center for Health Statistics
NCP	National Caries Program
NHANES	National Health and Nutrition Examination Survey
NHSC	National Health Service Corps
NIDCR	National Institute of Dental and Craniofacial Research
NIDR	National Institute for Dental Research
NIH	National Institutes of Health
NIST	National Institute of Standards and Technology
NOHI	new Oral Health Initiative
NOHSS	National Oral Health Surveillance System
NP	nurse practitioner
NQF	National Quality Forum
NRC	National Research Council
OHCC	Oral Health Coordinating Committee
OHI 2010	Oral Health Initiative 2010
OHPC	National Oral Health Policy Center
OHRC	National Maternal and Child Health Resource Center
OIG	Office of the Inspector General
PA	physician assistant
RDHAP	registered dental hygienist in alternative practice
SNODENT	Systematized Nomenclature of Dentistry
TEAM	training in expanded auxiliary management
URM	underrepresented minority
USCG	U.S. Coast Guard
USDA	U.S. Department of Agriculture
USPHS	U.S. Public Health Service
USPSTF	U.S. Preventive Services Task Force
VA	U.S. Department of Veterans Affairs
WHO	World Health Organization
WIC	Special Supplemental Nutrition Program for Women, Infants, and Children

Appendix B

Organizational Charts of the U.S. Department of Health and Human Services

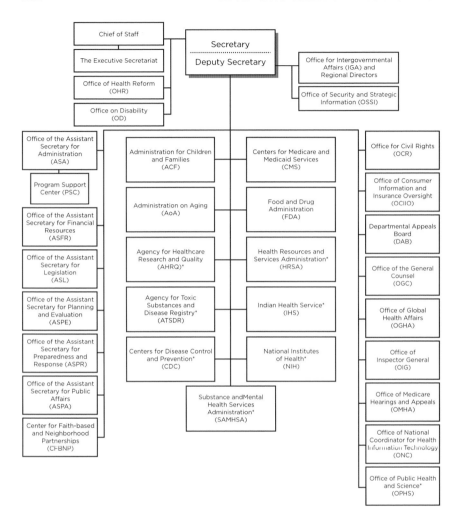

*Denotes members of the U.S. Public Health Service.

NOTE: The Office of Public Health and Science is now known as the Office of the Assistant Secretary for Health.

SOURCE: HHS. 2011. U.S. Department of Health and Human Services Organizational Chart. http://www.hhs.gov/about/orgchart/#text (accessed February 22, 2011).

KEY HHS OPERATING DIVISIONS FOR ORAL HEALTH

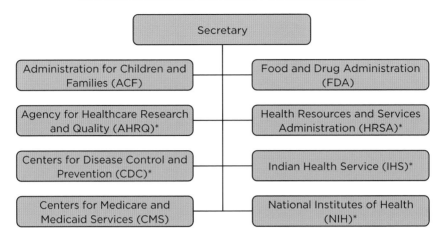

KEY HRSA OPERATING DIVISIONS FOR ORAL HEALTH

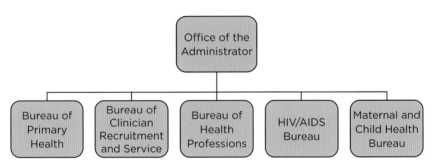

*Denotes members of the U.S. Public Health Service.

Appendix C

Workshop Agendas

MARCH 31, 2010—WORKSHOP FOR COMMITTEE
ON AN ORAL HEALTH INITIATIVE

Keck Center of the National Academies
500 Fifth Street, NW, Washington, DC 20001

11:45 AM   Welcome and Introductory Remarks
Richard Krugman, Committee Chair, University of Colorado

12:00 PM   Remarks from Study Sponsors and Discussion
Marcia Brand, Health Resources and Services Administration

1:30 PM   Position Statements—Professional Societies
David Halpern, Academy of General Dentistry
James Crall, American Academy of Pediatric Dentistry
Raymond Gist, American Dental Association
Ann Battrell, American Dental Hygienists' Association

2:20 PM   Behavioral Science and Public Health Interventions
Karen Glanz, University of Pennsylvania

2:45 PM   Implementing *Oral Health in America*—Lessons Learned
Dushanka Kleinman, University of Maryland

3:35 PM   The Current Oral Health "System" of Care
Beth Mertz, Center for the Health Professions, UCSF
Robert Weyant, University of Pittsburgh

4:05 PM   *Healthy People 2020*: Current Status and Future Direction
             Bruce Dye, Centers for Disease Control and Prevention

4:30 PM   Open Public Comment Period

5:00 PM   Concluding Remarks and Adjourn

JUNE 28, 2010—WORKSHOP FOR COMMITTEE ON AN ORAL HEALTH INITIATIVE

Keck Center of the National Academies
500 Fifth Street, NW, Washington, DC 20001

9:00 AM   Welcome and Opening Remarks
             Richard Krugman, Committee Chair

9:10 AM   *Workshop Session I—Education and Training*

             Critical Importance of HHS to Dental Training and
             Education
             Jack Bresch, American Dental Education Association

             Dental Hygiene Education—How It Will Evolve in the
             Future and the Role That HHS Can Play
             Laura Joseph, Farmingdale State College of New York

             Wanted—Physicians Who Understand Oral Health
             Wendy Mouradian, University of Washington

             Nursing Education and Research (Geriatrics)
             Rita Jablonski, The Pennsylvania State University

10:30 AM   BREAK

11:00 AM   *Workshop Session II—Literacy*

             The National Action Plan to Improve Health Literacy
             Cynthia Baur, Centers for Disease Control and Prevention

             Appropriate Health Literacy Materials Make a Difference
             Susan R. Levy, University of Illinois at Chicago

Communicating with Patients: A Survey of Dental Team Members
Linda Neuhauser, University of California, Berkeley

Health Literacy and Oral Health: Considering Proactive and Ameliorative Action
Rima Rudd, Harvard University

12:30 PM   LUNCH

1:30 PM   *Workshop Session III—HHS*

HHS Oral Health Initiative 2010
Mary Wakefield, Health Resources and Services Administration (HRSA)

The Oral Health Coordinating Committee
William Bailey, U.S. Public Health Service (USPHS)

Open Discussion
William Bailey, U.S. Public Health Service (USPHS)
Robin Brocato, Administration for Children and Families (ACF)
A. Conan Davis, Centers for Medicare and Medicaid Services (CMS)
Isabel Garcia, National Institute of Dental and Craniofacial Research (NIDCR)
Christopher G. Halliday, Indian Health Service (IHS)
William Kohn, Centers for Disease Control and Prevention (CDC)
Richard J. Manski, Agency for Healthcare Research and Quality (AHRQ)
Marian Mehegan, Office on Women's Health (OWH)
Rochelle Rollins, Office of Minority Health (OMH)
Mary Wakefield, Health Resources and Services Administration (HRSA)

3:30 PM   BREAK

3:45 PM   *Workshop Session IV—Discussants Panel*
               Burton L. Edelstein
               Ann LaBelle
               William Maas
               Vincent C. Mayher
               Lynn Douglas Mouden
               John P. Rossetti

4:45 PM   **PUBLIC COMMENT**

5:00 PM   **ADJOURN**

Appendix D

Committee and Staff Biographies

Richard D. Krugman, M.D. (*Chair*), is the first vice chancellor for health affairs for the University of Colorado at Denver. In this role, he supports the deans of the Schools of Dental Medicine, Pharmacy and Public Health, the College of Nursing, and the Graduate School for the Health Sciences. He oversees all clinical programs of the university at its five affiliated hospitals; the Center on Aging, the Center of Bioethics and Humanities, the Colorado Area Health Education (AHEC) system, and Risk Management also report to him. Dr. Krugman became dean of the University of Colorado School of Medicine in 1992 after serving as acting dean for 20 months. Dr. Krugman also has held a variety of administrative positions at the University of Colorado, including director of admissions and codirector of the child health associate program, director of the university's SEARCH/AHEC program, vice chairman for clinical affairs in the Department of Pediatrics, and director of the Kempe National Center for the Prevention of Child Abuse and Neglect. He is also president of University Physicians, Inc., the School of Medicine faculty practice plan. He is a member of the Institute of Medicine and currently serves on the boards of the University of Colorado Hospital and The Children's Hospital of Denver, among others. He earned his medical degree at New York University School of Medicine.

José F. Cordero, M.D., M.P.H., is dean of the Graduate School of Public Health at the University of Puerto Rico. Prior to that, he was an assistant surgeon general of the Public Health Service and the founding director of the National Center on Birth Defects and Developmental Disabilities (NCBDDD) at the Centers for Disease Control and Prevention. Dr. Cordero worked at the CDC for 27 years and has extensive public health experience in the fields of birth defects, developmental disabilities, and child health. He first joined the CDC as an Epidemiologic Intelligence Service officer within the Birth Defects Branch. In 1994, he was appointed deputy director of the National Immunization Program, one of the nation's most successful public health programs. Within a few years of being named the first director of the NCBDDD, it became a leading international institution devoted to research and prevention of birth defects and developmental disabilities. Dr. Cordero is also a former president of the Teratology Society, a professional research society devoted to the prevention of birth defects, where he promoted the eradication of rubella. His work has been published in many national and international journals. He obtained his medical degree from the University of Puerto Rico and his master's degree in public health from Harvard University.

Claude Earl Fox, M.D., M.P.H., is professor in the Department of Epidemiology and Public Health at the University of Miami, Miller School of Medicine, and the founding director of the Florida Public Health Institute. He was previously the first permanent director of the Johns Hopkins Urban Health Institute and professor of the Johns Hopkins Bloomberg School of Public Health, with joint academic appointments in the Johns Hopkins School of Nursing and School of Medicine. Prior to that, he served as the administrator of the federal Health Resources and Services Administration, overseeing the Ryan White HIV/AIDS program, the Office of Rural Health Policy, and all federally funded community health centers, transplant programs, and health professions training programs. While at HRSA, Dr. Fox made oral health an agency priority and also cochaired development and implementation of the Children's Health Insurance Program. From 1995 to 1997, he was deputy assistant secretary for health in the Office of Disease Prevention and Health Promotion at the Department of Health and Human Services. Before that, he served as HHS regional health administrator in Philadelphia, overseeing federal health and human programs in five states and the District of Columbia. He was Alabama's state health officer from 1986 to 1992 and Mississippi's deputy state health officer from 1983 to 1986. He has also served as president of the Association of State and Territorial Health Officials. He earned his medical degree from the University of Mississippi and his master's degree in public health from the University of North Carolina.

Terry Fulmer, Ph.D., R.N., FAAN, is Erline Perkins McGriff Professor, dean of the College of Nursing, and adjunct professor of medicine at the School of Medicine at New York University. She received her bachelor's degree from Skidmore College, her master's and doctoral degrees from Boston College, and her Geriatric Nurse Practitioner Post-Masters Certificate from New York University. She has previously held academic appointments at Boston College, the Harvard Medical School Division on Aging, Yale University, and Columbia University. Dr. Fulmer joined the faculty of New York University in 1995 and is currently a member of the Executive Committee for the new Medical School curriculum and also serves as an attending in nursing at the NYU Langone Medical Center. She is a codirector of the John A. Hartford Foundation Institute for Geriatric Nursing, and codirector of the Consortium of New York Geriatric Education Centers at New York University. She has spearheaded a number of innovative practice initiatives and research programs at the NYU College of Dentistry and serves as a member of the Santa Fe Group, a think tank that seeks to identify and implement effective solutions to significant problems in oral health and health care. She was a keynote speaker at the Second Annual Meskin Symposium, "Meeting the Oral Health Needs of the Aging Population: Education, Service & Advocacy." She has also served on previous panels with the Institute of Medicine, including *Violence in Families: Understanding Prevention and Treatment* (1998); *Abuse, Neglect, and Exploitation in an Aging America* (2003); and *Retooling for an Aging America: Building the Heath Care Workforce* (2007–2008). Dr. Fulmer's program of research focuses on acute care of the elderly and specifically elder abuse and neglect. She served on the National Research Council's panel to review risk and prevalence of elder abuse and neglect and has published widely on this topic. She is a member of the Institute of Medicine and has received the status of Fellow in the American Academy of Nursing, the Gerontological Society of America, and the New York Academy of Medicine. She has served as a member of the National Committee for Quality Assurance geriatric measurement assessment panel and is currently on the Veterans Administration Geriatrics and Gerontology Advisory Committee. She completed a Brookdale National Fellowship and is a Distinguished Practitioner of the National Academies of Practice. Dr. Fulmer was the first nurse to be elected to the board of the American Geriatrics Society and the first nurse to serve as the president of the Gerontological Society of America. She is a trustee of Skidmore College, Bassett Hospital, and the New York Academy of Medicine.

Vanessa Northington Gamble, M.D., Ph.D., is university professor of Medical Humanities and Professor of American Studies and Health Policy at The George Washington University. She is an internationally recognized expert on the history of American medicine and public health, racial and ethnic disparities in health and health care, cultural competence, and bioethics. Prior to her appointment at The George Washington University, Dr. Gamble was Director of the Tuskegee University National Center for Bioethics in Research and Health Care. She has also held positions as associate profes-

sor of History of Medicine and Family Medicine and founding director of
the Center for the Study of Race and Ethnicity in Medicine at the University of Wisconsin School of Medicine, vice president for Community and
Minority Programs at the Association of American Medical Colleges, and
associate professor and deputy director of the Center for Health Disparities
Solutions at the Johns Hopkins Bloomberg School of Public Health. She
chaired the committee that took the lead role in the successful campaign to
obtain an apology in 1997 from President Clinton for the infamous United
States Public Health Syphilis Study at Tuskegee. Dr. Gamble is a member of
the Institute of Medicine, National Academy of Sciences. A proud native of
West Philadelphia, Dr. Gamble received her B.A. from Hampshire College
and her M.D. and Ph.D. in the history and sociology of science from the
University of Pennsylvania.

Paul E. Gates, D.D.S., M.B.A., is chair of the Department of Dentistry
at Bronx-Lebanon Hospital Center. He is also an associate professor at
Albert Einstein College of Medicine. He has held teaching posts at Fairleigh
Dickinson University in both the School of Dentistry and the Institute of
Leadership Studies and Columbia University School of Dentistry. He is a
member of the Distinguished Practitioners of Dentistry in the National
Academies of Practice. He has been honored for his leadership and service
to the profession of dentistry by the American College of Dentists (Fellow),
and the National Dental Association Foundation. He is listed in *Who's
Who in Dentistry*, *Who's Who in the East*, *Who's Who in America*, *Who's
Who Among Black Americans*, and *Who's Who in Medicine and Health
Care*. He has published on oral health for the underserved and increasing
the numbers of minority faculty members in dental education. He holds a
dental degree from West Virginia University and an M.B.A. from Fairleigh
Dickinson University.

Mary C. George, R.D.H., M.Ed., is associate professor emeritus in the Department of Dental Ecology at the University of North Carolina at Chapel
Hill School of Dentistry. Her academic career has included directing an
undergraduate program in Dental Auxiliary Teacher Education, which was
one of the first programs in the country to educate dental hygiene, dental
assisting, and dental laboratory technology teachers; developing an M.S.
degree program for allied dental educators; and directing undergraduate
programs in dental hygiene and dental assisting. She has been involved
in funded demonstration and community service projects addressing oral
health among adults with disabilities and in access to care for local immigrant populations. Through the ADEA she was awarded the ADEA/
Sunstar Harry W. Bruce Jr. Legislative Fellowship; served as a member of

the Commission on Change and Innovation in Dental Education and the Commission on Improving the Oral Health Status of All Americans: Roles and Responsibilities of Academic Institutions. She was one of the 2004 recipients of the Pfizer/ADHA Award for Excellence in Dental Hygiene.

Alice M. Horowitz, R.D.H., Ph.D., is a research associate professor in the School of Public Health, University of Maryland, College Park. She is a retired senior scientist in the Division of Population and Health Promotion Sciences at the National Institute of Dental and Craniofacial Research. She served as the planning committee chairperson for the 1983 NIH Consensus Conference on Dental Sealants in the Prevention of Tooth Decay and cochairperson of the 2001 NIH Consensus Conference on the Management and Diagnosis of Dental Caries. Previously, she taught at the University of Iowa and worked as an education specialist at the USPHS Dental Health Center in San Francisco. In 1976 she joined the NIDCR in the National Caries Program, where she developed educational interventions for use in implementing school-based caries prevention regimens. She also collaborated in research on fluorides and sealants. Dr. Horowitz has served as president of the American Association of Public Health Dentistry, chair of the Intersectional Council and Oral Health Section of the American Public Health Association, and chair of the Science Transfer Committee of the International Association for Dental Research. Dr. Horowitz holds an R.D.H., B.A., and M.A. from the University of Iowa and her Ph.D. in health education from the University of Maryland.

Elizabeth Mertz, Ph.D., M.A., is an assistant professor in residence at the University of California, San Francisco, with a joint appointment in the Department of Preventive and Restorative Dental Sciences, School of Dentistry and in the Department of Social and Behavioral Sciences in the School of Nursing. She is affiliated with the UCSF Center to Address Disparities in Children's Oral Health and is research faculty at the Center for the Health Professions where she has worked since 1997. Dr. Mertz has researched, published, and lectured on a broad range of health professions workforce policy issues, including supply and demand of providers, health care regulation, state and federal workforce policy, access to care, and evolving professional practice models. She serves on the editorial board of the *Journal of Public Health Dentistry* and has served on advisory and planning committees for organizations such as the Health Resources and Services Administration, the California HealthCare Foundation, The San Francisco Foundation, the Pacific Center for Special Care, and the Institute of Medicine. She earned her M.A. from the Humphrey Institute of Public Affairs at the University of Minnesota and her Ph.D. in medical sociology from the University of California, San Francisco.

Matthew J. Neidell, Ph.D., is assistant professor in the Department of Health Policy and Management at the Mailman School of Public Health, Columbia University. His research interests include health and environmental economics, and he is the author of several papers on dental care and fluoridation. Dr. Neidell is a Faculty Research Fellow for the National Bureau of Economic Research. He received his doctorate in economics from the University of California, Los Angeles.

Michael Painter, J.D., M.D., is a senior program officer at the Robert Wood Johnson Foundation and a senior member of the RWJF Quality/Equality Team. He was a 2003–2004 Health Policy Fellow with the office of Senator William Frist. Prior to that, he was the chief of medical staff at the Seattle Indian Health Board, a community health center serving urban American Indians and Alaska Natives, where Painter led that clinic's award-winning diabetes team. He has a clinical faculty appointment with the University of Washington, Department of Family Medicine. Dr. Painter served as the cochair for the 2002–2003 Washington State Department of Health Collaborative on Adult Preventive Services; he also served as a medical educator and consultant for the Northwest AIDS Education and Training Center. He is a policy advocate at the national, state, and local levels regarding health care issues affecting urban American Indians and Alaska Natives. He is a member of the Cherokee Nation of Oklahoma, American Academy of Family Physicians, Association of American Indian Physicians, National Medical Association, and California Bar Association. Dr. Painter earned a J.D. from Stanford Law School and an M.D. from the University of Washington.

Sara Rosenbaum, J.D., is the Harold and Jane Hirsh Professor of Health Law and Policy and founding chair of the Department of Health Policy, The George Washington University School of Public Health and Health Services. Professor Rosenbaum's research and scholarship focus on the ways in which the law intersects with the nation's health care and public health systems, with an emphasis on health reform, health care quality, health care access, and health insurance coverage and managed care. She has been named one of the nation's 500 most influential health policy makers by McGraw-Hill; is a recipient of the Investigator Award in Health Policy from the Robert Wood Johnson Foundation; and has been recognized by the Department of Health and Human Services for distinguished national service on behalf of Medicaid beneficiaries. As a member of the White House Domestic Policy Council under President Clinton, she directed the drafting of the Health Security Act and oversaw the development of the Vaccines for Children program. She earned her law degree from the Boston University School of Law.

Harold C. Slavkin, D.D.S., is the founding director of the Center for Craniofacial Molecular Biology and a professor in the School of Dentistry at the University of Southern California. He served as dean of the School of Dentistry from 2000 to 2008. His expertise is in health promotion and disease prevention, access to health care for underserved populations, funding for health care, epidemiology, and craniofacial morphogenesis. He is the former director of the National Institute of Dental and Craniofacial Research (1995–2000), the lead agency on the surgeon general's report on oral health. He was the 2009 recipient of the American Dental Association's Gold Medal Award for Excellence in Dental Research. He also received the William J. Gies Award from the American College of Dentists. He has published more than 400 scientific papers in peer-reviewed journals. Dr. Slavkin is a member of the Institute of Medicine, a fellow in the American Association for the Advancement of Science, and a member of the American Dental Association. He earned his dental degree from the University of Southern California. He holds honorary science degrees from a number of universities, including Connecticut, Georgetown, Montreal, Maryland, New Jersey Medical and Dental, and Peking.

Clemencia M. Vargas, D.D.S., Ph.D., is associate professor at the University of Maryland Dental School. She served in the 1994 class of the Centers for Disease Control and Prevention's Epidemic Intelligence Service (EIS) at the National Center for Health Statistics, where she stayed for 4 more years. Dr. Vargas participated in the design of oral health objectives for *Healthy People 2010* and in the oral health component of national surveys. Dr. Vargas's research interest is socioeconomic inequalities in oral health, and she has published scientific articles and provided oral health data for publications and public health activities in this area of interest. Currently she is working on NIH-funded projects on the association between oral health of children and their mothers, early childhood caries prevention provided by physicians, and the association between beverages consumption and caries trends among preschoolers. Dr. Vargas holds degrees in dentistry and epidemiology from the Universidad de Antioquia, Colombia; after fulfilling the obligatory rural service, she worked in private practice, academia, and dental public health programs. She received a Ph.D. in medical sociology from Arizona State University.

Robert Weyant, D.M.D., Dr.P.H., is associate dean of Public Health and Outreach and professor and chair of the department of Dental Public Health and Information Management at the University of Pittsburgh School of Dental Medicine. He is also associate professor of epidemiology in the Graduate School of Public Health. Dr. Weyant is a former Navy dental officer and VA dentist. He has been a diplomate of the American Board of Dental Public Health since 1987 and is also a past president of the American Association for Public Health Dentistry. Dr. Weyant currently serves on numerous local, state, and national committees aimed at reducing oral health disparities, increasing the dental workforce, and improving access to oral care. His research involves general and social epidemiological research related to oral health disparities and oral disease etiology. He is presently the principal investigator (PI) or co-PI on several NIH-funded studies of oral disease etiology. Dr. Weyant also directs the Center for Oral Health Research in Appalachia (COHRA), and oversees the joint degree program in dentistry and public health. He received his master's degree in public health and his dental degree from the University of Pittsburgh and his doctorate in epidemiology from the University of Michigan.

INSTITUTE OF MEDICINE STAFF

Tracy A. Harris, D.P.M., M.P.H., is a senior program officer with the Institute of Medicine's (IOM's) Board on Health Care Services. Dr. Harris was trained in podiatric medicine and surgery and spent several years in private practice. In 1999, she was awarded a Congressional Fellowship with the American Association for the Advancement of Science and spent one year working in the U.S. Senate. Dr. Harris joined the IOM in 2004. Her most recent work has focused on aging and the health care workforce. She was the study director for the 2008 report *Retooling for an Aging America: Building the Health Care Workforce.* In 2009, she staffed a National Academies–wide initiative on the "Grand Challenges of an Aging Society" and directed a workshop on the oral health care workforce. Dr. Harris is the study director for this current report, a concurrent report to be issued by the Committee on Oral Health Access to Services, and director for an upcoming workshop on the allied health workforce. Dr. Harris has a doctor of podiatric medicine degree from Temple University and a master's degree in public health with a concentration in health policy, from George Washington University.

Ben Wheatley, M.P.P., serves as program officer at the Institute of Medicine (IOM). Since joining the organization in July 2005, he has been an author on a number of IOM reports, including *Emergency Medical Services at the Crossroads* (2006), *Knowing What Works in Health Care: A Roadmap for the Nation* (2008), and *Regionalizing Emergency Care* (2010). Prior to joining IOM, Mr. Wheatley served as senior manager for AcademyHealth, assisting states in developing programs to expand health insurance coverage for the uninsured. He provided direct technical assistance to states, authored numerous publications, and was a frequent presenter on Medicaid disease management programs. Prior to joining AcademyHealth, Mr. Wheatley worked at the National Rehabilitation Hospital Research Center where he conducted original research examining the consolidation of the rehabilitation hospital industry. Mr. Wheatley is a graduate of Georgetown University, where he received a master's degree in public policy with an emphasis in health care policy.

Meg Barry, J.D., M.P.H., is an associate program officer for the Board on Health Care Services. She joined the IOM in 2009. She has worked on two studies related to oral health and recently began working on a study of geographic variation in health care spending and promotion of high value care. Before joining the IOM, she worked on health care regulatory matters at a national law firm and reauthorization of the State Children's Health Insurance Program at the New America Foundation. Previously, she worked as a research scientist at Northwestern University. She is a graduate of the University of Michigan Law School and School of Public Health.

Amy Asheroff joined the IOM in 2009 as a senior program assistant for the Board on Health Care Services and the Board on Children, Youth, and Families. She is currently working on several projects: the Committee on an Oral Health Initiative, Committee on Oral Health Access to Services, Committee on the Mental Health Workforce for Geriatric Populations, and a workshop on the allied health workforce. Prior to joining the IOM, she completed a year of service in a safety net medical clinic in northwest Washington, DC, through AmeriCorps. She graduated from the University of California, Berkeley, with a bachelor's degree in the History of Art and Italian.

Roger C. Herdman, M.D., received his bachelor of science degree from Yale University in 1955, graduating Magna Cum Laude and Phi Beta Kappa. Dr. Herdman then graduated from Yale University School of Medicine and interned at the University of Minnesota. Dr. Herdman was a medical officer with the U.S. Navy from 1959 to 1961. Thereafter, he completed a residency in pediatrics and continued with a medical fellowship in immunology and nephrology at Minnesota. Between 1966 and 1979, Dr. Herdman held positions of Assistant Professor and Professor of Pediatrics, respectively, at the University of Minnesota and the Albany Medical College. In 1969, he was appointed Director of the New York State Kidney Disease Institute in Albany. From 1969–1977, he served as Deputy Commissioner of the New York State Department of Health and was responsible for research, departmental health care facilities, and the state's Medicaid program at various times. In 1977, he was named New York State's Director of Public Health. From 1979 until joining the U.S. Congress's Office of Technology

Assessment (OTA), Dr. Herdman was a Vice President of the Memorial Sloan-Kettering Cancer Center in New York City. In December 1983, he was named Assistant Director of OTA and then Acting Director and Director from January 1993–February 1996. After the closure of OTA, Dr. Herdman joined the National Academy of Sciences' Institute of Medicine as a senior scholar and directed studies on graduate medical education, organ transplantation, silicone breast implants, and the VA national formulary. On completing those studies, he was appointed Director of the IOM/NRC National Cancer Policy Board from August 2000 through April 2005. From May 2005 to September 2009, he initiated and directed the IOM National Cancer Policy Forum, which differed from the board by including as members federal and private sector agencies or organizations in addition to at large academic/industry members. In October 2007, Dr. Herdman was appointed Director of the IOM Board on Health Care Services in addition to his other duties. Also, from 1996 to date, he has worked on IOM relations with the U.S. Congress.